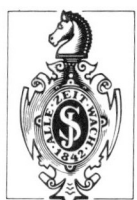

Treatment in Clinical Medicine

Series Editor: John L. Reid

Titles in the series already published:

Gastrointestinal Disease
Edited by C.J.C. Roberts

Rheumatic Disease
Hilary A. Capell, T.J. Daymond
and W. Carson Dick

The Elderly
W.J. MacLennan, A.N. Shepherd
and I.H. Stevenson

Forthcoming titles in the series:

Neurological and Neuro-psychiatric Disorders
J.D. Parkes, P. Jenner, D. Rushton and C.D. Marsden

Hypertension
B.N.C. Prichard and C.W.I. Owens

Respiratory Disease
Anne E. Tattersfield and M. McNicol

Endocrine and Metabolic Diseases
Edited by C.R.W. Edwards

A. Ross Lorimer · W. Stewart Hillis

Cardiovascular Disease

With 19 Figures

Springer-Verlag
Berlin Heidelberg New York Tokyo

A. Ross Lorimer, MD, FRCP
Consultant Cardiologist, Royal Infirmary,
Castle Street, Glasgow, Scotland, UK

W. Stewart Hillis, MB, FRCP
Senior Lecturer in Clinical Pharmacology
and Consultant Cardiologist,
Stobhill General Hospital,
Glasgow G21 2UW, Scotland, UK

Series Editor:

John L. Reid, MD, FRCP
Regius Professor of Materia Medica,
University of Glasgow, Scotland

ISBN 3–540–15426–4 Springer-Verlag Berlin Heidelberg New York Tokyo
ISBN 0–387–15426–4 Springer-Verlag New York Heidelberg Berlin Tokyo

Library of Congress Cataloging-in-Publication Data
Lorimer, A. Ross (Andrew Ross), 1937–   . Cardiovascular Disease.
(Treatment in clinical medicine)
Includes bibliographies and index.
1. Heart – Diseases. 2. Cardiovascular system – Diseases. I. Hillis, W. Stewart
(William Stewart), 1943–   . II. Title. III. Series.   [DNLM: 1. Cardiovascular
Diseases – therapy. WG 100 L872c]   RC681.L67   1985   616.1   85–26169
ISBN 0-387-15426-4 (U.S.)

© by Springer-Verlag Berlin Heidelberg 1985
Printed in Great Britain

Filmset by Herts Typesetting Services (1984) Ltd, Finchley, London N12
Printed by Henry Ling Limited, The Dorset Press, Dorchester.

2128/3916–543210

Series Editor's Foreword

'Cardiovascular Disease' is the fourth monograph in the series on management and treatment in major clinical subspecialties or patient groups. Each book is complete in its own right and has been prepared by practising physicians with specialist experience and a particular interest in treatment and management. The series has been prepared to fill a gap between standard textbooks of medicine and therapeutics and research reviews, symposia and original articles in specialist fields. The volumes aim to give authoritative, up-to-date advice on treatment and management which will be of use to both specialists and non-specialists and allow recent advances and developments to be seen in the context of contemporary clinical practice. The first three volumes dealt respectively with gastrointestinal diseases, rheumatic diseases and treatment in the elderly. Cardiovascular disease covers the range of common diseases affecting the heart and the circulation. In view of the importance of coronary heart disease as a cause of death and morbidity a substantial part of the book is devoted to description of the factors associated with coronary artery disease (hyperlipidaemia and hypertension) and their management by drug and non-drug means. A further five chapters are devoted to the clinical syndromes associated with coronary heart disease and their management. These not only consider acute 'in hospital' management, including surgery, but also address epidemiological questions, including approaches to secondary prevention of myocardial infarction. Other chapters deal with cardiac arrhythmias and the modern management of heart failure. In both of these areas, particularly the latter, there have been recent major therapeutic developments. Further chapters review the present status of rheumatic heart disease with regard to both acute rheumatic fever and chronic valvular disease and infective endocarditis. Finally cardiomyopathies and cor pulmonale (including pulmonary thromboembolism) complete the volume.

The authors are both active practising cardiologists in Glasgow. Dr. Lorimer is a consultant physician at the Royal Infirmary and honorary lecturer in the Department of Medical Cardiology in the University of Glasgow while Dr. Hillis is Pollok Senior Lecturer in the Department of Materia Medica and Therapeutics and honorary consultant cardiologist at Stobhill Hospital and the Royal Infirmary. They are well qualified to cover aspects of pathogenesis, investigation, management and drug treatment of patients with cardiovascular disease. The volume should provide not only a useful guide to treatment but also an easy reference to drug interactions and adverse reactions. It should be particularly useful for the young hospital doctor in training for higher qualifications and the more experienced general physician or general practitioner who wishes to keep up to date with developments in cardiology.

Glasgow, August 1985   John L. Reid

Preface

Cardiovascular disease ranks high as a worldwide cause of death and disability. Advances in treatment have emphasised the need for an appreciation of basic aspects of pharmacokinetics and their modification by disease.

Treatment of established disorders is important but there are now increasing areas where prevention has become feasible. For this reason this book presents our views as clinical cardiologists on aspects of primary prevention in terms of lipid disorders as well as reviewing and outlining the management of many cardiac problems. Sudden death has been considered both as a primary event and as a sequel to acute myocardial infarction. There are now exciting areas of possible myocardial salvage after infarction and these have been dealt with in detail.

The management of angina and heart failure has changed dramatically in recent years. The advent of new therapeutic strategies involving β-adrenoceptor blocking compounds, calcium channel blockers and now converting enzyme inhibitors has resulted in major changes in our pharmacological approach to these problems.

The considerable developments in cardiac surgery have made close co-operation between physician and surgeon even more important. The timing of surgery and the rate of medical therapy before and after operation have been considered in detail and the need for a joint approach emphasised.

Rheumatic heart disease is less prevalent but remains a considerable clinical problem and we have felt it important to review both its management and that of complications such as infective endocarditis. The management of some rarer conditions such as the cardiomyopathies has also been included since current treatment requires detailed consideration of the clinical pharmacology of various treatment regimes.

In each chapter we have tried to define pathophysiology with an emphasis on a logical pharmacological approach.

We regard this book as suitable for registrars anxious for background information in pharmacology, as an update for practising physicians and as a useful aid for primary care practitioners looking for a text to provide helpful background to the logical treatment of cardiovascular disease.

Acknowledgement

We are extremely grateful to Mrs. Jacqueline Clark and Mrs. Elma Gordon for all the time and effort put into typing the manuscript. We would also like to acknowledge the support of our families in allowing us the time to write this text.

A. Ross Lorimer
W. Stewart Hillis

Contents

1 Pharmacokinetic Properties of Cardiovascular Drugs

In the last three decades there has been a great increase in the number of drugs available to treat cardiovascular diseases. Patients have a wide spectrum of clinical presentation and can provide complex management problems. They may require emergency treatment using drugs by a parenteral route or long-term oral therapy during which time many clinical parameters are changing. The therapeutic and toxic effects of drugs depend on the available concentration at the site of action, and in general the drug concentration in plasma or whole blood correlates well with the pharmacological response. The development of sensitive and specific analytical methods to measure drugs in blood and/or urine has greatly enhanced our knowledge of their pharmacokinetic behaviour (Mayer et al. 1980).

Pharmacokinetics

Pharmacokinetics describes the processes which a drug undergoes following its administration, and includes:

1. Absorption
2. Distribution
3. Metabolism
4. Excretion

Pharmacodynamics

Pharmacodynamics is the study of drug effects and their mechanism of action. Mathematical models are useful to predict drug concentrations in plasma and body tissues in relation to the dose, route of administration and time. Such information allows the development of dosing schedules to maintain drug concentrations within the optimum or therapeutic range. This concentration range is that within which drugs exhibit their therapeutic action with few or no adverse effects.

Drug Absorption

The rate of absorption of a drug affects the duration and intensity of action. In many cardiovascular diseases clinical needs demand a rapid onset of drug action and predictable plasma levels and duration of effect. The route of administration is therefore of considerable importance (Fenster and Perrier 1982). This may either be enteral (predominantly oral) or parenteral.

Oral Administration

This is the safest, most convenient and economical method of administration. Absorption from the gastrointestinal tract is affected by the physicochemical properties of each drug. Compounds which are soluble in aqueous solution are more rapidly absorbed. Drug disintegration and dissolution are important and influenced not only by solubility but also by polarity — the more polar the drug, the better it is absorbed. Variation in tablet formulation may lead to enhanced or decreased absorption, with a resulting modification in bioavailability (Lindenbaum et al. 1971). Changes in the absorption may lead to toxicity, particularly in compounds with a narrow therapeutic range and a small therapeutic index, such as the cardiac glycosides.

Absorption from the gastrointestinal tract usually follows first order or linear kinetics and the rate is proportional to the concentration of the drug. After ingestion the high local concentration allows rapid absorption over a high concentration gradient. With a decrease in concentration, the rate of absorption is reduced.

Absorption across the gut wall can be affected by gut motility. In diarrhoeal states, rapid transit may reduce absorption. If reduced motility is present, the duration of contact of the drug with gastric acid is prolonged and may lead to drug decomposition. Malabsorptive states also reduce drug absorption, as may mucosal oedema secondary to cardiac failure. In the latter situation reduced bioavailability can cause apparent diuretic resistance and a considerable diuresis may follow subsequent intravenous administration.

The presence of other agents may lead to drug interactions affecting absorption (see pp.10–13).

Drugs with rapid absorption and a short half-life require frequent administration to maintain therapeutic levels, which may contribute to reduced compliance. In some situations slow-release formulations have been developed to prolong absorption and improve compliance (e.g. procainamide for the treatment of arrhythmias) (Giardina et al. 1980).

First Pass Hepatic Metabolism. Some drugs, although well absorbed from the gastrointestinal tract, are subject to extensive metabolism during the first pass through the liver. This is determined by (a) hepatic clearance of the drug, and (b) hepatic blood flow. Such metabolism results in a decrease in the systemic availability of the drug. For example propranolol has a high hepatic clearance, with only 30%–40% of an oral dose reaching the systemic circulation. Hepatic metabolism and blood flow also explain why lignocaine is not given orally. There is a high first pass metabolic effect with formation of metabolites which have no anti-arrhythmic effect but do have toxic properties. In addition, plasma levels are inversely related to hepatic blood flow. In cardiac failure this is reduced and standard infusion regimes require modification to prevent toxicity. High first pass metabolism may not be important if the therapeutic index is wide (Wilkinson and Shand 1975).

Parenteral Administration

When parenteral routes are used the gastrointestinal tract is bypassed and the drug reaches the systemic circulation directly. Drugs may be given by injection (subcutaneous, intramuscular or intravenous), percutaneously (as creams or ointments) or by inhalation.

Intravenous

The intravenous route is used to obtain therapeutic drug concentrations with minimal delay. Infusions can be controlled and stopped instantly if adverse effects occur. The rate of administration can be controlled for long periods using slow infusions with constant infusion apparatus. The intravenous route is useful if there is a narrow therapeutic ratio or if rapid excretion of a drug occurs. It is used routinely in emergency management of unconscious patients or patients who are uncooperative during their acute illness.

Intravenous therapy is not innocuous. A rigid aseptic technique is required. Poor technique may result in damage to the vascular wall, with local venous thrombosis and perhaps embolism. If drugs are given too rapidly, then circulatory collapse may result owing to the bolus of concentrated drug. Anaphylactoid reactions occasionally occur. In patients with cardiac failure, the volume of fluid administered should be carefully controlled.

Intramuscular

With intramuscular administration, absorption is a function of blood flow. Aqueous solutions are usually absorbed in some 10–30 min, depending on the vascularity of the site, the lipid solubility of the drug and its volume and osmolality. In shock or cardiac failure, muscle blood flow may be significantly reduced and slow absorption may initially occur. If the haemodynamic status improves, a large volume may be rapidly absorbed, which can cause adverse effects, e.g. as may occur with intramuscular lignocaine in the early stage of myocardial infarction.

Subcutaneous

Subcutaneous injections are simple to administer, but absorption is slower as blood flow is less in these tissues. Percutaneous or transdermal administration of drugs may be used with absorption following local diffusion of creams or ointments.

The use of inert organic solvents facilitates drug penetration. This route of administration is best suited to drugs with a high lipid solubility. Chronic administration of nitrates has recently been performed by this route.

Bioavailability

Bioavailability is the term used to describe the proportion of administered drug that reaches the systemic circulation in unchanged form. It is obtained by comparing the total area under the serum concentration/time curves following oral and intravenous administration

$F = AUC_o/AUC_{iv}.$

The rate of absorption may be obtained by measuring the time to peak serum concentration (t_{max}). If no intravenous formulation is available, different oral formulations can be studied and the relative rather than the absolute bioavailability may be obtained by comparing the serum concentration/time curves.

Drug Distribution

Following intravenous or oral absorption, a drug is available for body tissue distribution. If all tissues and fluids took up the drug at the same rate, the body would behave as a single homogeneous unit and the serum concentration/time curve would be described by a mono-exponential equation.

Such a one compartment model describes the drug concentration following a single intravenous bolus dose (Fig. 1.1). The time course of drug concentration in plasma is such that in a particular time interval, the concentration will fall to half of its initial value. Each time interval is the half-life. Approximately 90% of the dose is removed in three half-lives and some 97% in five half-lives. The first order or exponential decay of concentration can be linearised by plotting the logarithm of the concentration versus time or by plotting the data on semi-

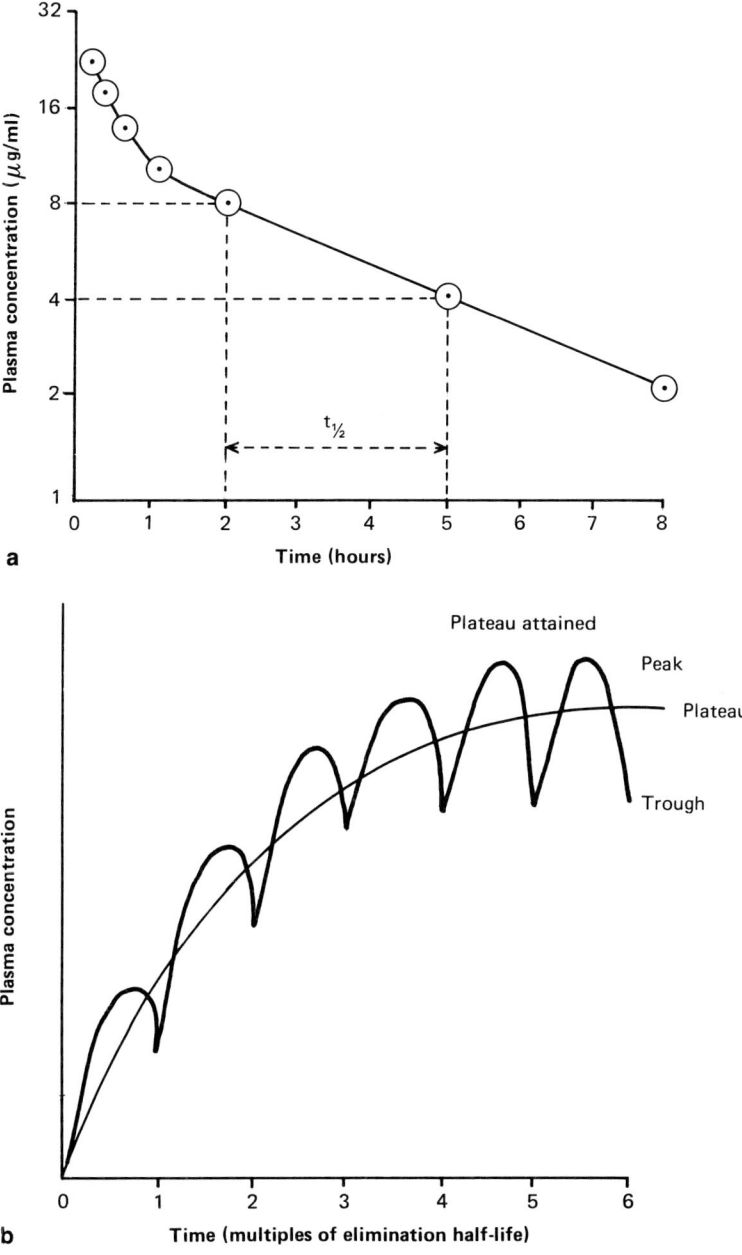

Fig. 1.1. a One compartment model of drug concentration following a single intravenous bolus dose. **b** Pharmacokinetic relationship for repeated administration of drug. *Solid line* represents equivalent level achieved by constant infusion. Peak and trough values proportional to dosage interval/half-life are avoided by intravenous infusions, blunted by slow absorption.

logarithmic graph paper. Drug half-life determines the dosage schedule. Most drugs demonstrate rapid distribution equilibrium, reflecting cardiac output and regional blood flow. The heart, liver, kidney and brain receive the highest early dose. Other tissues take up the drug more slowly and the serum concentration time profile is better described by multi-exponential equations, the simplest being $C = Ae^{-\alpha t} + Be^{-\beta t}$. A and B are coefficients and α and β first order rate constants. These are a function of (a) dose, (b) volume of distribution and (c) the rate constant for distribution and elimination.

Pharmacological effects generally correlate with serum levels measured during the terminal log linear phase, which reflects distribution equilibrium. Plasma levels measured before this phase will not necessarily correlate with pharmacological effects. In therapeutic drug monitoring, careful note must be made of the dose, time of administration and time of sampling. Therapeutic drug monitoring should be performed after three or four half-lives into the post-absorption, post-distribution phase of the plasma concentration time curve.

Volume of Distribution

This is a proportionality constant relating the amount of drug in the body to serum concentrations. It is not usually a measure of a real physiological space but may be determined from the formula $V_d = Cl_s/\beta$.

Cl_s = total body clearance of the drug and is equal to the i.v. dose/AUC; β = the terminal disposition rate constant and is related to the half-life (t1/2) by the equation $\beta = 0.693/_{t\frac{1}{2}}$. The volume of distribution is dependent on the relative serum and tissue binding of a drug. Lipid-insoluble drugs permeate membranes poorly and tend to be restricted in their distribution and potential sites of action. The drug may also be limited by binding to plasma proteins. Accumulation in a specific tissue may serve as a reservoir and prolong the drug action at a distal site.

Drug Elimination

The primary routes of drug elimination are hepatic metabolism and renal excretion. Hepatic metabolism usually creates substances which are more polar and thus are more soluble and more easily excreted. Clinically it is important to know the contribution of hepatic metabolism to the elimination of the drug and to be aware of any pharmacological activity of the resulting metabolites.

Activity in the hepatic enzyme systems may be affected by factors such as smoking, genetics, age, specific disease states and the co-administration of other drugs. There is considerable patient variability.

Hepatic Microsomal System

The microsomal enzymes catalyse glucuronide conjugations and also most oxidative reactions, including:

1. N-O alkyl dealkylation
2. Side chain hydroxylation
3. N-oxidation and N-hydroxylation
4. Sulphoxide formation
5. Deamination and desulphuration

Glucuronides are generally inactive and are usually rapidly excreted. Some compounds which are eliminated in the bile may be hydrolysed and the liberated drug reabsorbed by the intestine. This leads to an enterohepatic circulation, which may prolong drug action. Drug interactions may lead to inhibition or reduction of microsomal drug metabolism (see below).

Genetic Modification of Drug Biotransformation

Conjugation of aromatic primary amines or hydrazines involves several N-acetyl transferases, with acetyl co-enzyme A as the acetyl donor. Genetic polymorphism may be exhibited, with slow or fast acetylation being evident. This metabolic route is bimodally distributed in the population. Rapid acetylators metabolise a greater proportion of any drug dose than do slow acetylators. Slow acetylators may have toxic effects due to higher levels of the parent compound while fast acetylators may have adverse effects due to high concentration of metabolites. Hydralazine and procainamide are metabolised by the acetyl transferase system. Slow acetylators are more apt to develop the lupus-like syndrome while on chronic treatment (Drayer and Reidenberg 1977).

Drug Excretion

Drugs are excreted either unchanged or as metabolites. Polar compounds in general are more efficiently eliminated than substances with high lipid solubility. Renal excretion is the most important route of elimination. Metabolites formed in the liver may pass into the intestinal tract via the bile and either be excreted in the faeces or, as is more common, reabsorbed into the blood and ultimately excreted in the urine. Creatinine clearance is a reasonable index of renal drug elimination, e.g. digoxin clearance is linearly related to creatinine clearance. Excretion of drugs and metabolites in the urine in general involves three processes: glomerular filtration, active tubular secretion and passive tubular reabsorption (Kristensen et al. 1974). Changes in renal function may also alter drug distribution secondary to a change in serum proteins and/or the tissue binding of highly bound drugs (Oie and Tozer 1979).

Total Body Clearance

Total body clearance (Cl_s) is defined as the volume of serum totally cleared of a drug per unit time by all organs of elimination. It is equal to the sum of the clearances for each process of administration. Most drugs are eliminated by a combination of hepatic and renal mechanisms and $Cl_s = Cl_h + Cl_r$

The clearance by an individual organ is a function of:

1. The blood flow to the organ of elimination (Q)
2. The proportion of drug free or unbound in blood (α)
3. The intrinsic clearance of the free drug (Cl_l)

Some drugs have a high intrinsic clearance, e.g. propranolol and lignocaine clearance is primarily dependent on the blood flow. Conversely, the clearance of digitoxin is primarily dependent on protein binding and intrinsic clearance.

The half-life of a compound is often used as an index of drug elimination; however, it is a function not only of elimination but also of distribution. This is shown by the relationship $t_\frac{1}{2} = 0.693\ V_d/Cl_s$. Changes in drug distribution can therefore produce a change in the drug half-life.

Chronic Drug Administration

Most patients receive a drug over a period of time and chronic administration may be performed as a continuous infusion or by a series of oral doses. When given by constant infusion, the drug concentration gradually increases to a plateau level at a rate that is determined by the half-life. During one half-life, constant infusion reaches 50% of the final, plateau value, and in four half-lives, 90%. When the plateau is reached, a steady state situation occurs where the rate of drug administration is equal to the rate of drug elimination and there is no net change in drug concentration. Steady state concentration (C_{ss}) is given by the equation

$$C_{ss} = \frac{\text{infusion rate}}{Cl_s} = \frac{\text{infusion rate } t_\frac{1}{2}}{0.693\ V_d}$$

When drugs have a long half-life an initial loading dose may be needed to obtain an early therapeutic response. When a drug has been given by constant infusion an appropriate intravenous loading dose can be calculated from the equation $dose_1$, $= C_{ss} V_c$, where V_c is the volume of the central or rapidly equilibrating compartment. $V_c = $ i.v. $dose/C_o$, where $C_o = A + B$.

After the administration of a single oral dose, drug levels increase, reach a peak and then decline. A second dose is generally given before the first dose is completely eliminated and therefore the dosage regime can be considered from a pharmacokinetic point of view to be the equivalent of intermittent infusions. With oral dosing, plasma concentrations fluctuate between a maximum and a minimum value during the dosage interval. The magnitude of the fluctuation is a function of the absorption rate of the drug and its half-life. There is an increase in concentration with successive doses and accumulation will continue until the rate of drug elimination reaches the rate of drug administration. The average steady state concentration is dependent upon the maintenance dose ($dose_m$), the dosing interval (τ), the fraction of the dose which is absorbed (F) plus the distribution and the elimination characteristics of the drug. The relationship is shown in the equation

$$C = \frac{F\ dose_m}{Cl_s\ \tau} = \frac{F\ dose_m t_{\frac{1}{2}}}{0.693\ V_d \tau}$$, and is illustrated in Fig. 1.1b.

Plasma concentration fluctuation during a dosage interval may have important clinical effects. Many anti-arrhythmic drugs have a low therapeutic to toxic ratio (therapeutic index) and it is often undesirable to allow drug concentration to fluctuate by more than a two- to threefold range during the dosing interval. Such drugs with narrow therapeutic indices and short half-lives should be given by intravenous infusion.

Influence of Organ Disease on Drug Disposition

The treatment regimes of many cardiovascular drugs are based on a combination of clinical experience and general pharmacokinetic principles. For many patients general guidelines will be adequate. The presence of other disease states may have major clinical implications.

1. *Renal disease.*   The effects of renal disease are dependent on the fraction of the drug dose, which is normally eliminated unchanged in the urine. The use of common indices of renal function, e.g. creatinine clearance, may allow guidelines to be established for dose adjustment in patients who have renal dysfunction. Nomograms have been devised for several drugs, e.g. digoxin.

2. *Cardiac failure.*   Alterations in cardiac output and regional organ blood flow may result. Drugs with high hepatic (blood flow sensitive) clearances such as lignocaine or propranolol may show great changes in disposition. Intestinal congestion may also influence absorption by the oral route (see above).

3. *Protein binding.*   The free concentration of drug unbound to plasma proteins determines the concentration that most closely reflects receptor site

concentration and pharmacological response. For most drugs, the free concentration is a constant fraction of the total. In drugs which are highly protein bound (> 90%) a decrease in this protein will increase the free fraction considerably and may lead to adverse effects.

Drug Interactions

Drug interactions occur when there is modification of the effect of one drug by another by direct or indirect means. Such interactions are common in patients with cardiovascular disease. Multiple drugs and prolonged treatment are often required. The use of therapeutic drug monitoring has identified many drug interactions which may be potentially detrimental (Tables 1.1–1.7). Care must be taken to assess the clinical significance of such laboratory observations. Drug interactions may be beneficial by combined use of compounds with complementary mechanism of action which lead to an advantageous pharmacological result, e.g. antihypertensive compounds.

Drug interactions may be pharmacodynamic or pharmacokinetic (Beeley 1984).

Pharmacodynamic

Pharmacodynamic drug interactions occur as the result of competition at the receptor site or when both drugs act on the same physiological system. Competing drugs often have agonist or antagonist properties and interaction can usually be predicted from the known pharmacology. Other compounds may be

Table 1.1. Drug interactions involving anti-arrhythmic drugs (after Beeley 1984)

Drug affected	Drug interacting	Effect
Anti-arrhythmic drugs	Drugs used in combination therapy	Myocardial depression or conduction defects
Disopyramide Quinidine	Diuretics	Hypokalaemia, which may cause toxicity
	Amiodarone	Possible risk of ventricular arrhythmias
Lignocaine Mexiletine Tocainide	Diuretics	Hypokalaemia, which reduces activity
Lignocaine Mexiletine	Cimetidine, propranolol	Increased risk of lignocaine toxicity
	Atropine, opioid analgesics	Delayed absorption
	Antacids	Increased plasma concentration, reduced urinary excretion
Verapamil	β-Adrenoreceptor blocking drugs	Hypotension, conduction defects, asystole

classified within a drug group but have ancillary properties and non-specific actions, e.g. phenothiazines show vasodilating activity secondary to α-adrenergic antagonistic properties.

Table 1.2. Drug interactions involving antihypertensive drugs (after Beeley 1984)

Drug affected	Drug interacting	Effect
All antihypertensive drugs	Non-steroidal anti-inflammatory compounds, carbenoxolone, corticosteroids, oestrogen and oral contraceptives	Reduced efficacy
	Alcohol, antidepressants, hypnotics, sedatives, tranquillisers, levodopa, vasodilators	Increased effect
Bethanidine Guanethidine	Sympathetic amines, tricyclic antidepressants	Antagonism
Captopril	Potassium sparing diuretics, potassium supplements	Hyperkalaemia
Clonidine	β-Adrenoreceptor blocking drugs	Enhanced clonidine withdrawal with hypertension
	Tricyclic antidepressants	Antagonism

Table 1.3. Drug interactions involving β-adrenoreceptor blocking drugs (after Beeley 1984)

Drug affected	Drug interacting	Effect
All β-adrenoreceptor blocking drugs	Ergotamine	Peripheral vasoconstriction
	Indomethacin	Reduced efficacy
	Nifedipine	Hypotension
	Sympathetic amines	Severe hypertension
Labetalol	Cimetidine	Reduced metabolism, possibly leading to potentiation
Propranolol	Cimetidine	Reduced hepatic metabolism, possibly leading to potentiation

Table 1.4. Drug interactions involving cardiac glycosides (after Beeley 1984)

Drug affected	Drug interacting	Effect
All cardiac glycosides	Carbenoxolone, diuretics	Hypokalaemia, leading to toxicity
	Cholestyramine, colestipol	Reduced absorption
Digitoxin	Phenobarbitone	Inhibition
Digoxin	Amiodarone, quinidine	Enhanced levels. Maintenance dose may require reduction
	Nifedipine, verapamil	Potentiation may occur

Table 1.5. Drug interactions involving diuretics (after Beeley 1984)

Drug affected	Drug interacting	Effect
All diuretics	Non-steroidal anti-inflammatory agents	Antagonism
	Carbenoxolone, corticosteroids, corticotrophin, oestrogens	Antagonism
Loop diuretics and thiazides	Carbenoxolone, corticosteroids, corticotrophin	Hypokalaemia
Indapamide Carbenoxolone	Diuretics	Hypokalaemia

Table 1.6. Drug interactions involving aldosterone antagonists (after Beeley 1984)

Drug affected	Drug interacting	Effect
Amiloride Triamterene	Captopril, potassium supplements	Hyperkalaemia
Heparin	Aspirin, dipyridamole	Potentiation

Table 1.7. Drug interactions involving oral anticoagulants (after Beeley 1984)

Drug affected	Drug interacting	Effect
Warfarin	Barbiturates, carbamazepine, oral contraceptives, primidone, rifampicin, vitamin K	Reduced efficacy
	Alcohol, amiodarone, anabolic steroids, aspirin, bezafibrate, chloramphenicol, cimetidine, clofibrate, co-trimoxazole, danazol, disulfiram, dextrothyroxine, dipyridamole, erythromycin, metronidazole, miconazole, neomycin, oxyphenbutazone, phenylbutazone, sulphinpyrazone, sulphonamides, thyroxine	Potentiation
	Allopurinol, mefenamic acid, cholestyramine, dextropropoxyphene, indomethacin, nalidixic acid, paracetamol, phenytoin, tetracyclines	Potentiation may occur
Phenindione	Oral contraceptives, vitamin K	Inhibition
	Anabolic steroids, aspirin, bezafibrate, cholestyramine, clofibrate, dipyridamole, neomycin, thyroxine	Potentiation

Pharmacokinetic

Pharmacokinetic drug interactions occur when a drug alters the absorption, distribution, metabolism or excretion of another. This may lead to enhancement or inhibition of activity or there may be no significant clinical result. The internal environment may be affected by drugs altering pH or electrolyte balance, e.g. long-term diuretic use. Drug-induced changes in hepatic or renal function may also alter drug activity.

Interactions Affecting Absorption

Interactions may occur prior to absorption into the systemic circulation. Drug resins such as cholestyramine have an adsorbent capacity and may form complexes with steroids such as cardiac glycosides. Alteration in gastric or intestinal motility may inhibit or enhance the rate or extent of absorption. Reduced absorption of mexiletine and other anti-arrhythmics may occur after opioid analgesics. Antibiotic administration may alter the gut flora, with reduced vitamin K production. This may enhance the efficacy of vitamin K antagonists such as warfarin, with an associated risk of bleeding. Neomycin may reduce the absorption of fat-soluble drugs.

Interactions Affecting Distribution

Plasma protein binding may lead to drug interaction affecting compounds which are highly protein bound. A minor change in the proportion of bound drug may lead to a major rise in concentration of free drug. This is of clinical importance in compounds which are > 90% protein bound. Warfarin levels may be increased following concomitant administration of barbiturates or analgesics, and interactions may also occur with various anti-arrhythmic compounds.

Interactions Affecting Metabolism

Variable effects on metabolism may occur when some cardiovascular drugs are given together. Inhibition of hepatic metabolism of a drug may lead to high plasma concentration with increased effects and risk of complications. Conversely, the rate of metabolism may be increased by the induction of the hepatic microsomal enzyme system. This may lead to decreased effective plasma concentration, requiring an increase in maintenance dosage. Withdrawal of the inducing agent may then lead to increased concentration and potential toxicity. Warfarin may be affected in this way by barbiturates and other anti-epileptic compounds.

Interactions Involved in Excretion

Drugs are excreted by glomerular filtration and active tubular secretion. Interactions may accompany the administration of drugs competing for active transport systems in the proximal tubule. This mechanism may be used to advantage with Probenecid to give enhanced antibiotic levels in the treatment of bacterial endocarditis.

References

Beeley LN (1984) Drug interactions. British National Formulary
Drayer DE, Reidenberg M (1977) Clinical consequences of polymorphic drugs. Clin Pharmacol Ther 22: 251–258
Fenster PE, Perrier D (1982) Applications of pharmacokinetic principles to cardiovascular drugs. Med Concs Cardiovasc Dis 57: 91–96
Giardina EGV, Fenster PE, Bigger JT Jr, Mayersohn M, Perrier D, Marcus FI (1980) Efficacy, plasma concentrations and adverse effects of a new sustained release procainamide preparation. Am J Cardiol 46: 855–862
Kristensen M, Molholm Hansen J, Kampmann J, Lumholtz B, Siersback Nielson K (1974) Drug elimination and renal function. J Clin Pharmacol 14: 307–308
Lindenbaum J, Mellow MH, Blackstone MO, Butler VP (1971) Variation in biological availability of digoxin from four preparations. N Engl J Med 285: 1344–1347
Mayer SE, Melman KL, Gilman KG (1980) General principles. In: Gilman AG, Goodman LS, Gilman A (eds) The pharmacological basis of therapeutics. Macmillan, New York, pp 1–27
Oie S, Tozer TN (1979) Effect of altered plasma protein binding on apparent volume of distribution. J Pharm Sci 68: 1203–1205
Wilkinson GR, Shand DG (1975) A physiologic approach to hepatic drug clearance. Clin Pharmacol Ther 18: 337–390

2 Atherosclerosis and Hyperlipoproteinaemia

Coronary heart disease (CHD) remains the leading cause of death in many countries. The fact that it may be declining in some areas (e.g. United States, Australia) allows no grounds for complacency. It is estimated that still more than 1.25 million Americans suffer a heart attack each year (Levy 1981), and in Scotland in 1977 the death rate from coronary disease was 800 per 100 000 population.

Pathophysiology

Clinical CHD — angina, myocardial infarction and sudden death — is related to atherosclerotic thickening and narrowing of coronary arteries. The development of atherosclerotic lesions follows a well defined pattern, although the initiating factors have not been fully established. The theory of Ross and Glomset (1976) seems acceptable at present. This postulates that the initiating event is a break in the continuity of the endothelial cell layer lining the inner vessel wall. This "injury" may be due to a variety of insults, including anoxia, cigarette smoking, hypertension, raised cholesterol and catecholamines. Such damage is probably frequent and usually repaired. However, if it occurs on a repeated or severe basis the normal cycle of damage/repair may be interrupted. It seems likely that platelet interaction with the vessel wall may help with repair but can also be associated with underlying tissue response to the damage. Platelets adhere to the site of injury. Platelet-derived growth factor (PDGF) causes excessive growth and migration of medial smooth muscle cells towards the subendothelial area. Further development of the lesion probably involves the deposition of macromolecules such as collagen, elastin and mucopolysaccharides as well as the accumulation of blood components such as fibrinogen and lipoprotein. The atherosclerotic plaque may then be complicated by ulceration, haemorrhage and superimposed thrombus formation.

Aetiology of Atheroma

It seems likely that the aetiology of atheroma is multifactorial. Although genetic predisposition is certainly involved in a significant number of patients, atherosclerosis is also modified by environmental influences. Some risk factors (defined as factors which increase the risk of CHD measured over a set period) have been identified, and more probably remain to be discovered. These risk factors include cigarette smoking, hypertension, lack of exercise, obesity, male sex, raised plasma cholesterol and low values of high density lipoprotein (HDL) cholesterol. High plasma cholesterol has been well identified as a definite risk factor. Gordon et al. (1977) have shown that the risk of developing CHD is proportional to the initial plasma cholesterol level in men aged 30–60 and women up to the age of 50.

Since the bulk of plasma cholesterol is in the low density lipoprotein (LDL) fraction it seems likely that the level of LDL might be related to the incidence of CHD. This has been confirmed, although the predictive value is no better than that of total plasma cholesterol. There has also been much recent interest in the association of HDL and CHD. In direct contrast to LDL, HDL correlates negatively with CHD and is thought to be a protective factor if present in high enough concentration (Miller and Miller 1975). Raised plasma triglyceride may also be associated with the subsequent development of CHD, although this relationship is much less established than with cholesterol.

Lipoprotein Metabolism

Blood lipids are hydrophobic and circulate in the plasma as lipid–protein complexes — lipoproteins. These particles exist in a dynamic system whose function is the intercellular transport of lipid (Fig. 2.1). Lipoprotein classes can be separated mainly on the basis of density.

1. Chylomicrons — primary products of the absorption of intestinal dietary fat.
2. Very low density lipoprotein particles (VLDL) — triglyceride-rich particles produced by the liver.
3. Intermediate density lipoprotein particles (IDL) — intermediate in the metabolism of VLDL to LDL.
4. Low density lipoprotein (LDL) — which makes cholesterol available to cells throughout the body.
5. High density lipoprotein (HDL) — which mediates cholesterol transport to the liver.

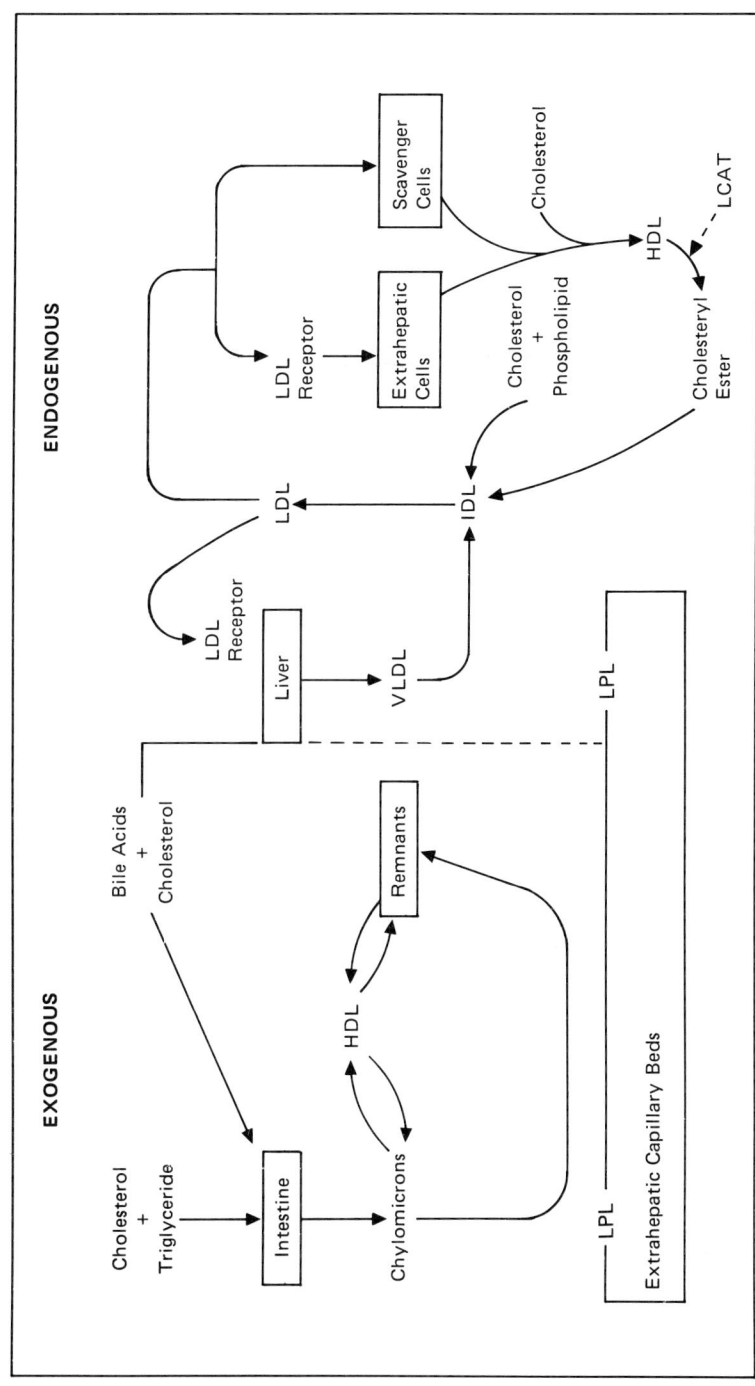

Fig. 2.1. Lipoprotein transport in man.

Associated with these lipids are a number of specific polypeptides — the apolipoproteins — which determine the metabolism of the particles. Each day the average man ingests around 120 g of fat, containing 0.5–1.0 mg cholesterol. The mucosal cells of the upper gut synthesise this into large triglyceride-rich particles which are secreted into the intestinal lymphatics and plasma. These chylomicrons interact with lipoprotein lipase located on the endothelial surfaces of capillary beds. The particles become progressively depleted of triglyceride and the remnants are avidly accumulated by the liver. The net result is rapid transfer of dietary triglyceride to peripheral storage and utilisation sites and the transfer of cholesterol to the liver. In the postabsorptive phase the liver acts to maintain the availability of lipid in the circulation. It secretes triglyceride-rich VLDL particles whose catabolism occurs by a mechanism similar to that of chylomicrons. Interaction with lipoprotein lipase converts them to smaller IDL particles. This remnant particle is transformed to LDL in a process during which cholesteryl ester is lost so that the final LDL contains 45% cholesterol, with its sole protein component being apolipoprotein B. LDL transports the bulk of cholesterol in human plasma and supplies cholesterol not only for the physiological needs of the cell but also for any developing atherosclerotic lesion. LDL is catabolised in at least two ways. The first process is mediated by a cell surface receptor which recognises apolipoprotein B and binds it with high affinity. The LDL/receptor complex is then taken into the cell and transferred to the lysosomal apparatus, where the LDL is degraded and its cholesterol either stored or transferred within the cell for use. The receptor can then be recycled to the cell surface. LDL can also be catabolised by a scavenger mechanism in which the reticuloendothelial system and associated phagocytes are involved. There is no feedback control to the scavenger pathway.

Of all the lipoprotein classes, least is known of the in vivo function of HDL. It participates in dynamic exchange of components with other lipoproteins and is likely to be involved in cholesterol transport from the periphery to the liver.

Metabolic Defects in Hyperlipoproteinaemia

A molecular defect can now be attached to each of Frederickson's phenotypic variants (Fredrickson et al. 1967).

Type I   — Persistence of chylomicrons in fasting plasma — defect in tissue lipoprotein lipase.

Type II   — Familial hypercholesterolaemia. There is a defect in the receptor mechanism for LDL catabolism so that LDL accumulates in the plasma. In familial combined hypercholesterolaemia there is overproduction with accumulation of both cholesterol and triglyceride in the plasma.

Type III   — This defect has recently been shown to derive from a single point mutation resulting in the substitution of cysteine for arginine in the apolipoprotein E of affected subjects. The IDL is raised in plasma, with the appearance of cholesterol-rich particles in VLDL.

Type IV — This is poorly understood. There is probably both overproduction and undercatabolism of VLDL, with a consequent rise in plasma levels of VLDL and triglyceride.

Type V — There is accumulation of both exogenous and endogenous triglyceride-rich particles, probably due to defective clearance.

It should be emphasised that not all lipoprotein disorders predispose to premature vascular disease. This has been shown to be an effect of types II, III and possibly IV.

Clinical Associations of Hyperlipoproteinaemia

The rationale for lowering plasma lipids has been based on correlations between raised plasma lipids and the risk of developing clinical CHD. The evidence rests on clinical studies (e.g. of familial hypercholesterolaemia), comparisons of populations in terms of cholesterol level and evidence of CHD, and correlation of coronary disease demonstrated at angiography with lipid levels (Murray et al. 1975). The question of whether or not a reduction in lipids, especially cholesterol, can reduce the incidence of CHD has been answered by The Lipid Research Clinics, Coronary Primary Prevention Trial results (1984a,b). The three major trials that first reported gave grounds for cautious optimism (Editorial 1975), but subsequent results were disappointing. This was especially true with regard to the clofibrate study, which set out to assess the long-term effect of clofibrate on cholesterol values and the incidence of CHD in apparently healthy volunteers (Committee of Principal Investigators 1978). From the cities of Edinburgh, Budapest and Prague were recruited 15 745 men aged between 30 and 59 years at entry. Three groups were studied.

1. Treatment group. Clofibrate was given to a randomly chosen 50% of those whose cholesterol value was in the upper third of the distribution of those tested.
2. A control group of 5000 men with similar cholesterol levels, who were given a placebo.
3. A second control group of 5000 men drawn from those whose cholesterol level was in the lower third of the distribution of those studied.

A cholesterol reduction of 15% was planned, but the actual reduction achieved was only 9%. The overall incidence of CHD was reduced by 20% due mainly to a reduction in non-fatal infarctions. However, the overall effect was adverse in that the number of deaths and crude death rates were higher in the treated group. More disquieting results have recently been reported (1980). The period of observation was 9.6 years — 5.3 in the trial and 4.3 afterwards. There were 25% more deaths in the clofibrate-treated group than in the high cholesterol control group. This occurred in all three participating centres. Mortality from all causes was higher, with no particular disease accounting for the increase. This was not an effect of continuing to take clofibrate, since less than 2% of subjects continued on the drug after the trial officially ended. Clofibrate therefore does not appear to be indicated for general use, although it is possible that it will continue to have a role in the treatment of specific hyperlipoproteinaemias.

The results reported by Hjermann et al. (1981) are more encouraging. They selected 1232 healthy normotensive men at high risk of CHD for a 5-year randomised trial to establish whether lowering of serum lipids and stopping smoking could reduce the incidence of CHD. Thus those in the intervention group were recommended to lower their blood lipids by a change of diet and to stop smoking. Mean cholesterol levels were approximately 13% lower during the trial in the intervention than in the control group, while tobacco consumption decreased by 45% more in the intervention than in the control group. At the end of the study the incidence of myocardial infarction (fatal and non-fatal) and sudden death was 47% lower in the intervention group than in the control group. This reduction correlated with the reduction in total cholesterol and to a lesser extent with reduced smoking.

The case for primary prevention of CHD has been strongly reinforced by the report of The Lipid Research Clinics (1984 a,b). This multicentre, randomised and double-blind clinical study was set up to test the effect of cholesterol lowering in reducing the risk of CHD in 3806 asymptomatic middle-aged men with type II hyperlipoproteinaemia (primary hypercholesterolaemia). The treatment group received the bile acid sequestrant cholestyramine resin and the control group a placebo for an average of 7.4 years. Both groups favoured a moderate cholesterol-lowering diet. The cholestyramine group achieved an average plasma total cholesterol reduction of 13.4%. This group also experienced a 19% reduction in risk ($P<0.05$) of the primary end-point — definite CHD death and/or definite non-fatal myocardial infarction —, reflecting a 24% reduction in definite CHD death and a 19% reduction in definite non-fatal myocardial infarction. The reduction of CHD incidence seemed to have been mediated principally by a reduction in total cholesterol and LDL cholesterol levels. These results provide strong evidence for the need to identify and treat those with significantly raised lipid values. It is not suggested that all will require drug treatment. This will be reserved for the most severely affected who do not respond to dietary cholesterol restriction.

The relationship between increasing levels of plasma cholesterol and the prevalence of CHD in a population has led to it being regarded as reasonable to attempt to lower increased cholesterol levels in affected individuals. A number of countries have proposed dietary advice aimed at lowering cholesterol levels in the population. It is possible to add drug therapy to initial dietary advice, but this should not be entered into lightly for, as with any pharmacological intervention, there are associated risks. Therefore the physician must carefully assess and review all relevant risk factors in the individual before embarking on what may well be lifelong therapy. There is certainly no indication for indiscriminate use of lipid-lowering agents in the population. These should be reserved for those with raised levels who have not responded to measures of weight reduction and dietary control. The falling incidence of CHD in the United States and Canada is of great interest. The reasons are unknown but could well be related to recognition of risk factors and alteration of life-style in terms of exercise, diet and weight. The evidence that treatment of raised lipid values can slow the rate of femoral atherosclerosis is potentially very important (Duffield et al. 1983).

In patients with CHD there would appear to be a case for a general dietary recommendation:

1. Correction of obesity
2. Reduction of dietary fat to 25%–30% of food energy
3. Roughly equal proportions of polyunsaturated and saturated fats.
4. Reduced cholesterol intake (dairy produce, liver, shellfish)

Management of Hyperlipoproteinaemia

The basis of treatment is always dietary and close liaison with the Nutrition Department is essential. Drug administration is an adjunct to diet and never a substitute. Drug treatment to lower lipid values should only be considered after the underlying anomaly has been accurately classified and the effect of diet assessed. Overall, relatively few patients will require drug treatment.

The commonest abnormalities are types IIA, IIB and V. Types I, III and V are uncommon.

Type I

Management is by control of dietary fat intake. A clofibrate analogue (see below) may be required.

Type IIA

Drug treatment is required only if raised cholesterol values persist after achieving a satisfactory body weight and after an adequate trial of low cholesterol diet.

First-line therapy is a bile acid sequestrant resin such as cholestyramine or colestipol. Cholestyramine (Questran) is available as 4-g sachets whose contents are then made up to 50–100 ml with water (or another suitable vehicle) and taken in a dose of three to six sachets per day. The taste is unpleasant and alimentary upset, especially constipation, can occur. Colestipol (Colestid) is an alternative. It is taken in a similar way to cholestyramine, in a dose of 15–30 g per day. Alimentary side-effects do occur but are said to be less marked than with cholestyramine.

Second-line therapy is usually a nicotinic acid derivative such as nicrofuranose (Bradilan) or a clofibrate analogue, such as bezafibrate (Bezalip). The starting dose of nicrofuranose is 250 mg t.i.d., increasing if necessary and if tolerated. This is an effective drug which would be more widely used but for its side-effects of flushing, sweating and diarrhoea. It is usually worthwhile persevering with, since side-effects may at times become less troublesome.

The use of clofibrate (Atromid-S) or newer analogues such as bezafibrate and gemfibrozol has declined since their initial widespread use and popularity. Clofibrate (Atromid-S 500 mg) is taken as three or four capsules daily. Alimentary side-effects are rare. Occasionally transitory increases in hepatic enzymes occur, and gallstones are a well recognised complication. Bezafibrate has a shorter half-life and is taken as 200 mg t.i.d. Side-effects are few, and gallstones do not seem to be a problem. Bezafibrate is also said to increase HDL levels, which may be of benefit (although this is not proven) in CHD.

Consideration may also need to be given to probucol (Lurselle) as second-line therapy (250 mg t.i.d.). The mode of action is uncertain; however, cholesterol levels are lowered, with reductions in both LDL and HDL — a fact which may reduce long-term clinical benefits.

Type IIB

Dietary control of weight and a reduction in cholesterol-containing foods are important and may be all that is needed. A clofibrate analogue and/or a nicotinic acid derivative are the most effective drugs, with additional use of a bile acid sequestrant resin to be considered.

Type III

Management is predominantly by a low fat, carbohydrate-controlled diet. The drug of choice is a clofibrate analogue. This can be extremely effective, leading to the disappearance of xanthomata and return of lipids to virtually normal values.

Type IV

Many subjects have a raised triglyceride value because they eat and drink to excess. Weight and alcohol control will often return triglyceride values to normal. Lipid-lowering drugs should not be given unless the patient co-operates in this way. In those whose triglyceride levels remain high, a clofibrate analogue or a nicotinic acid preparation is indicated.

Type V

This is a rare abnormality again often associated with alcohol excess. Management is predominantly by diet, although a clofibrate analogue may be required.

Mode of Action of Lipid-Lowering Drugs

Clofibrate

This is the ethyl ester of P-chlorophenoxyisobutyric acid (CPIB). It is absorbed relatively slowly, and after hydrolysis by intestinal and plasma hydrolases reaches a peak concentration after 3–6 h. The CPIB is 96% protein bound to albumen. This is important since it means a restricted volume distribution of 6–10 litres and a plasma half-life between 12–15 h. There may also be displacement of less firmly bound but potent therapeutic agents such as phenytoin and warfarin, so that the dosage of these compounds has to be reduced when they are given in association with clofibrate. The long plasma half-life means it is possible to maintain effective blood levels by giving 1 g b.i.d. There has been considerable controversy over the mechanism of action. It was initially thought that clofibrate displaced other metabolically active compounds such as androsterone or thyroxine from their binding sites and thus potentiated their action. In fact it now seems likely that clofibrate and a number of recently introduced analogues such as bezafibrate achieve their lipid-lowering effect through the stimulation of lipoprotein lipase found on capillary endothelium and responsible for initiating VLDL triglyceride hydrolysis. Clofibrate can reduce free fatty acid output from adipose tissue but its principal effect is to increase the rate of VLDL utilisation at the periphery. Clofibrate also causes a suppression of cholesterol synthesis, apparently by inhibiting hepatic HMG CoA reductase. There is a reduction in sterol synthesis and an increase in efflux from tissues. The increase in faecal sterol excretion does, however, supersaturate the bile and increase the risk of gallstone formation. The CPIB derivatives are most effective in hypertriglyceridaemic patients. VLDL reduction begins within 2–5 days of starting treatment. A reduction of 20%–30% in plasma triglyceride can be achieved. The cholesterol response depends on the pre-treatment triglyceride value. In patients with pronounced hyper-triglyceridaemia the clofibrate-induced reduction in VLDL is often associated with a rise in both LDL and HDL cholesterol. Thus although VLDL cholesterol falls during treatment, this effect may be offset by the rise in LDL and HDL cholesterol so that overall plasma cholesterol levels may be little changed or even rise. However, in subjects whose plasma triglyceride is initially normal, LDL levels usually fall, suggesting that clofibrate and its analogues also accelerate LDL catabolism, possibly through activation of the high affinity LDL receptor pathway.

Analogues such as bezafibrate, ciprofibrate and gemfibrozil may have additional benefits in that they raise HDL. However, they have not yet been subjected to rigorous clinical trials to assess their effect on mortality or the extent of their side-effects.

Nicotinic Acid

Nicotinic acid is unique among lipid-lowering agents in being able to produce substantial lowering of both plasma cholesterol and triglyceride in most recipients. It has had varying popularity, mainly due to its side-effects of flushing and gastrointestinal irritation. Virtually all is absorbed from the gut and blood levels peak within 1 h of ingestion. It is nicotinic acid itself that is the active agent and most is excreted unchanged in the urine. The dose is 2–3 g per day in divided doses.

The primary action of nicotinic acid is on the flux of free fatty acids to the liver. These fatty acids are generated by the hydrolysis of triglyceride in peripheral adipose tissue mediated by hormone-sensitive lipase. Nicotinic acid suppresses lipoprotein lipase activity and reduces the plasma free fatty acid level below that required to maintain normal hepatic VLDL synthesis and secretion. As a result triglyceride and VLDL levels fall, with the level of reduction being a function of the initial triglyceride level. The influence of nicotinic acid on VLDL metabolism leads to a secondary reduction in the synthesis of LDL. There may also be an inhibitory effect of nicotinic acid on cholesterol synthesis through an effect on HMG CoA reductase.

The overall average fall in triglyceride values is around 40%, although the range is large, being 15% to 94%. In patients with type IIA hyperlipoproteinaemia the cholesterol level may fall by up to 15%. The recent resurgence of interest in nicotinic acid partly reflects the finding that it produces a rise in the possible anti-atherogenic HDL. However, much more long-term work is needed to establish the value of these various additional actions.

Bile Acid Sequestrant Resins

Bile acid sequestrant resins, such as cholestyramine and colestipol, function by binding to bile acids in the intestinal lumen and preventing their enterohepatic circulation.

Each day 10–20 g of cholesterol and its derivatives passes through the intestine and liver in an enterohepatic circulation. Cholesterol is secreted by the liver into bile; it then mixes with dietary sterol and is extensively reabsorbed. Bile acids are formed from cholesterol in a biosynthetic sequence initiated by cholesterol-7-hydroxylase. These bile acids are conserved by an active uptake mechanism in the terminal ileum.

Reabsorption of bile acids can be reduced by oral administration of high molecular weight ion exchange resins which bind large quantities of bile acids irreversibly and prevent their uptake by mucosal cells. These compounds are polymers of styrene and divinylbenzene (cholestyramine) and tetraethylenepentamine and epichlorohydrin (colestipol). They alter the activities of several important hepatic enzymes whose function is normally regulated by the reabsorbed bile acids. The rate-limiting enzyme in bile acid synthesis is activated and initiates the conversion of cholesterol to bile acids, which increases the drain on the hepatic cholesterol pool. As might be expected, there are compensatory mechanisms to counteract the decline. Endogenous cholesterol synthesis increases, and LDL cholesterol assimilation by the liver is also increased. Overall, bile acid sequestrants have a marked hypocholesterolaemic action, lowering the plasma LDL by 20%–30%. In general there is little overall effect on triglyceride levels, though they may rise transiently.

Total HDL cholesterol remains unchanged. Overall these compounds seem to be relatively free of the complications that have occurred with other cholesterol-lowering drugs. However, because of their bulk and general unpalatability (nausea and diarrhoea are not uncommon) many patients find compliance a problem. Cholestyramine is taken as four to eight sachets daily, suspended in water or orange juice. Colestipol has similar actions but less side-effects and is well worth trying in those who cannot tolerate cholestyramine.

Probucol

The chemical structure of probucol, a recently introduced compound, differs completely from that of other lipid-lowering agents. It is sulphur containing bisphenol [4,4'-(isopropyl-idene dithio)bis(2,6-di-tert-butylphenol]. It is only sparingly water soluble, which results in little absorption from the gut and substantial retention in body fat stores. It has few side-effects and seems well tolerated in the long term. Probucol lowers plasma cholesterol by 10%–20% without affecting triglyceride levels, but there is no good evidence as to its mechanism of action. It possibly inhibits release of lipoproteins by the liver. It has been shown that both LDL and HDL cholesterol levels fall. The reduction in LDL cholesterol varies from 8% to 16%, while that of HDL is around 25%.

While the significance of these lipid changes for the long-term prophylaxis of CHD is unclear, it is suggested that probucol should at present be reserved for those individuals who, when given a trial of the drug, exhibit (a) a fall in plasma cholesterol due primarily to the fall in LDL cholesterol and (b) a minimal fall in HDL cholesterol. The dosage is 250–500 mg twice daily.

The uses and modes of action of lipid-lowering drugs in frequent use are given in Table 2.1

Table 2.1. Lipid-lowering drugs

Non-proprietary name	Proprietary name	Postulated primary action	Effective in hyperlipoproteinaemia types
Nicotinic acid derivatives	Bradilan Ronicol	Inhibit lipolysis Reduce transport of fatty acids to liver	IIA IV V
Bile acid sequestrant resins	Questran Colestid	Bind bile acids in gut: Interrupt enterohepatic circulation of bile acids	IIA
Clofibrate Bezafibrate Fenofibrate Ciprofibrate Gemfibrozil	Atromid-S Bezalip	Decrease VLDL synthesis Increase VLDL catabolism	} IIB IV V
Probucol	Lurselle	? Inhibits lipoprotein synthesis	IIA

Conclusion

The evidence that a raised cholesterol level contributes to premature CHD is convincing in situations such as familial hypercholesterolaemia, where marked increases in LDL are found and both homozygote and heterozygote subjects present with early CHD, and is probable in other hyperlipoproteinaemias with polygenic or multifactorial causes. The evidence for triglyceride as a risk factor remains controversial.

Raised lipid values may thus be associated with early CHD but does treatment to lower them mean a corresponding reduction in the number of clinical events or the extent of atherosclerosis? The answer to both questions is possibly but not certainly yes. The Oslo study (Hjermann et al. 1981) indicated that in initially healthy men who were at increased risk of CHD, advice with regard to smoking and diet significantly reduced the incidence of the first event of myocardial infarction and sudden death. Conflicting evidence has arisen from other studies (WHO European Collaborative Group 1983; MRFIT Research Group 1982), where only a slight benefit apparently resulted from lowering of lipid levels. In terms of regression of atherosclerosis following treatment of hyperlipoproteinaemia, Olsson et al. (1982), in an open study, reported beneficial effects of femoral atheroma. Duffield et al. (1983) have now reported a randomised control trial of the effect of treatment of hyperlipoproteinaemia in subjects with symptomatic femoral atherosclerosis. Atherosclerosis in those treated advanced much more slowly than in those left untreated.

The management of hyperlipoproteinaemia depends on individual clinical assessment. It is only one of the known risk factors, albeit an important one. Our approach is to modify all possible risk factors — such as cigarette smoking, hypertension and hyperlipoproteinaemia — in an attempt to lessen the chance of early clinical CHD or to improve the subsequent prognosis.

References

Committee of principal investigators (1978) A co-operative trial in the prevention of ischaemic heart disease using clofibrate. Br Heart J 40: 1069

Duffield RGM, Lewis B, Miller NE, Jameson CE, Brunt JNH, Colchester ACF (1983) Treatment of hyperlipidaemia retards progression of symptomatic femoral atherosclerosis. Lancet II: 639–642

Editorial (1975) Lipids and ischaemic heart disease. Lancet II: 398

Fredrickson DS, Levy RI, Lees RS (1967) Fat transport in lipoproteins — an integrated approach to mechanisms and disorders. N Engl J Med 276: 34, 94, 148, 215, 272

Gordon T, Castelli WP, Mjortland MC, Kannel WB, Dawber TR (1977) Predicting coronary disease in middle-aged and older persons. The Framingham Study. JAMA 238: 497

Hjermann I, Velve Byre K, Holme I, Leren P (1981) Effect of diet and smoking intervention on the incidence of coronary heart disease. Lancet II: 1303–1310

Levy RI (1981) Lipoproteins, apoproteins and heart disease. Present status and future prospects. Clin Chem Acta 27: 653

Miller GJ, Miller NE (1975) Plasma high density lipoprotein concentration and development of ischaemic heart disease. Lancet I: 16

MRFIT Research Group (1982) Multiple risk factor intervention trial: risk factor changes and mortalitiy results. JAMA 248: 1465–1477

Murray RG, Tweddel A, Third JLHC, Hillis WS, Hutton I, Lorimer AR, Lawrie TDV (1975) Relation between extent of coronary artery disease and severity of hyperlipoproteinaemia. Br Heart J 37: 1035

Olsson AG, Carlson LA, Erikson U, Helmius G, Hemmingsson A, Ruhn G (1982) Regression of computer estimated femoral atherosclerosis after pronounced serum lipid lowering in patients with asymptomatic hyperlipidaemia. Lancet I: 1311

Ross R, Glomset JA (1976) The pathogenesis of atherosclerosis. N Engl J Med 295: 420

The Lipid Research Clinics Coronary Primary Prevention Trial Results (1984) I. Reduction in incidence of coronary heart disease. JAMA 251: 351

The Lipid Research Clinics Coronary Primary Prevention Trial Results (1984) II. The relation of reduction in incidence of coronary heart disease to cholesterol. JAMA 251: 365

WHO European Collaborative Group (1983) Multifactorial trial in the prevention of coronary heart disease. 3. Incidence and mortality results. Eur Heart J 4: 141–147

3 Angina Pectoris

Clinical Presentation

Angina pectoris is a symptom complex due to reversible myocardial ischaemia. The diagnosis must not be made casually. The symptoms are those of chest pain or tightness which can radiate to either or both arms, throat or back. Pain is brought on by effort or emotion or may occur spontaneously at rest.

Patients with angina pectoris can be divided into clinical subsets by symptoms. Those with stable angina have a reproducible pattern in terms of intensity and duration of pain and precipitating factors. Unstable angina includes those with recent onset of symptoms (less than 6 months) or a changing pattern often involving spontaneous pain at rest or with crescendo worsening of symptoms.

Differential Diagnosis

A detailed history and physical examination are required. Patients complain of chest pain which may or may not be cardiac in origin. Other causes of pain may arise from the alimentary tract or respiratory system, or be of musculoskeletal origin (Table 3.1). The commonest cardiac cause of angina is atherosclerosis of the major coronary arteries. Cinical examination may suggest other factors such as aortic stenosis, systemic hypertension, anaemia and arrhythmia.

Table 3.1. Causes of chest pain

Cardiac			Non-cardiac		
Angina		Non-anginal, e.g. pericardial	Alimentary	Musculo-skeletal	Other
Coronary athero-sclerosis	± Aortic valve disease Anaemia Dysrhythmia (brady- or tachycardia) Thyroid dysfunction (hyper- or hypothyroidism)		Hiatus hernia Gall bladder disease	Cervical spondylosis	Functional

Investigations

Since angina pectoris is a symptom complex, objective confirmatory evidence of the diagnosis is sought. The main investigation remains electrocardiography. The resting electrocardiogram may show evidence of ischaemia or infarction in 50% of patients. Exercise electrocardiography using treadmill or bicycle ergometer is useful in establishing the degree of disability and increasing the diagnostic yield by about 35%. Additional techniques to localise reversible myocardial ischaemia include radionuclide assessment of perfusion (exercise thallium scintigraphy). Selective coronary arteriography is the ultimate investigation to provide information on the coronary anatomy and the extent of atherosclerotic disease. This investigation is usually performed in patients with stable angina who are refractory to medical treatment or in subjects with unstable angina with a view to performing coronary artery bypass surgery.

Pathophysiology

Angina pectoris results from an imbalance of myocardial oxygen supply and demand. There is a transient lack of oxygen available for myocardial needs. Until recently our concept of the pathogenesis of angina was based on an underlying stenotic lesion of one or more coronary arteries. Symptoms occur when myocardial oxygen demand is increased above that level which can be supplied. The factors which influence demand are listed below:

Heart rate
Contractility
Wall tension (determined by systolic blood pressure)
Left ventricular volume

The concept that dynamic coronary obstruction, most commonly due to coronary vasoconstriction (spasm), is a potential cause of angina has recently been re-emphasised and highlighted, especially by the work of Maseri and his colleagues (1978, 1980). Spasm occurs most often in association with underlying coronary atherosclerotic narrowing, but can also occur in a normal vessel, where it may be an exaggeration of normal tone. Coronary spasm has been well documented, but other causes of dynamic obstruction may occur, such as platelet aggregation possibly related to prostaglandin imbalance with increased thromboxane A_2 levels. Dynamic and fixed obstruction may both contribute to a variable extent in individual patients. Subjects with stable angina have predominantly, although not exclusively, coronary atherosclerotic obstructive disease, while those with unstable angina are more likely to have a combination of atherosclerotic and dynamic obstruction. Occasionally dynamic obstruction or spasm may be solely responsible.

Management

Treatment is directed towards improvement in the quality of life by relief of symptoms. Hopefully prognosis may also be improved, although this has not yet been convincingly established. The steps to be taken include:

1. Relief of pain
2. Control or correction of risk factors such as cigarette smoking, systemic hypertension and hyperlipoproteinaemia

Reduction in cigarette smoking is especially important since smoking can impair the response to β-blockers such as propranolol by altering their metabolism.

Clinical Aspects of Drug Use

Patients who present with angina pectoris due to CHD can be considerably improved by medical management. Each patient requires detailed evaluation and consideration of their individual problems. Recent developments in management indicate it is now possible to select compounds that may act in one or several ways:

1. By reducing myocardial oxygen needs
2. By increasing myocardial blood flow by coronary vasodilatation
3. By the combination of reduced myocardial needs and increased flow

In terms of reduction of myocardial oxygen needs, there are compounds which will:

1. Predominantly reduce preload by venous or capacitance vessel dilatation — *nitrates*
2. Act on the heart to reduce heart rate and blood pressure — β *receptor antagonists*
3. Predominantly reduce afterload by dilatation of arterioles or resistance vessels — *calcium channel blockers*

These compounds can be used singly or together to produce additive effects.

Increased Myocardial Blood Flow

Coronary vasospasm has been shown to be a significant factor in many patients. It usually occurs in association with underlying fixed (atherosclerotic) coronary disease, but can occur spontaneously in apparently normal vessels. Nitrates and calcium channel blockers have proven effective in abolishing spasm, dilating coronary arteries and improving flow. The haemodynamic effects of the main anti-anginal drugs are illustrated in Table 3.2.

In patients with stable exertional angina it is logical to use a quick acting nitrate for relief of pain or as a prophylactic before effort known from experience to cause pain. β-Adrenoreceptor antagonists should be used in adequate doses as maintenance therapy. The choice of a non-selective or a selective compound will depend on the individual patient's needs. Many will benefit from a long acting preparation which reduces the need for frequent dosing. Further developments in medical management are likely. The prostacyclin analogues may well become useful (Bergman et al. 1981). Such compounds decrease platelet aggregation and cause coronary and systemic vasodilatation. Conversely, agents to antagonise or reduce platelet aggregating properties of

Table 3.2. Haemodynamic effects of the main drugs used in angina

	β-blockers	Calcium antagonists	Nitrate	Combination
Heart rate	↓	→ ↑	↑	↓
Blood pressure (afterload)	↓	↓	↓	↓
Preload	→ ↑	↓	↓ ↓	↓
Contractility	↓	→ ↓	↑	↓ →
Coronary blood flow	?	↑	↑	↑

thromboxane synthetase may well also be developed (Editorial 1981). These compounds, however, have not yet been fully evaluated and cannot be recommended for routine use.

Step Care Management

The management of angina pectoris is essentially a matter of personal experience and choice. The policy outlined below is ours, but others are equally valuable.

1. Avoid precipitating factors, e.g. exertion after a meal, exposure to cold and wind.
2. Control adverse factors, i.e. hypertension, smoking, obesity and high lipid levels (especially of cholesterol).
3. Rapid acting preparation for relief of pain or as prophylaxis before effort known to evoke pain. The following preparations may be used: glyceryl trinitrate, buccal nitrate spray, chewable isosorbide and nifedipine capsule (to be bitten rather than swallowed).
4. Maintenance therapy with β-adrenoceptor blocking compounds such as atenolol 50–100 mg daily or metoprolol 50 mg t.i.d. One should aim for a resting heart rate of 60. Occasionally there may be a need to check inhibition of exercise heart rate to ensure the dose is adequate.
5. If angina is not controlled or if β-adrenoceptor blockage is contraindicated add either:
   a) A calcium channel blocker — either nifedipine or verapamil
   b) A nitrate
   Triple therapy should be used if required to control symptoms, though it often offers little in addition to double therapy.
6. Those whose quality of life is significantly impaired should be considered for investigation for coronary artery bypass surgery.

General Measures

A most important step is to inform the patient of the cause of his symptoms, and involve him in their management. The lay interpretation of angina pectoris is that of inevitable eventual sudden death from myocardial infarction. It should be emphasised that this is not necessarily so. Explanation should be given as to the cause of pain, its transitory nature and the benefits and rationale of treatment. An overall individual management plan should be developed, care being taken to explain the importance of the development of a changing pattern of symptoms. Large meals, demanding and tense business schedules or unaccustomed severe exercise may produce symptoms and should be avoided or amended. A change of occupation may or may not be appropriate. This depends on the type of work and the precipitating factors of angina. Obviously a man engaged in heavy labour may find himself unable to continue in this and require to seek lighter work. Those with emotionally induced pain may benefit from a reorganisation of activities. It should always be remembered, however, that lighter work may imply a considerable reduction in salary. The physician's attitude should always be positive and directed towards what can be done rather than be negative and prohibitory.

Exercise

Exercise is regarded as helpful both psychologically and physiologically. The possible benefits of exercise include:

1. A slower heart rate both at rest and on exercise
2. A slight reduction in blood pressure
3. Increased output and physical work capacity
4. Lower low density lipoprotein and triglyceride
5. An increase in high density lipoprotein

Physiological improvement with training has been found in patients with angina (Redwood et al. 1972; Kennedy 1976). There is increasing interest in exercise programmes and this aspect of management may become more commonly used. Exercise should be graded to the patient's fitness, his surroundings and his background. A possible training programme would be:

1. Establish exercise tolerance
2. On several occasions in the next 2–3 weeks exercise just short of this level
3. Reassess exercise tolerance after 2–3 weeks. Increase or maintain the exercise level as indicated

Adverse features may occasionally accompany exercise. These, however, are predominantly musculoskeletal rather than cardiac. Exercise should be limited in those with significant obesity, chronic obstructive airways disease or arrhythmia. Any increase in symptoms should be noted and the exercise programme curtailed.

Relief of Pain

Patients quickly learn that exertional angina can be relieved by slowing down or standing still. The erect position leads to venous pooling in the legs, with a reduction in venous return and consequently diminished cardiac work and oxygen requirements.

Drug Treatment

In terms of management of angina it is now possible to identify the main sites of pharmacological activity that will produce benefit (Table 3.3).

Table 3.3. Sites of action of anti-anginal treatment

A. Action on capacitance vessels to produce reduction in preload by venous dilatation, e.g. nitrates
B. Action on myocardium by reduction in heart rate, blood pressure and myocardial contractility, e.g. β-adrenoceptor blockade
C. Action on resistance vessels to produce reduction in afterload by arteriolar dilatation, e.g. calcium channel blockers
D. Relief of coronary spasm by vasoactive compounds, e.g. nitrates, calcium channel blockers

Nitrates

Nitrates have been and remain a mainstay in the management of angina pectoris. Inorganic nitrates and organic nitrites and nitrates are all active. The smooth muscle of arterioles and veins is relaxed by a direct dose-related effect. As already noted, angina may be due to increased myocardial demands, as occurs with exercise, or to a sudden reduction in coronary flow, as occurs with coronary spasm. In the former situation reduction in myocardial oxygen demand is more likely to meet with success than attempts to augment coronary flow. When spasm is present, removal of the vasoconstriction and a consequent increase in flow will relieve pain, although reduction in myocardial oxygen needs remains a major factor. Nitrates have both actions. Their main therapeutic effect is to reduce myocardial oxygen needs by their action on the peripheral circulation in reducing preload by means of venous dilatation while in addition, though to a lesser extent, they reduce afterload by arteriolar dilatation. Sublingual glyceryl trinitrate (GTN) should be taken to relieve pain and also prophylactically before effort known from experience to cause symptoms. It is usually taken as a 0.5 mg tablet, although other concentrations are available. The beneficial effects last for 45–60 min and can be repeated as required, although persistence of pain is an indication to seek further help. Tolerance does not develop nor is the beneficial effect reduced by concomitant therapy with isosorbide (Lee 1978). Rapid relief of symptoms can also be obtained by other preparations. Isosorbide dinitrate is widely used, especially as chewable tablets again aimed at absorption from the buccal mucosa. The dose is 5–10 mg. An aerosol inhaler is available for administration of a metered dose and is claimed to be effective in providing rapid pain relief.

Longer Acting Nitrates

The use of longer acting nitrates is an area of considerable controversy, claim and counterclaim. There have been recent innovations in terms of administration and metabolism, but more time is needed for these to be evaluated.

Isosorbide dinitrate, swallowed as 10 mg tablets, has been used for years in the maintenance management of angina. Improvement in exercise tolerance has been claimed for 4–6 h. It has also been suggested that an increase in the dose to 20 mg t.i.d. may be useful in prolonging the action. Especially in patients with nocturnal angina there would appear to be a place for sustained release preparations. Recent interest has centred on the system of delivery. Should this be an ointment or should it be via an impregnated pad? The ointment has been available longer. The nitrate is absorbed through the skin and can be applied anywhere although, probably for psychological reasons, many patients prefer the precordial area. The method seems strange initially, with dosage starting at 2 cm of ointment and increasing to 5 cm, but patient acceptance is good. The ointment must be covered to prevent loss by volatilisation. The site should be changed and the occlusive dressing least likely to cause skin irritation selected. The more recently introduced transdermal slow release preparation also shows promise. Sustained release preparations of oral nitrates are available and preferred by some patients. There is no doubt they are effective but the duration of action is uncertain. A sustained release preparation which is absorbed over a period of hours from the buccal mucosa has recently been introduced. Early claims seem promising but not enough data are yet available. The development of tolerance seems possible.

Side-effects

The major side-effect of nitrates is headache due probably to vasodilatation. The headache can be severe and pounding and is intolerable to some. Care should always be taken to tell the patient that this is an anticipated side-effect and is a reflection of the action of the drug. It is said that the headache eventually becomes less troublesome while the pain relief persists. Palpitation and flushing may also occur due to reflex tachycardia and vasodilatation. These may be persistent but not so clamant as the headache. Table 3.4 gives examples of nitrate preparations.

Clinical Pharmacology

Glyceryl Trinitrate (GTN). In the healthy animal GTN dilates arteries, and it exerts a similar effect on healthy and vasoconstricted segments of human coronary arteries. In angina due to increased metabolic demands for oxygen the effect of GTN is dominated by its action on the peripheral circulation. Pooling of blood in capacitance vessels by venodilator action leads to a fall in venous return and a fall in left ventricular end-diastolic pressure (which

Table 3.4. Examples of currently used nitrate preparations

Generic name	Proprietary name	Usual dose
Glyceryl trinitrate (GTN)		
tablets	–	0.5 mg sublingually
GTN spray	Nitrolingual	0.4 mg
GTN slow release lozenge	Suscard Buccal	1–5 mg
GTN slow release tablets	Sustac Nitrocontin	2–10 mg t.i.d.
GTN ointment	Percotol	1–3 cm b.i.d. or t.i.d.
GTN skin patch	Transidern-Nitro	1 patch (25 mg) per 24 h
Isosorbide dinitrate tablets	Cedocard, Isordil Sorbitrate	10–20 mg t.i.d.
Isosorbide slow release		
tablets	Cedocard Retard, Isordil	
	Tembids	40–160 mg b.i.d.
Isosorbide solution	Cedocard I.V. Isoket	5–30 mg/h i.v.
Isosorbide mononitrate		
tablets	Elantan, Ismo 20 Monit	20–40 mg t.i.d.

increases at the onset of an anginal attack). There is a slight fall in systemic blood pressure, a decrease in forearm vascular resistance and a reflex tachycardia. The development of radionuclide techniques for studying myocardial perfusion has given further information: The majority of chronically underperfused but non-infarcted areas of the left ventricle demonstrate an improvement in local contraction after GTN. This improvement in regional function is probably attributable to two actions: (a) an indirect extracardiac mechanism such as reduction of preload and possibly also afterload; (b) a possible shunting of blood to the ischaemic subendocardial zone. In coronary vasoconstriction the beneficial effects are related both to vasodilatation of the constricted segment or segments and to the peripheral action.

GTN is moderately volatile whereas nitrates of higher molecular weight compounds such as isosorbide dinitrate are solid and non-volatile. For rapid effects the drug should be chewed or allowed to dissolve slowly in the mouth. This permits rapid achievement of peak blood concentrations — often within a few minutes — and a rapid onset of action and pain relief.

Longer Acting Nitrates. The initial studies of potentially longer acting nitrates were not convincing. Needleman (1972) showed there was considerable first pass hepatic degradation of organic nitrates. However, the dosages used in these studies may have been inadequate and higher dosages have shown measurable plasma levels of active compound several hours after oral administration. Prolongation of action may be possible by saturation of enzymatic degradation processes. Thus 20 mg of oral isosorbide has been shown to have haemodynamic effects and to improve exercise tolerance for up to 4 h after administration (Markis et al. 1979). There is considerable variation in what is an effective dose. This should be assessed individually since the required dose may be 15, 30 or even 60 mg. It is known that the dinitrate is biotransformed in man by glutathione-5-transferase to the 2- and 5-mononitrate and to isosorbide. It is probable that the mononitrate metabolites, especially the 5-isomer, contribute to the beneficial action and a prolonged effect. Isosorbide-5-mononitrate is now available for clinical use. Reports are so far scanty, but certainly the compound would seem to have the benefit of prolonged action because of high plasma levels and no first pass hepatic metabolism.

Other formulations of nitrates have been introduced. Topical sustained release preparations applied as an ointment circumvent the portal circulation and thus avoid first pass hepatic metabolism. Blumenthal et al. (1977) demonstrated approximate equivalence in the plasma nitrate levels achieved with oral sustained release preparation and with ointment. It should, however, be noted that the assay of nitrate is complicated, involving gas chromatography with electron capture, and cannot yet be regarded as completely reliable and reproducible. Further methods of assessment of individual preparations have involved physiological markers of pharmacological activities. Such markers include the left ventricular ejection time (LVET) measured from systolic time intervals, the filling pressure of the left ventricle derived from measurement of pulmonary capillary wedge pressure and the duration of exercise before pain. Other methods of administration include nitrate-impregnated discs for prolonged absorption through the skin and a buccal spray. Sustained release tablets for buccal absorption are now also available, although their role has not yet been established. Some years ago the nitrates could have been regarded as a static area of clinical cardiology, but they have recently enjoyed a renaissance in terms of new indications, new formulations and new information as to the mode of action.

Intravenous Nitrates.   Stable preparations of nitrates for parenteral use are now available. They include nitroglycerine and isosorbide dinitrate. These drugs can be given intravenously or, if necessary, directly into the coronary circulation during angiography. If coronary vasoconstriction occurs during angiography, nitrate given into the coronary artery will relax the spasm and restore coronary flow. Intravenous use of nitrate can be extremely effective in relieving angina of both stenosis and spasm by its rapid and major peripheral effect on capacitance vessels, with a reduction in preload and thus in left ventricular end-diastolic pressure. Patients with unstable angina may be treated for prolonged periods (days if necessary) by continuous intravenous isosorbide. Dose schedules for the use of nitrates are shown in Table 3.4.

Calcium Channel Blockers

Although calcium channel blockers have been available in Europe for more than 15 years, it is only recently that their diverse pharmacological effects and the range of their clinical applications have been appreciated. Calcium channel blockers reduce transmembrane transport of calcium ions on which vascular (and other) tissue depends for contraction or impulse formation. Although these compounds may have a similar effect, they also have widely varying formulae and variable actions on smooth muscle, pacemaker and myocardial tissue. Each drug has a different pharmacological profile. In the management of angina the most frequently used compounds are nifedipine (popular), verapamil (popular) and diltiazem (recently introduced); perhexilene has now been withdrawn following reduction in its use (Table 3.5). There are many other compounds under assessment at present.

Table 3.5. Examples of currently used calcium channel blockers

Generic name	Proprietary name	Usual dose
Nifedipine capsules	Adalat	10–30 mg t.i.d.
Nifedipine slow release tablets	Adalat Retard	20–40 mg b.i.d.
Verapamil	Cordilox	80–120 mg t.i.d.

Mode of Action

For many years Ca^{2+} ions have been known to play a major role in the development of the action potential and the contraction of the myocardial cell. There are thought to be three mechanisms for increasing the intracellular Ca^{2+} content:

1. A slow inward current of Ca^{2+}, important in the development of the action potential (plateau phase, phase 2).
2. An exchange of Na^+ and Ca^{2+} ions across cell membranes which is independent of the slow channel.
3. Release of larger amounts of intracellular Ca^{2+} from the sarcoplasmic reticulum by the inward movements of small amounts of Ca^{2+} across the cell membrane. Similar ion movements occur in smooth muscle cells in the arterial wall, playing an important part in the degree of contraction or tone of arteries. Calcium channel blockers reduce the movement of Ca^{2+} ions as outlined above.

Calcium channel blockers depress myogenic activity and the responsiveness to vasoconstrictor stimuli of smooth muscle cells in the precapillary vessels. Their inhibitory effect on the contractile responses of vascular smooth muscle cells of arteries reduces vasospasm. By inhibition of the constrictor responses of the splanchnic capacitance vessels there is a reduction in preload.

Calcium channel blockers vary in their site and extent of action and have major differences in tissue selectivity which reflect differences in their pharmacodynamic and pharmacokinetic properties. Thus verapamil has a greater negative inotropic action and slows A-V conduction more than does nifedipine.

Haemodynamic Effects

Calcium channel blockers can have considerable haemodynamic effects. By their action on ion fluxes in myocardial cells they can depress myocardial contractility, while their action on peripheral vessels causes vasodilatation, which may affect coronary and peripheral vessels. Verapamil, diltiazem, perhexilene and nifedipine, in that order, have a negative inotropic action. Because of peripheral vasodilatation, nifedipine produces a reflex response resulting in a slight increase in heart rate which counterbalances the direct negative effect on the myocardium. Verapamil, on the other hand, causes a slight reduction in heart rate. Verapamil is less potent as a peripheral vasodilator (although it is effective in relieving coronary spasm) but has a more pronounced negative inotropic action and greater electrophysiological effect in terms of reducing conductivity in, for example, the A-V node.

There are several mechanism by which calcium channel blockers may be effective in angina pectoris.

1. Reduction in afterload by peripheral vasodilatation, leading to reduced oxygen requirements, the main action.
2. Depression of myocardial contractility, reducing myocardial oxygen requirements, probably of little importance.
3. Dilatation of coronary vessels to increase myocardial oxygen supply, when coronary vasoconstriction is prominent.

Nifedipine

Nifedipine is a dihydropyridine derivative. It is rapidly and almost completely absorbed after oral or sublingual administration and appears in plasma within 2–3 min with a peak concentration after 1–2 h. First pass extraction by the liver is not high and systemic bio-availability is approximately 65%. Nifedipine is metabolised to inactive forms, with about 80% being excreted in the urine and 15% eliminated via the gut. It is about 90% bound to plasma proteins. Assay methods (isotopic, gas chromatographic and fluorimetric) are unreliable and difficult and perhaps because of this, data correlating nifedipine plasma concentrations with simultaneous drug effects are rare.

Nifedipine has been shown to improve ST segment depression in exercise-induced angina both in single dose studies and in studies carried out over several weeks. It reduces the frequency of angina on exercise and increases exercise tolerance (Lynch et al. 1980). It also reduces myocardial oxygen consumption as measured by the double product of rate times pressure. It seems likely that its main beneficial effects are on the peripheral circulation, the rise in heart rate being insufficient to offset the decreases in afterload and peripheral resistance. In a review of data from several study centres, Ebner and Dunschede (1975) reported that even in rather low doses of 10 mg t.i.d., nifedipine reduced the frequency of attacks in patients with chronic exertional angina by 60%. In the management of stable exertional angina, nifedipine is given in 10 mg doses initially and is usually given 3 times a day. The dose may be increased in amount or frequency depending on response. Although dramatic falls are unlikely, blood pressure should be monitored as a rough guide to drug effect. Increases in dose above 60 mg daily are more likely to be associated with side-effects.

In general the drug is well tolerated and safe. A review of more than 5000 patients (Ebner and Dunschede 1975) cited headache (5.9%) as the most frequent side-effect. Other side-effects were also related to the vasodilatory properties of nifedipine and included feelings of warmth and flushing. Ankle swelling may occur but this is a reflection of vasodilatation and not necessarily of heart failure. Care should, however, be taken when large doses of β-adrenoceptor blocking drugs are being given concomitantly, since occasionally heart failure is precipitated.

Verapamil

Verapamil is a papaverine derivative that undergoes extensive biotransformation in man. The only metabolite that appears to possess significant pharmacological activity is the N-demethylated form (nor-verapamil), which in dogs at least, has about 20% of the activity of the parent compound as a coronary vasodilator. After oral administration, absorption is rapid and virtually complete. Because of its extensive hepatic first pass extraction, bioavailability is only of the order of 10%–20%. Most of the drug is excreted in the urine as conjugated metabolites (70%), with less than 5% being eliminated unchanged. During long-term administration, accumulation has only rarely been reported (McAllister 1982).

Verapamil is gaining acceptance as a useful compound in the management of stable exertional angina. Balasubramanian et al. (1982) have shown that it is as effective as both propranolol and nifedipine and is associated with fewer side-effects. The dosage initially recommended was 40 mg t.i.d., but this may have been too low; thus a dosage of 120 mg t.i.d., can be given if needed.

There has been controversy over the combined use of verapamil and β-adrenoceptor blocking compounds. It was suggested that considerable myocardial depression might occur since both have a predominantly depressant action on the myocardium. This was not a major problem in the series reported by Balasubramanian et al. (1982), but we have seen profound bradycardia develop and use the combination cautiously. The combination of β-blockade and intravenous verapamil should definitely be avoided because of both negative chronotropic and negative inotropic effects. Severe bradycardia and heart block can occur.

Side-effects are usually attributable to predictable pharmacological activity or are relatively non-specific, including dizziness, nausea, headache and constipation.

Diltiazem

Diltiazem is a benzothiazepine derivative. Pharmacokinetic data are scanty. There appears to be rapid absorption with a prominent hepatic first pass metabolism involving primarily deacetylation, but a significant proportion may be excreted unchanged. The bio-availability would seem to be around 13%.

Diltiazem is now available for routine use in the treatment of patients with angina pectoris. It has anti-arrhythmic activity and may occupy an intermediate position in clinical practice between nifedipine and verapamil.

Perhexilene

Perhexilene should not be considered as a first choice drug in angina pectoris. It may be a calcium channel blocker but has additional actions. It is metabolised by the liver. Significant side-effects have been reported in up to 3% of patients, and these may be serious, including papilloedema, peripheral neuropathy and hepatocellular dysfunction. It is no longer used in our clinical practice.

β-Adrenoceptor Blocking Compounds

Adrenoceptor Theories and Pharmacology

Catecholamines modulate many diverse responses in man. These are initiated by the interaction of catecholamines with discrete receptor sites located on the plasma membrane of cells. Noradrenaline is primarily the neurotransmitter released from sympathetic terminals, while adrenaline is the circulatory hormone released from the adrenal medulla. These catecholamines initiate target cell responses by binding to specific recognition sites, the adrenergic receptors, which are the initial decoders of extracellular messages. The existence of two primary types of adrenergic receptor has long been postulated (Ahlquist 1948), as has the existence of β-adrenergic subtypes (Lands et al. 1967). These workers provided evidence for two types of β-adrenergic receptor, β_1 and β_2. β_1-receptors include those that mediate the positive inotropic actions of catecholamines on the heart and are those at which adrenaline and noradrenaline are approximately equipotent. β_2-receptors are those at which adrenaline is markedly more potent than noradrenaline and include bronchial smooth muscle receptors. These differences probably reflect structural dissimilarities in the receptors. β-Adrenoceptors are also subdivided into pre- and postsynaptic subtypes. The excitation of presynaptic (prejunctional) β-receptors facilitates the release of endogenous noradrenaline, whereas their blockade has the converse effect.

α-Adrenergic Receptor Subtypes

More recent studies have indicated the existence of α-receptor subtypes (Hoffman and Lefkowitz 1980). Although noradrenaline release from adrenergic nerve terminals is primarily controlled by the rate of firing of the neurone, it is now known that there are α-receptors that regulate, in an auto-inhibitory fashion, the release of noradrenaline. These α-receptors (α_2) may be localised

Presynaptic   **Postsynaptic**

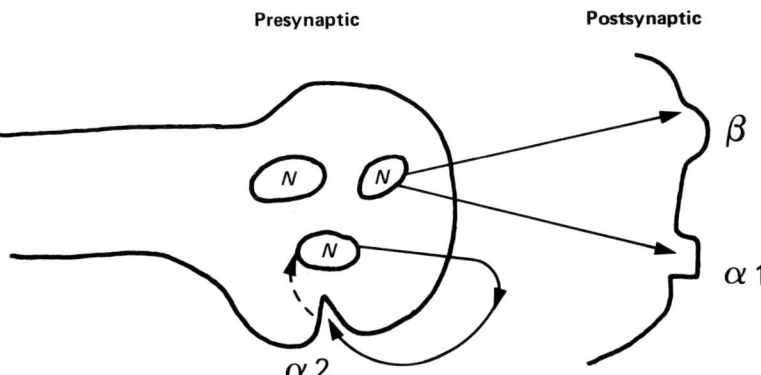

β

α 1

α 2

Fig. 3.1. Schematic representation of sympathetic neurone synapse with effector cell. Stimulation of presynaptic α_2-receptors inhibits noradrenaline release from the nerve terminal, whereas drugs that block α_2-receptors enhance noradrenaline release. *Unbroken arrows*, stimulation; *broken arrow*, inhibition.

to presynaptic sites on the nerve ending itself and reduce the amount of noradrenaline released by nerve impulses when stimulated by noradrenaline on the synaptic cleft. Thus when high concentrations of noradrenaline are present, subsequent impulses inhibit its release (Fig. 3.1).

Since 1975 these receptors have been studied by using radioactive-labelled hormone and drug derivatives known as radioligands (Motulsky and Insel 1982). The radioligands typically bind to the receptor in a saturable manner. The specific binding approaches a maximum (B_{max}) that represents the total quantity of receptors present. Radioligand techniques have been extremely valuable in clarifying the types of adrenergic receptors. In radioligand binding studies α_1- and α_2-adrenoceptors can each be directly identified with subtype-specific radioligands such as [^{3}H] prazosin and yohimbine. There are no such selective radioligands for β_1- and β_2-receptors, although they can be differentiated in competitive binding experiments using a non-selective radioligand and a relatively selective competitor. With appropriate analysis these experiments can determine the relative proportion of each receptor subtype present.

The second messengers mediating the various receptor responses are distinct. Both β_1- and β_2-receptors activate adenylate cyclase and thereby increase cellular levels of adenosine $3'5'$-monophosphate (cyclic AMP). α_1-Receptors increase intracellular calcium levels and often increase phosphoinositol hydrolysis. α_2-Receptors inhibit adenylate cyclase activity and in turn decrease cellular cyclic AMP levels.

Down Regulation and Desensitisation

Continued exposure to an agonist can lead to a blunted response to that agonist. This is termed desensitisation, tolerance or tachyphylaxis. Experimentally this phenomenon is often accompanied by a decrease in the affinity of the receptor for the hormone (uncoupling) and can be followed by a decrease in the number of receptors (down regulation).

Supersensitivity and Up Regulation

Animal studies during depletion of catecholamines by adrenergic antagonists have suggested a supersensitivity of the tissues to catecholamines and an up regulation of the receptor number. Possible up regulation of human β-adrenoceptors has been studied during the administration and withdrawal of propranolol, but results are conflicting and indecisive.

The β-adrenoceptor blocking compounds possess substantial affinity for the receptors, so that these become blocked (by competitive inhibition) and inaccessible to the endogenous neurotransmitter. A drug receptor complex is formed without giving rise to receptor activation as occurs with an agonistic compound. The inaccessibility of the receptors for endogenous catecholamines considerably reduces or even abolishes the influence of the sympathetic nervous system although, of course, it remains intact.

Ancillary Properties (Table 3.6)

All β-adrenoceptor blocking agents used in clinical practice block β_1 receptors, and it is this action that is largely responsible for their therapeutic effect. Certain of the β-blocking compounds also substantially block β_2 receptors, and this may give rise to side-effects such as peripheral vasoconstriction and bronchoconstriction. Other properties of these compounds include (a) a membrane-stabilising action (local anaesthetic effect), (b) intrinsic sympathomimetic activity (ISA) and (c) cardioselectivity.

Membrane-Stabilising Action. Various β-adrenoceptor blocking compounds have a direct effect on the cell membrane and reduce membrane permeability to ions such as Na, K^+ and Ca^{2+}. This action has nothing to do with β-blockade. In the standard therapeutic dose range the compounds with this property have

Table 3.6. Ancillary properties of β-adrenoceptor blocking drugs

Drug	β_1-selectivity	Membrane stabilisation	ISA
Acebutolol	$\beta_1 > \beta_2$	−	+
Alprenolol	$\beta_1 + \beta_2$	±	+
Atenolol	$\beta_1 >> \beta_2$	−	−
Metoprolol	$\beta_1 >> \beta_2$	−	−
Oxprenolol	$\beta_1 + \beta_2$	±	++
Pindolol	$\beta_1 + \beta_2$	−	+++
Practolol	$\beta_1 >> \beta_2$	−	++
Propanolol	$\beta_1 + \beta_2$	+	−
Sotalol	$\beta_1 + \beta_2$	−	−
Timolol	$\beta_1 + \beta_2$	−	−

little membrane-stabilising action, and it is doubtful if such an action contributes in any way to anti-anginal effects. It should be noted that there is dissociation of MSA and β-blockade. Thus both optimal isomers of propranolol possess MSA but only the *l* form produces β-blockade.

Intrinsic Sympathomimetic Activity. Since β-blockers form a drug-receptor complex, all possess affinity towards the β-receptor. Certain of them, such as pindolol and oxprenolol, show a degree of agonist activity. The receptor is blocked and inaccessible to endogenous catecholamines, while oxprenolol and pindolol slightly stimulate the β-receptor. This is classified as partial agonist activity or intrinsic sympathomimetic activity.

Cardioselectivity. There has been considerable interest in developing drugs with preferential affinity towards β_1-receptors. Examples such as metroprolol and atenolol are currently available but it should be remembered that while the expression β_1-selectivity is acceptable, cardiospecificity is not, since such compounds will still affect β_2-receptors, albeit to a lesser extent.

Pharmacokinetic Properties

The β-adrenoceptor blocking drugs have similar pharmacological properties but display considerable differences in their pharmacokinetic properties, including variability in gastro-intestinal absorption, the extent of first pass hepatic metabolism, protein binding, lipid solubility, brain penetration, pharmacological activity of metabolic products and renal clearance. All or some of these properties may affect their clinical use. In general, those metabolised by the liver have short half-lives while those excreted by the kidney have long half-lives and actions. When taken orally, compounds with extensive hepatic first pass metabolism can undergo so much biotransformation that relatively little reaches the systemic circulation. When active metabolites are produced, the total pharmacological effect will depend on both the amount of drug given and the proportion of metabolites. The presence of protein binding has also to be considered since changes in protein levels may influence pharmacological actions. Finally, many side-effects, such as drowsiness, depression and vivid dreams, may at least in part be due to lipophilicity and penetration into the brain (Table 3.7).

Attempts have also been made to establish a relationship between oral dose, plasma levels and pharmacological effect, but this has proved extremely difficult. After administration of a given dose of β-adrenoceptor blocker (especially one subject to hepatic metabolism) there are large differences between individuals in terms of plasma drug levels and large differences between plasma concentration and therapeutic effect. The reasons are uncertain but include (Frishman 1981):

1. Individual differences in sympathetic tone
2. Clinical effects lasting longer than indicated by the plasma half-life

Table 3.7. Properties of commonly used β-adrenoceptor antagonists

Metabolism	Compound	Selective or non-selective	Plasma half-life (h)	Daily dose (mg)	Long-acting preparation available	Proprietary name
Lipid soluble						
All extensive first pass metabolism in liver	Propranolol	NS	1–6	60–480	Yes	Inderal
	Oxprenolol	NS	1–3	60–480	?? Effective	Trasicor
May have active metabolites	Metoprolol	S	2–4	100–400	Yes	Betaloc, Lopresor
Lower dose in liver disease	Timolol	NS	4–6	15–45	No	Blocadren, Betim
	Alprenolol	NS	2	200–600	No	Aptin
	Acebutolol	PS	3	600–1200	No	Sectral
Lipid insoluble						
Excreted by kidneys	Atenolol	S	6–9	100–200	Long acting	Tenormin
	Nadolol	NS	16–24	40	Long acting	Corgard
	Sotalol	NS	15–18	240–480	Long acting	Beta-Cardone, Sotacor

3. Failure or inadequacy of assay to measure active drug and/or metabolites

There are still considerable gaps in our knowledge of the action of β-adreno-ceptor blocking drugs. However, they have been a major therapeutic advance and are very widely used.

Choice of β-Adrenoceptor Antagonist

The effectiveness of β-adrenoceptor blockade in the management of angina pectoris is well established. Around 70% of patients are improved. The reason for non-response is uncertain. It may be that the dosage is inadequate to control exercise tachycardia or that unopposed vasoconstriction may contrib-ute. However, the addition of an α-blocker does not necessarily result in improvement. It terms of β-adrenoceptor blockade, there is little to choose between compounds, and the choice depends on additional factors such as cardioselectivity (Table 3.7) and patient compliance. The need for improved compliance has been responsible for the introduction of long acting once daily treatment — either by compounds with a long half-life or by slow release formulations. The important clinical decision is whether or not to introduce β-blockade. The question of selectivity and type of preparation comes next. The majority of patients will do well with either a non-selective or a selective compound; however, some require a cardioselective agent and for a few β-blockade should not be used.

Side-effects

Side-effects are mainly due to the pharmacological actions of the β-adrenocep-tor antagonist concerned and are largely predictable.

Respiratory Function.   Airways resistance is influenced by both adrenergic and cholinergic receptors. The adrenergic system is probably more important, with β-stimulation causing bronchial dilatation and conversely $β_2$-blockade causing bronchial constriction.

All β-adrenoceptor antagonists adversely affect lung function. Johnsson et al. (1975) administered metoprolol, propranolol and placebo in random order to subjects with a history of airway disease. Two hours later the FEV_1 was 2.15 litres after placebo, 1.70 litres after propranolol and 1.78 litres after metoprolol.

Cold Hands and Feet.   Many patients with angina pectoris due to coronary disease will also have impaired peripheral circulation. A fall in cardiac output or increased vasoconstriction will make this worse. A complaint of cold hands or cold feet is common and occurs with all β-adrenoceptor antagonists, although to a lesser extent with cardioselective compounds. McSorley and Warren (1978), for example, found that propranolol, unlike metoprolol, reduced skin and resting muscle blood flow.

Muscle Pains and Fatigue.   Muscle ache, fatigue and a reduction in exercise capacity can occur with β-blockade. Lundborg et al. (1981) compared the effect of propranolol and metoprolol on carbohydrate and lipid metabolism in six volunteers undergoing prolonged exercise. Both compounds reduced exercise capacity. However, at an equivalent degree of β-blockade, all subjects could exercise for longer after the cardioselective compound (placebo 152 ± 10 min, propranolol 88 ± 9 min and metoprolol 117 ± 6 min). Free fatty acids increased most with placebo and least with propranolol, suggesting that a reduction in substrate availability could be responsible for reduced exercise capacity.

Provided patient selection is adequate, the incidence of side-effects of β-blockade is low at around 5% (Greenblatt and Koch-Weser 1973), and patient acceptance is usually excellent. Sexual dysfunction, usually impotence, occurs in approximately 5%, although higher levels of 13% have been reported in a recent study in treatment of mild hypertension (MRC Working Party on Mild to Moderate Hypertension 1981). The development of congestive heart failure with β-adrenoceptor blockade has been overemphasised. This is a matter of clinical common sense: Those with a history of heart failure or who have cardiomegaly should be treated by diuretic, vasodilator and digoxin if appropriate. Subsequent cautious introduction of β-blocking compounds may then, but *only* then, at times be feasible. Theoretically, compounds with intrinsic sympathomimetic activity should be less likely to produce heart failure, but this has not been the general experience.

Emergency or Elective Surgery

There may be a need for surgery in patients already receiving β-blockade. In general it is preferable to continue the treatment rather than to withdraw it abruptly, since this may cause its own problems. It is important that the surgeon and anaesthetist be aware that β-adrenoceptor blocking compounds are being given, because of their effect on heart rate and blood pressure and the reduced heart rate response to blood loss. General policy should always be to withdraw β-blocking compounds gradually, although the fears of Miller et al. (1975) that rapid withdrawal would cause worsening angina and possible myocardial infaction have not been realised. It has been suggested that there may be a rebound release of catecholamines or that the β-receptor population is increased. The evidence is not completely convincing in either direction.

Compliance

β-Adrenoceptor antagonists initially required to be given several times daily. It was recognised that compliance was poor with such regimes, and therefore long acting preparations have been developed. This has been achieved either by the development of compounds with a long half-life, such as atenolol, nadolol and sotalol, or by special formulation to prolong half-life, as has been done with metoprolol, propranolol and oxprenolol. The results seem successful for propranolol (McIlmoyle et al. 1979), atenolol (Jackson et al. 1980) and metoprolol

(Uusitalo and Keyrilainen 1979), but there remains doubt as to whether long acting oxprenolol is any more effective than standard release oxprenolol (Bobik et al. 1979).

Unstable Angina

There are several possible definitions of unstable angina. A satisfactory one includes:

New onset angina
Sudden increase in severity
Occurrence at rest or minimal activity

On assessment the findings include:

1. No new Q wave development
2. Transient ST (either elevation or depression) or T wave changes
3. No significant rise in cardiac enzymes

As a general rule, underlying coronary atherosclerosis is present and precipitating factors may include platelet aggregation or platelet factors leading to coronary vasoconstriction due to increased vasomotor time. This is often described as coronary spasm. It usually occurs in association with coronary disease but can develop in otherwise normal vessels.

Management

Treatment should initially be medical, although early assessment for surgery may be required.

The patient should be assessed clinically with careful electrocardiographic monitoring, and a formal ECG should be performed if the patient has episodes of pain at rest. If pain persists for more than 48 h, coronary arteriography is indicated. If the pain settles, the patient should be considered for elective coronary arteriography later. In the initial stages treatment consists of nitrates and/or a calcium channel blocker. Nitrates may be given in various ways, being used both if pain occurs and for continuing control. They may be given:

1. As a buccal spray or sublingually
2. Topically (transdermally)
3. Orally
4. Intravenously

Verapamil and nifedipine have also both been shown to be effective. The combination of nitrate and calcium channel blocking compounds will reduce preload and afterload and relieve spasm. There are caveats to the use of β-adrenoceptor blocking compounds since unopposed α-effects may cause deleterious effects by coronary vasoconstriction. The use of anticoagulants should be considered, using heparin if the patient does not settle; the possible use of thrombolytic therapy should also be taken into account, although its role remains uncertain at present.

It has been suggested that early investigation and coronary angioplasty if appropriate might be useful treatment. This has not yet been established. In the long term, many of those who initially settle will continue to have pain later, and around 30%–40% will require surgery within 2 years and thereafter have a good prognosis (83% survival at 10 years). All patients with unstable angina should therefore be carefully followed.

The natural history of pure coronary spasm has been studied by Bott-Silvermann and Heupler (1983). They investigated 59 patients who had coronary spasm but an underlying normal coronary angiogram: 64% had ST elevation, 17% had ST depression and 19% developed myocardial infarction. There were no deaths.

Waters et al. (1983) followed up 100 patients with variant angina (episodes of pain associated with ST elevation). Coronary angiography was normal in 52, and abnormal in 48. Remission without therapy occurred in 45, remission on therapy, in 37. There was persistent angina in 18 (coronary arteries often normal).

The hypothesis has been put forward that enhanced platelet reactivity is causally related to some of the complications of coronary disease. The effect of aspirin on unstable angina was investigated by Lewis et al. (1983). Patients were assessed within 48 h of admission and acute myocardial infarction excluded as far as possible. Suitable male patients were randomly allocated to aspirin (324 mg daily) or to the control group and followed for 12 weeks. There were 31 deaths in the aspirin-treated group and 65 in the control group. In terms of myocardial infarction, there were 21 in the aspirin-treated group and 44 in the control group. This is an interesting study that opens further approaches to management.

Unstable angina continues to pose considerable problems, although management guides have certainly become clearer.

References

Ahlquist RP (1948) A study of the adrenotropic receptors. Am J Physiol 153: 586
Balasubramanian V, Lamiri A, Sivam P, Raftery EB (1980) Anti-anginal action of verapamil – a controlled study. Am J Cardiol 45: 389 (ABS)
Bergman G, Atkinson L, Richardson PJ, Daly K, Rothman M, Jackson G, Jewitt DE (1981)

Prostacyclin: Haemodynamic and metabolic effects in patients with coronary artery disease. Lancet I: 569–572

Blumenthal HP, Fung ML, McNiff EF, Yap SK (1977) Plasma nitroglycerin levels after sublingual, oral and topical administration. Br J Clin Pharmacol 4: 241–242

Bobik A, Jennings GL, Korner PI, Ashley P, Jackman G (1979) Absorption and excretion of rapid and slow release oxprenolol and their effects on heart rate and blood pressure during exercise. Br J Clin Pharmacol 7: 545–549

Bott-Silverman C, Heupler FA (1983) Natural history of pure coronary spasm in patients treated medically. J Am Coll Cardiol 2: 200–205

Ebner F, Dunschede HB (1976) Haemodynamics, therapeutic mechanism of action and clinical findings of Adalat use based on world wide clinical trials. In: Domingos A, Lichtlen PR (eds) Third International Adalat Symposium. Excerpta Medica, Amsterdam Oxford, p 283

Editorial (1981) Prostacyclin in therapeutics. Lancet I: 643

Greenblatt DJ, Koch-Weser J (1973) Adverse reactions to propranolol in hospitalised medical patients: a report from the Boston collaborative drug surveillance program. Am Heart J 86: 478–484

Hoffman BB, Lefkowitz RJ (1980) Alpha adrenergic subtypes. N Engl J Med 302: 1390–1396

Jackson G, Schwartz J, Kates RE, Winchester M, Harrison DC (1980) Atenolol: once daily cardioselective beta blockade for angina pectoris. Circulation 61: 555–560

Johnsson G, Svedmyr N, Thiringer G (1975) Effects of intravenous propranolol and metoprolol and their interaction with isoprenaline on pulmonary function, heart rate and blood pressure in asthmatics. Eur J Clin Pharmacol 6: 175–180

Kennedy CC (1976) One year graduated exercise program for men with angina pectoris. Mayo Clin Proc 51(4): 231–236

Lands AM, Adnold A, McAuliff JR, Ludvena FP, Brown TG (1967) Differentation of receptor systems activated by sympathomimetic amines. Nature 214: 597–598

Lee G, Mason DT, De Maria AN (1978) Effects of long term oral administration of isosorbide dinitrate on the anti-anginal response to nitroglycerin: absence of nitrate cross tolerance and self tolerance shown by exercise testing. Am J Cardiol 41: 82–87

Lewis HD, Davis JW, Archibald DG, Steinke WE (1983) Protective effects of aspirin against acute myocardial infarction and death in men with unstable angina. Results of a Veterans' Administration Cooperative Study. N Engl J Med 309: 396–403

Lundborg P, Astrom H, Bengtsson C, Fellenius E, Von Schenr H, Suensson L, Smith U (1981) Effect of adrenoceptor blockade on exercise performance and metabolism. Clin Sci 61: 299–305

Lynch P, Dargie H, Krikler S, Krikler D (1980) Objective assessment of antianginal treatment: A double blind comparison of propranolol, nifedipine and their combination. Br Med J 281: 184–187

Markis JE, Gorlin R, Hills M, Williams RA, Schweitzer P, Ransil BJ (1979) Sustained effect of orally administered isosorbide dinitrate on exercise performance of patients with angina pectoris. Am J Cardiol 43: 265–271

Maseri A (1980) Pathogenic mechanisms in angina pectoris. Br Heart J 43: 648–660

Maseri A, Severi S, DeNes M et al. (1978) "Variant" angina: one aspect of a continuous spectrum of vasospastic myocardial ischaemia. Am J Cardiol 42: 1019–1035

McAllister RG (1982) Clinical pharmacology of slow channel blocking agents. Prog Cardiovasc Dis 25: 83–102

McIlmoyle EL, Blair ALT, Calvert HWA, Boyle DMc, Shanks RG, Leaney W, Barber JM (1979) Studies with a slow release formulation of propranolol in angina. J Irish Med Assoc 72: 27–28

McSorley PD, Warren DJ (1978) Effects of propranolol and metaprolol on the peripheral circulation. Br Med J II: 1598–1600

Miller RR, Olson HG, Amsterdam EA, Mason DT (1975) Propranolol – withdrawal rebound phenomenon. N Engl J Med 293: 416–418

Motulsky HJ, Insel PA (1982) Adrenergic receptors in man. N Engl J Med 307: 18

MRC Working Party on Mild to Moderate Hypertension (1981) Adverse reactions to bendrofluazide and propranolol for the treatment of mild hypertension. Lancet II: 539–543

Needleman P, Lang S, Johnson EM (1972) Organic nitrates: relation between biotransformation and rational angina pectoris therapy. J Pharmacol Exp Ther 181: 489–497

Redwood DR, Rosing DR, Epstein SE (1972) Circulatory and symptomatic effects of physical training in patients with coronary artery disease and angina pectoris. N Engl J Med 286: 959–965

Uusitalo AS, Keyrilainen O (1979) Slow release metoprolol in angina pectoris. Ann Clin Res II: 199–203

Veterans' Administration Co-operative Study (1983) Protective effects of aspirin against acute myocardial infarction and death in men with unstable angina. N Engl J Med 309: 396–403

Waters DD, Bouchard A, Theroux P (1983) Spontaneous remission is a frequent outcome of variant angina. J Am Coll Cardiol 2: 195–197

4 Sudden Death

Coronary heart disease (CHD) can present as angina pectoris, myocardial infarction or sudden death. Reduction of this latter presentation remains one of the most important challenges in cardiology. Sudden death is now recognised as a distinct entity and has been variously defined. A practical definition is "unexpected cardiac death occurring without symptoms or with symptoms of less than 1 hour's duration". Two-thirds of all deaths associated with CHD occur outside of hospital without prior symptoms or with symptoms of very short duration. Sudden cardiac death is the leading cause of mortality in 20–64 year olds. The mode of death is arrhythmic and it may occur in the absence or associated with evidence of acute myocardial infarction (Cobb et al. 1980).

Ventricular fibrillation is the usual arrhythmia evident when fortuitous monitoring is being performed at the time of sudden death or when cardiac arrest is seen in the coronary care unit (Gradman et al. 1977). *Asystole* may occasionally be encountered, but this is usually an agonal rhythm found when death has occurred at some indeterminate time and when there has been a substantial delay in obtaining an electrocardiogram. In sudden cardiac death 75% of subjects have evidence of CHD. Other cardiac causes include cardiomyopathies, valvular disease, prolonged QT interval, hypokalaemia and pre-excitation syndromes. Myocarditis may rarely be present. Normal hearts are rare (1%–2%) (Reichenbach et al. 1977).

Asystole may also be the terminal arrhythmia associated with other severe medical conditions — severe pulmonary, metabolic or vascular catastrophes. Death in these circumstances is seldom instantaneous, however, and other bradyarrhythmias or electromechanical dissociation may be present.

Ventricular fibrillation may occur without frank pathological evidence of acute myocardial infarction. Survivors of cardiac arrest and sudden death infrequently show evidence of myocardial infarction, with new Q waves being evident in some 19% and with elevation in the LDH isoensyme in less than 40%. Post-mortem myocardial histology often shows areas of myocytolysis, with scattered focal changes similar to those seen following catecholamine infusions in experimental animal models (Cobb et al. 1978).

The precipitation of ventricular fibrillation appears to be the end-result of an interplay of electrical and mechanical factors related to myocardial ischaemia. Acute myocardial ischaemia in animal models is associated with local anoxia and extracellular acidosis and a resultant delay in membrane depolarisation and conduction. Inhomogeneous depolarisation may be accentuated by sympathetic or parasympathetic discharge, leading to ventricular arrhythmias with a re-entry mechanism (Han 1969). In patients who have had previous ischaemic incidents, mechanical factors such as dyskinetic segments may play a role in precipitating arrhythmias. Increased wall stress may lead to local enhanced myocardial oxygen consumption and local ischaemia may precipitate electrical instability (Gibson et al. 1978).

Community Emergency Care Systems

Following the recognition that most coronary heart deaths occur outside of hospital, but that the fatal arrhythmia is potentially reversible, the modern techniques of cardiopulmonary resuscitation and defibrillation have been applied in an attempt to reduce this community mortality. This has been possible by the development of emergency care systems. Pantridge and his Belfast associates pioneered a hospital physician-based system using a suitably equipped ambulance in the treatment of early myocardial infarction. Following early gratifying results with successful resuscitation, many other systems have been developed. These have not necessarily been exclusively physician manned, but have involved specially trained paramedics, emergency medical technicians and ambulance men (Partridge and Geddes 1967; Cobb et al. 1976).

The most developed community care programme has been that in Seattle, Washington — a metropolitan area of some 92 square miles with a population of 500 000. The Medic One advanced life support system based on the fire service has been developed to cover the acute treatment of sudden illness. This includes an early response to patients with sudden collapse, heart attacks, trauma, drowning accidents, etc.

Paramedical staff have been trained in cardiopulmonary resuscitation (including endotracheal intubation), in arrhythmia recognition and in the use of emergency drugs and cardiac defibrillation. Using fire service vehicles and with the local motorway system, the response time from despatch to arrival at a patient is less than 3 min. This response system has been allied to a training programme of resuscitation techniques for the community, with some 225 000 individuals having undertaken a 45-min resuscitation programme. This has enabled bystanders to initiate resuscitation procedures in approximately 35% of sudden deaths (Thompson et al. 1979). In this population some 350 subjects are treated yearly for ventricular fibrillation by the paramedical team. Successful resuscitation is achieved in about 60%, with some 30% being stabilised and able to be discharged home.

The results of prehospital management of patients with acute myocardial infarction in other centres has been variable and this may be related to geography and the delay before acute care is delivered. Following initial resuscitation, patients are transferred to the coronary care unit for monitoring and treatment, as for acute myocardial infarction. Particular attention is paid to continued arrhythmias, hypotension and left ventricular dysfunction.

Long-Term Prognosis

There remains a significant mortality after successful out-of-hospital resuscitation with a 1-year mortality of 26% which rises to 36% at 2 years. Seventy-five per cent of this mortality is secondary to further cardiac arrest and recurrent sudden death. Factors influencing this mortality include the presence or absence of transmural acute myocardial infarction. The prognosis of ventricular fibrillation associated with a completed transmural myocardial infarction is good with a mortality of about 2%. This increases to 20% if the infarction is subendocardial rather than transmural. This suggests that the predisposing factors to arrhythmogenesis remain in these patients. Independent determinants of recurrent sudden death include a previous history of proven myocardial infarction, prior congestive cardiac failure with marked left ventricular dysfunction, the presence of complex ventricular arrhythmias and extensive coronary artery disease (Cobb et al. 1975). A significant morbidity may result from neurological sequelae of cardiac arrest, varying from a degree of retrograde or anterograde amnesia to the development of a frank neurological deficit with focal neurological signs. The incidence of these complications is greatly reduced if cardiopulmonary resuscitation is initiated by trained bystanders (Caronna and Finklestein 1978).

Long-term Management

Patients are screened to determine subsets who have a high risk of recurrent ventricular fibrillation. Exercise testing and 24-h ambulatory monitoring are performed, and anti-arrhythmic therapy introduced if appropriate. If angina occurs then early coronary arteriography is indicated, with consideration being given to coronary artery bypass surgery.

Cardiac Arrest

Cardiac arrest occurs when there is sudden and often unexpected cessation of spontaneous circulation and respiration. Cardiac arrhythmias associated with CHD are the usual cause; other causes include trauma, asphyxiation, electrocution and poisoning.

Cardiac arrest causes ineffective mechanical activity, reduced cardiac output and cerebral hypoperfusion. In the presence of acute myocardial infarction, cardiac arrest does not necessarily reflect serious or irreversible myocardial damage. The patient sustaining a cardiac arrest can return to a near normal life expectancy by rapid restoration of normal cardiac rhythm following supportive cardiopulmonary resuscitation. If commenced within 3–5 min of cessation of the circulation, irreversible cerebral and cardiac damage may be prevented. *Early diagnosis and resuscitative measures are mandatory.*

In the hospital setting all personnel should be trained in these methods so that the procedure may be commenced and maintained until trained medical staff can be called to the patient. Emergency resuscitation trolleys containing essential drugs and equipment required during cardiac arrest (Tables 4.1, 4.2) should be stationed at all areas within a hospital where cardiac arrest may occur, e.g. in the coronary care unit, the casualty department, general wards and departments where diagnostic X-ray investigations using radiographic medium or invasive techniques, e.g. endoscopy or cardiac catheterisation of any kind, are performed. In addition they must be available in all areas where anaesthetics are being administered. A trained team able to undertake endotracheal intubation, defibrillation and cardiopulmonary resuscitation should be available throughout the 24-h period.

Diagnosis

Cardiac arrest must be assumed to be the diagnosis in the presence of:

1. Any clinical situation of sudden collapse
2. Unconsciousness in a patient known to have been well a short time before
3. Sudden onset of cyanosis with respiratory stridor
4. Sudden convulsive seizure in a patient at risk of cardiac arrest

Table 4.1. Equipment used in the treatment of cardiac arrest

1. Mobile trolley	a) Portable defibrillator and defibrillator paddles
	b) Battery-operated electrocardiographic machine and ECG straps
	c) Electrode gel
2. Ventilation tray	a) 1 Ambu bag with associated masks
	b) Brook airways 2, 3, 4
	c) Laryngoscope — 1 curved blade, 1 straight blade
	d) Endotracheal tubes 8, 8.5, 9, 9.5
	e) Introducer
	f) Magill forceps (1)
	g) Artery forceps (2)
	h) Angled connectors and corrugated black rubber connections
	i) KY jelly
	j) Gauze swabs
	k) Tape
	l) Syringes

Table 4.2. Drug list for a cardiac arrest trolley

	Preparation
Anti-arrhythmics	
Lignocaine (P.F.S.)	100 mg
Tocainide	750 mg
Disopyramide	50 mg
Mexiletine	250 mg
Digoxin	0.5 mg
Verapamil	5 mg
Bretylium	100 mg
Amiodarone	150 mg
Flecainide	150 mg
Adrenaline	1/1000
Atropine	0.5 mg
Isoprenaline	0.2 mg
Calcium chloride	10 ml (10%)
Metoprolol	5 mg
Practolol	10 mg
Naloxone	0.4 mg
Nikethamide	500 mg
Diazepam	10 mg
Frusemide	50 mg
Dexamethasone	8 mg
Dexamethasone Shock Pack	100 mg
Dextrose	50 ml (50%)
Intravenous fluids	
Sodium bicarbonate	8.4% (200 ml)
Dextrose	5% (500 ml)
Lignocaine/dextrose	1 g/500 ml

Upon discovery of a patient with suspected cardiac arrest, action depends on the circumstances. If in a general ward or diagnostic area, trained staff must be summoned utilising a telephone code system. The central telephone exchange should be alerted using an easily dialled code (222 or 999) with access to the switchboard by a direct line. The site and nature of the emergency should be clearly stated. Trained staff should be alerted using a radio-page system or hospital Tannoy.

Other causes of sudden collapse should be considered, including:

1. Stokes-Adams attacks
2. Vasovagal syncope
3. Convulsive seizure
4. Haemorrhage
5. Cerebrovascular accident

When in doubt as to the cause, resuscitative procedures should be commenced; a decision may be taken to discontinue them if the procedure subsequently proves inappropriate to an individual patient's diagnosis.

Initial Clinical Assessment

Clinical examination should be rapid but thorough, confirming the usual clinical findings in patients sustaining cardiac arrest.

1. *Colour.*   The patient appears extremely pale or may be cyanosed.
2. *Conscious level.*   Following collapse, rapidly deepening unconsciousness develops.
3. *Arterial pulse.*   The pulses are absent even over the major arterial sites (carotid and femoral), and the heart sounds are absent.
4. *Respiration.*   Spontaneous respiration may continue for several minutes, but the rate slows and the volume is usually too low for adequate oxygenation.
5. *Dilated pupils.*   This occurs as a late sign following cerebral hypoxia; however, it may not be apparent following the administration of opiates in the early stage of acute myocardial infarction when pupillary constriction will be retained.

Cardiopulmonary Resuscitation

The essential measures to be undertaken in resuscitation are:

1. *External cardiac massage.*   The patient should be placed on his back on a hard surface. A board may be placed on or under a bed mattress. If the bed is not boarded, then the patient should be transferred to the floor. A sharp, firm blow should be applied to the sternum. This will occasionally be enough to initiate electrical activity or may even defibrillate the heart. A similar mechanical stimulus may be given by raising the legs to promote venous return. The heel of one hand is placed on the sternum just above the xiphoid, the heel of the other hand is placed on top, and firm pressure is applied sufficient to move the sternum about 4 cm downwards. Adequacy of technique may be judged by the presence of a carotid or femoral pulse and pupillary constriction in response to massage. A rate of 70–80 compressions should be performed per minute.

2. *Artificial ventilation.*   A clear airway must be ensured. Dentures or obstructing food or vomit should be removed. The tongue should be swept forward and the head should be tilted backwards and maintained in a hyper-extended position with the mandible pushed forward using pressure at the angle of the jaw. Ventilation may be maintained spontaneously, although artificial ventilation is usually required. A Brooke airway should be used. If ventilation is impaired, a cuffed endotracheal tube must be inserted and oxygen administered. An Ambubag should be used with air or 100% oxygen. If delay occurs before endotracheal intubation, mouth-to-mouth artificial respiration should be employed by forcibly blowing into the mouth while keeping the nose closed by pinching the nostrils. Exhalation occurs passively. Observation of chest movement will determine whether ventilation is adequate by this

method. Once the airway is clear and artificial ventilation established, if resuscitation is commenced by a single individual, then every 15 external cardiac compressions should be followed by two ventilations. When an adequate team is available, four or five external compressions are followed by a single ventilation. These combined measures must be continued during transport and until definitive therapy is given and the patient's condition stabilised.

3. *Diagnosis and treatment of arrhythmia.* In almost all patients the cardiac rhythm at the time of cardiac arrest is ventricular fibrillation. If a DC defibrillator is available, immediate defibrillation should be performed without waiting for electrocardiographic diagnosis. The earlier defibrillation is performed, the more likely is restoration of sinus rhythm. Delay may lead to further ischaemia, anoxia and acidosis, which make defibrillation more difficult. External cardiac massage and ventilation should be maintained until successful defibrillation and restarted immediately afterwards until sinus rhythm with adequate mechanical activity and cardiac output is achieved. Electrode jelly or jelly pads should be placed over the sternum and over the cardiac apex to ensure good contact is achieved with no loss of current. Alternatively, a flat electrode paddle should be placed under the mid-thorax of the patient. A DC shock of 200 J should be given, increasing to 400 J if initially unsuccessful. Cardiac massage should be maintained between shocks while the defibrillator is being recharged. Further anti-arrhythmic therapy depends on the rhythm established after defibrillation.

4. *Venous cannulation.* A port of entry for the administration of intravenous drugs must be available. The site should be a large vein if possible. During cardiac arrest arm and leg veins may be collapsed and the jugular or subclavian route may be utilised.

5. *Drug treatment.* During cardiac arrest, metabolic acidosis becomes firmly established, and intravenous sodium bicarbonate ($NaHCO_3$) is administered. 100 ml of 8.4% solution (100 mmol) is immediately infused. For each further minute of cardiac arrest, a further 10 mmol should be given up to 200 mmol. Continuing therapy depends on blood gas measurements and acid-base balance. Parenteral administration of drugs depends on the arrhythmias encountered and the resulting haemodynamic status of the patient. If defibrillation is unsuccessful, then anti-arrhythmic therapy should be given using a class I anti-arrhythmic agent, followed by a further attempt at defibrillation. The agents and their standard preparations are shown in Table 4.2.

Treatment of Asystole

Asystole may represent an agonal end-stage rhythm following ventricular fibrillation. In other circumstances it may be the result of massive cardiac damage and resuscitative measures are often unsuccessful. Treatment should be initiated with external cardiac massage and artificial ventilation; stimulation with pharmacological agents or electrical methods may be attempted but is seldom effective.

Cardiostimulant Drugs.   Atropine 0.5–1.5 mg is given intravenously and cardiac massage maintained. If no activity results, 1 g calcium chloride (10 ml of 10% solution) plus 1 mg adrenaline should be given intravenously (these drugs may also be given by intracardiac injection). An isoprenaline infusion may also be commenced (5 mg in 500 ml of 5% dextrose). The infusion rate will depend on the resulting rhythm and rate. As a result of administration of these pharmacological agents, sinus rhythm may be restored or other arrhythmia may supervene. Supraventricular, junctional or ventricular rhythms may occur and should be treated by electrical cardioversion or standard anti-arrhythmic therapy. Ventricular fibrillation may supervene and defibrillation should then be performed.

Pacing.   If asystole persists, or if a ventricular rhythm with an inadequate rate and output occurs, then cardiac pacing should be considered. This can be technically difficult during resuscitation. External cardiac massage should be maintained. Radiological visualisation of the pacemaker electrode is ideal, but may not be available or may be difficult to perform. External massage may need to be temporarily stopped until the pacemaker crosses the tricuspid valve. The internal jugular, subclavian, femoral or antecubital approach may be used in accordance with the experience of the physician. In the absence of X-ray screening facilities, flotation balloon catheters with pacing electrodes are useful. An intracardiac electrocardiogram may also be required to localise the electrode position.

Direct ventricular puncture may be performed using a sub-xiphoid approach. Aspiration of blood confirms intracardiac positioning and a bipolar catheter (Elecath) may be inserted. In our hands this technique has seldom been successful for more than a brief period, but it may allow time for a transvenous pacing catheter to be inserted. If pacing is established and a regular rhythm maintained, continuing therapy is aimed at achieving an adequate cardiac output.

Post-resuscitation Aftercare

After stabilisation, standard aftercare is given. Patients are transferred to the intensive or coronary care unit. A firm diagnosis should be sought. Heart rate, blood pressure and urinary output are monitored. Urinary catheterisation is necessary if output is impaired (< 10 ml/h). Haemodynamic monitoring may be required by the introduction of a flotation catheter. Haemodynamic abnormalities should be treated in the standard fashion. Although many patients will be fully conscious and orientated after resuscitation, there may be cerebral oedema if resuscitation has been prolonged. This is managed by an osmotic diuretic such as mannitol (200 ml of 20%) and followed by corticosteroids in the form of dexamethasone 10 mg intravenously with 4 mg 6 hourly, reducing the dose over the following few days.

References

Caronna JJ, Finklestein S (1978) Neurological syndromes after cardiac arrest. Curr Concepts Cerebrovasc Dis 13: 9–14

Cobb LA, Baum RS, Alvarez H, Schaffer WA (1975) Resuscitation from out-of-hospital ventricular fibrillation: 4 year follow-up. Circulation 51, 52 [Suppl III]: 223–228

Cobb LA, Alvarez H, Copass MK (1976) A rapid response system for out-of-hospital cardiac emergencies. Med Clin No Amer 60: 283–290

Cobb LA, Hallstron AP, Weaver WD, Copass MK, Haynes RE (1978) Clinical predictors and characteristics of the sudden cardiac death syndrome. The Proceedings of the USA/USSR First Joint Symposium on Sudden Death. DHEW Publication No. (NIH) 78–1470, pp 99–116

Cobb LA, Werner JA, Teobaugh J (1980) Sudden cardiac death. Mod Concepts Cardiovasc Dis XLIX 6: 31–36

Gibson DG, Doran JH, Traill TA, Brown DJ (1978) Regional abnormalities of left ventricular wall movement during isovolumic relaxation in patients with ischaemic heart disease. Eur J Cardiol 7 [Suppl]: 251–264

Gradman AH, Bell PA, De Busk RF (1977) Sudden death during ambulatory monitoring. Circulation 55: 210–211

Han J (1969) Ventricular vulnerability during acute coronary occlusion, Am J Cardiol 24: 857–864

Pantridge JF, Geddes JS (1967) A mobile intensive care unit in the management of myocardial infarction. Lancet II: 271–273

Reichenbach DD, Moss NS, Meyer E (1977) Pathology of the heart in sudden cardiac death. Am J Cardiol 39: 865–872

Thompson RG, Hallstrom AP, Cobb LA (1979) Bystander-initiated cardiopulmonary resuscitation in the management of ventricular fibrillation. Ann Intern Med 90: 737–740

5 Acute Myocardial Infarction

Acute myocardial infarction develops when myocardial ischaemia occurs for a sufficient time to cause necrosis of a localised area of myocardium. The initial reduction in myocardial blood flow may be secondary to:

1. Coronary artery spasm or increased vasoconstrictor tone in normal or severely stenosed coronary arteries (Maseri et al. 1978)
2. Platelet aggregation in the presence of severe atheroma, leading to reduced flow
3. Subintimal haemorrhage with bleeding into an atheromatous plaque
4. Intracoronary thrombosis (Davies et al. 1976)

Infarction may occur without total coronary artery occlusion when coronary flow falls due to severe hypotension. This can be associated with haemorrhage, trauma, severe dehydration or shock accompanying any other condition.

The extent and site of the myocardial necrosis depend on:

1. The anatomical distribution of the occluded coronary artery
2. The presence of coronary collaterals
3. The presence of previous coronary arterial occlusion

Coronary Artery Anatomy

There are two main coronary arteries in the human (Fig. 5.1). The right coronary artery is dominant on anatomical grounds, i.e. it supplies the posterior portion of the interventricular groove in 60% of subjects, while the left coronary artery is of major importance in clinical terms. The left coronary artery divides into the left anterior descending and circumflex branches, thereby developing a triple-vessel anatomical relationship. The anterior descending branch runs down the interventricular groove to the apex of the heart and supplies the anterior portion of the right ventricle, the interventricular

RIGHT CORONARY ARTERY   LEFT CORONARY ARTERY

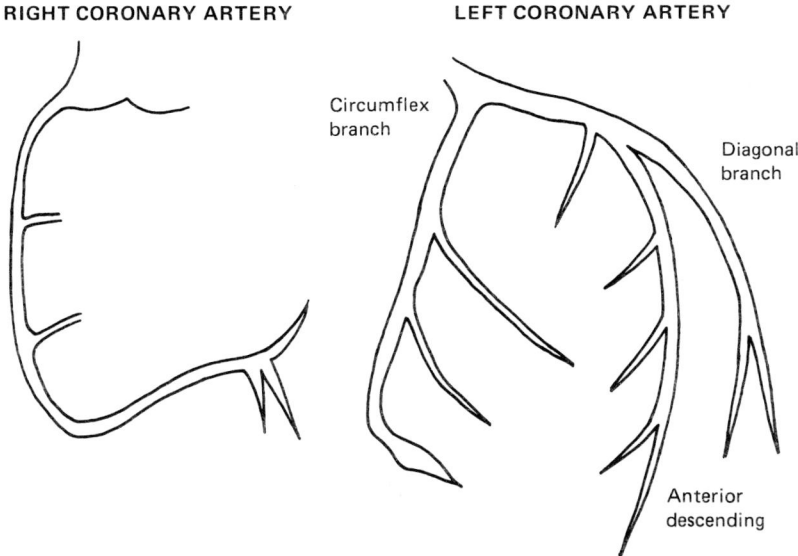

Fig. 5.1. Schematic representation of the coronary arteries showing the major branches.

septum and, most importantly, the anterior and apical portions of the left ventricle. The circumflex artery runs posteriorly between the left atrium and the left ventricle, supplying the upper lateral and posterior portions of the left ventricle. The right coronary artery runs between the right atrium and right ventricle into the interventricular groove and supplies the anterior right ventricle and the inferior portion of both ventricles. Occlusion of the left anterior descending branch leads to anterior myocardial infarction. Occlusion of the circumflex branch leads to anterolateral necrosis, while right coronary artery occlusion leads to infarction of the postero-inferior portion of the left ventricle. The anterior papillary muscle is supplied by the anterior descending artery, its diagonal branches or the circumflex branch of the left coronary artery. The posterior papillary muscle is supplied by the right or circumflex branches of the coronary system. The sino-atrial node is supplied by the right coronary artery (55%) or circumflex branch (45%). The atrioventricular node is also supplied by the right coronary artery (90%) or the circumflex artery (10%). These anatomical relationships are of major importance in regard to the haemodynamic sequelae, complications and conduction defects occurring in the course of acute infarction.

Clinical Presentation

It is often unclear which factors, if any, precipitate an acute infarction. Unaccustomed physical effort may precede an attack. Emotion may be influential and adverse life events such as bereavement, loss of work or domestic strife may precipitate the episode. Change of environmental temperature may be important. Severe physical exertion after a meal and in a cold environment may be particular predisposing circumstances.

Symptoms

Premonitory symptoms are common but their origin is often unrecognised. Unstable angina as manifested by an alteration in the pattern of established angina, by recent onset of symptoms and particularly by crescendo features may occur in more than 33% of patients who subsequently present within hours or days with acute myocardial infarction.

The pain of myocardial infarction is similar to that of angina pectoris in its quality and radiation but results from irreversible myocardial ischaemia. The pain does not subside with rest or glyceryl trinitrate and may last for several hours. The pain is usually severe although its character may be difficult to describe. Its intensity gives no indication of the severity of the infarction. A proportion of patients with acute myocardial infarction will present with atypical symptoms without pain. Particularly in the elderly, myocardial infarction may be "silent" and masked by non-cardiac events. Accompanying symptoms may include nausea, weakness and faintness, sweating, light-headedness, palpitation, syncope, dyspnoea, orthopnoea and wheezing.

Signs

The physical findings may be highly variable during the early stages of myocardial infarction. The patient usually appears ill, is cold, clammy, sweating and obviously in pain. In the early hours following onset of symptoms, parasympathetic effects may predominate, with bradycardia and hypotension evident (Adgey et al. 1968). Sympathetic effects may be present, with tachycardia and hypertension (Valori et al. 1969). In patients with acute infarction and mild to moderate haemodynamic effects, no abnormal findings may be evident. In a severe episode tachypnoea may be obvious. The pulse may be weak and the heart sounds soft (tic tac) in quality. A triple rhythm (either 3rd or 4th heart sounds) may be present, representing ventricular dysfunction with altered compliance. Distended neck veins, pulmonary crepitations or even pulmonary oedema may occur. The blood pressure may be normal or even elevated in the acute stage, although profound hypotension and shock may accompany the most severe attack. Pericardial friction may be present in those cases with epicardial involvement, occurring in 10%–30% between the 2nd and 5th days. This may be transient. Rhythm disturbances and conduction defects may produce abnormal signs in the early stages. Moderate fever is often present on the 1st to 3rd days.

Laboratory Findings

A transient polymorphonuclear leucocytosis occurs during the first few days. The ESR rises after 24–48 h and gradually returns to normal over 4–6 weeks. Serial estimations of cardiac enzymes are also of major importance in confirming the presence of myocardial necrosis in patients with doubtful symptoms and indeterminate electrocardiographic changes; this is especially so in the presence of left bundle branch block pattern or when previous myocardial infarction has occurred. Serial estimations of AST, ALT, LDH and CPK are routine during the first 48–72 h of infarction.

The characteristic changes of acute myocardial infarction are fairly specific and evolve with sequential or serial changes occurring during the acute attack. It is important to remember that an electrocardiogram (ECG) recorded during the earliest stage of symptoms may not show diagnostic changes or may even be normal. Serial tracings are required to demonstrate sequential change.

ST elevation occurs early in the evolution of the infarction and tends to return towards the isoelectric time during the first 48 h, with development of symmetrical T wave inversion. Leads facing the surface of the infarction show pathological Q waves which are pathognomonic of infarction. The distribution of the Q wave depends on the occluded artery and the resulting site of infarct.

Differential Diagnosis

Many conditions may make the diagnosis of acute myocardial infarction difficult. The differential diagnosis includes chest pain of both cardiac and non-cardiac origin (Table 5.1).

Table 5.1. Differential diagnosis of myocardial infarction: causes of chest pain

Cardiac	Non-cardiac	
	Thoracic	Extrathoracic
Pericarditis	Cervical spine	Acute pancreatitis
Pulmonary embolism	Thoracic spine disease	Cholecystitis
Dissecting aortic	Hiatus hernia	Perforation
aneurysm	Pneumothorax	
	Mediastinal emphysema	
	Herpes zoster	

Management

Treatment is initially aimed at relieving the associated symptoms and then the management of complications. Early studies identified that the mortality from acute myocardial infarction occurs in two phases:

1. An early mortality secondary to arrhythmic events, especially ventricular fibrillation occuring shortly after the onset of symptoms or even as the first symptom (see Chap. 4)
2. A later mortality secondary to the results of myocardial damage following arterial occlusion with major haemodynamic consequences

The management of acute myocardial infarction may therefore be divided into three periods:

1. Early or prehospital phase of acute myocardial infarction (Pantridge and Adgey 1969)
2. The hospital management of acute myocardial infarction, performed within the coronary care unit
3. Long-term rehabilitation and secondary prevention

Prehospital Phase

If no community emergency service is available, then the out-of-hospital mortality will be high and the impact of treatment using modern therapeutic interventions will be reduced. Several inherent delays occur between the onset of symptoms of myocardial infarction and admission to a coronary care unit:

   1. Delay between onset of symptoms and notification of medical personnel (1–2 h). This delay may be shortened by lay education programmes to recognise symptoms and to seek early medical attention.

   2. Delay prior to arrival of medical services. It is in this area that most impact can be made by the early attendance of the primary care physician or practitioner.

   3. The transport delay from home to hospital. The practitioner is required to wait during this time to ensure that no specific complications have occurred.

   4. Intrahospital delay between the acute admission area and the coronary care unit; this delay can be improved by a direct admission policy.

The mean time of hospital admission in many general hospitals is often some 4 h after onset of symptoms, and recognition that the period of highest risk has passed by the time of patient admission has suggested that in specific subsets of patients, long-term prognosis would be as good if the patients were treated at home. This has led to several studies comparing the home and hospital management of acute myocardial infarction. Three studies in the United Kingdom are worthy of detailed examination. Mather and his colleagues (1976) studied patients in the Bristol area. The study was confined to males less than 70 years old who had suffered acute myocardial infarction within the previous 48 h. Of 1203 such patients, only 28% (343) were randomised. This resulted in 77% being treated in hospital and only 23% being treated at home. Significant difference in mortality was noted in the randomised group at 28 days (home 10%, hospital 14%). The median interval from onset of symptoms to arrival of the primary care physician was 4 h and was hence after the time of maximum risk. In those patients seen within the first hour, prognosis was better in the hospital-treated group (41% of those treated at home, vs. 29% of those treated in hospital). Thereafter a progressive decrease in mortality occurred in both groups with each succeeding hour. This study suggests that for a minority of patients seen late after the onset of acute myocardial infarction, hospital admission produces no benefit.

Colling and his co-workers (1976) performed a non-randomised study on Teesside. Of some 2000 patients with suspected acute myocardial infarction, 43% died before being seen by their practitioner. Those who survived were treated at home, in a coronary care unit or in a general medical ward. Of those patients who died, 75% succumbed within 3 h. In those with confirmed acute myocardial infarction, 8.8% treated at home died, 12.9% treated in the coronary care unit and 18.7% treated in the general medical wards. The median interval between onset of symptoms and assessment was twice as long (at 2.6 h) in those treated at home as in those referred to hospital (1.3 h). More patients were at highest risk in the hospital group. From this study it was suggested that coronary care units may have little to offer patients after the first 3 h of acute myocardial infarction (Dellipiani et al. 1977).

A randomised 4-year study was conducted in Nottingham using a hospital-based physician team which responded to calls from G.P.s to patients with suspected acute myocardial infarction (Hill et al. 1978). The hospital physician made the diagnosis and provided emergency treatment. Patients with overt complications were excluded from randomisation. After a 2-h period of observation, patients were randomised to home or hospital management. At 6 weeks similar mortality was reported in both groups (home 13%, hospital 11%). Almost 60% of patients contacted their physician during the early high-risk period of symptoms, however, the average time of physician arrival was some 3 h and a further period of 2 h of observation meant that the patients were randomised when they were in a low-risk phase. Before the hospital team arrived, some 14 subjects died, and a further seven developed ventricular fibrillation after the team's arrival. The subjects were successfully resuscitated, emphasising the usefulness of resuscitation procedures within a domestic setting.

In summary, it appears that after the very acute phase of myocardial infarction, i.e. after 5 or 6 h of symptoms, the mortality in uncomplicated infarction is similar whether patients are treated at home or in the coronary care unit. The success of community emergency services such as the Seattle Medic One group emphasises that the highest return of successful resuscitation and the biggest impact on community death results from early intervention by trained observers and staff. Home management should be considered in those patients with an uncomplicated clinical course who are seen after the first 6 h from onset of symptoms, particularly in the elderly and when the coronary care facilities are so distant as to make transportation difficult. It should also be considered when the patient's inclination is to stay at home and when their environment is good and adequate nursing back-up is available.

Home management usually requires that the primary care physician performs an ECG to confirm the diagnosis and pays twice daily home visits during the first 2 or 3 days, with daily visits during the first week of recovery. This may be difficult for those with a busy clinical practice. The treatment of female patients at home in the absence of supportive female relatives is particularly difficult.

Hospital Phase

The general care of the patient involves the careful observation of vital signs and the early management of complications. Coronary care units have been developed to allow careful monitoring of the patient during the early high-risk phase when electrical instability predisposes to ventricular fibrillation. The patients are nursed in individual cubicles. Each cubicle should have basic fitments, including oxygen supply, suction points, adequate electrical points for supplying electrical equipment, bedside monitors and overhead facilities for carrying i.v. infusion sets. The design should allow observation of each cubicle from a central nursing console, and the monitored electrocardiographic signal from each patient should be conveyed to this central observation point. The ECG should be clearly presented to allow easy scanning by a trained observer. Audiovisual alarms should be available with preset high and low triggers, and there should be a replay facility to allow review of individual arrhythmic events. A portable defibrillator should be easily available and an emergency trolley with basic cardiac resuscitation equipment and cardiac drugs (Tables 4.1, 4.2) should be to hand. X-ray screening equipment should also be available, either as portable equipment which may be taken to an individual room or, alternatively, based in a nearby procedure room. Pressure monitoring equipment should also be available to measure pulmonary artery pressure, left ventricular filling pressure and arterial pressure if necessary.

The coronary care unit groups patients at high risk within the hospital and also localises specialised facilities and nursing and medical staff trained in resuscitative procedures. In this setting nursing staff play a major role in the observation and identification of cardiac arrhythmias and conduction defects. With adequate supervision and training, the nursing staff take on an extended role in regard to administration of cardioactive drugs and initiation of resuscitation procedures, including defibrillation.

Treatment policies should be clearly identified and administration organised on a team basis with regular discussions and meetings of the medical and nursing staff to discuss (a) therapeutic approaches and (b) morbidity and mortality in the unit.

In view of the high intensity nature of the activities of such units, adequate staffing levels must be maintained and rest facilities should be available for medical and nursing staff. The development of the coronary care unit concept has led to the reduction in hospital mortality from some 30% to 10%–15%.

General Management

Following admission, the monitored ECG tracing must be obtained and an indwelling venous cannula inserted to allow rapid administration of necessary medications. Patency should be maintained by intermittent heparinised saline flushes. The patient's confidence should be developed by careful explanation of the role of the coronary care unit and the investigations and procedures being performed. In addition, full discussion of the patient's symptoms and any anxieties should be discussed.

Rehabilitation can be greatly encouraged by early explanation and discussion of the probable duration of the stay in the coronary care unit, the total period of hospitalisation, mobilisation and return to normal living activities, and potential time to return to work. In the case of patients who are distressed at the time of admission, such discussion should be deferred until the patient is stabilised.

Analgesia

Adequate analgesia, with reduction in central sympatho-adrenal discharge, affords symptomatic relief and may also influence the incidence of ventricular arrhythmias and reduce myocardial infarct size by lowering myocardial oxygen requirements. The ideal analgesic for use in acute myocardial infarction has a rapid onset of action, a relatively short duration of action as the pain of infarction is usually self-limiting, no deleterious haemodynamic effects and few side-effects.

The opioid agonist morphine has high affinity for mu (μ) opioid receptors which are stereo-specific, saturable and widely distributed in brain and the nervous system. It has agonist activity and remains the standard analgesic compound for comparison with developmental agents. In view of the dependence problem associated with morphine, other opioid analgesics have been developed with mixed agonist/antagonist activity (Table 5.2). In general these compounds have been developed by substituting at the 3, 6 or 17 carbon positions on the morphine molecule. Mixed agonist/antagonist opioids have varying affinity and actions at the postulated three types of opioid receptors. They bind to the μ receptor but exert either no or little agonist activity.

Morphine

Although readily absorbed from the gastrointestinal tract, morphine is subject to a high first pass metabolism and its analgesic effects may be delayed; thus the oral route is unsuitable for the treatment of patients with acute myocardial infarction. Used parenterally, it may be administered by the subcutaneous,

Table 5.2. The opioid agonist/antagonist used in the treatment of acute myocardial infarction; chemical structures, dose and duration of action are noted

Opioid	Chemical radicals and carbon positions			Dose (mg)	Duration of action (h)
	3	6	17		
Morphine	-OH	-OH	-CH$_3$	10	4–5
Diamorphine	-OCOCH$_3$	-OCOCH$_3$	-CH$_3$	2–5	3–4
Pentazocine^a	-OH	–	-CH$_2$ CH = C$<$CH$_3$ / CH$_3$	20–40	3
Buprenorphine	-OH	-OCH$_3$	-OCH$_2$—▽	0.3–0.4	6
Nalbuphine	-OH	-OH	-CH$_2$—◇	10	3–6

a Pentazocine is a benzo-morphan derivative: the 5, 6, 7 and 8 atoms of the morphine molecule are absent

Table 5.3. Haemodynamic changes following the administration of the opioid agonist/antagonist analgesics used in the treatment of acute myocardial infarction

	Morphine (8 mg)	Pentazocine (48 mg)	Buprenorphine (0.3 mg)	Nalbuphine (10 mg)
Heart rate	No change	↑13%	↓7%	↓15%
Aortic pressure: systolic	↓9%	↑12%	↓14%	No change
diastolic	↓3%	↑10%	↓8%	No change
mean	–	–	–	–
Pulmonary pressure: systolic	↓12%	↑31%	↓9%	No change
diastolic	No change	↑41%	No change	No change
mean	–	–	–	–
Systemic vascular resistance	↑4%	↑11%	–	↑19%
Pulmonary vascular resistance	↑8%	↑75%	–	↑27%
Left ventricular end-diastolic pressure	↑24%	↑17%	–	–
Cardiac index	↓12%	↑8%	–	↓10%
Stroke volume index	↓11%	↑4%	–	↑3%
Myocardial oxygen consumption	↓12%	↑5%	–	–

intramuscular or intravenous route, the latter being the route of choice. It may be given by slow intravenous injection in dose increments from 2.5–15 mg. Dosing by this route may be repeated at 15–20-min intervals.

Cardiovascular Effects.   When administered in therapeutic doses to supine patients, morphine has little effect on heart rate, cardiac rhythm or arterial pressure. Analgesia is obtained, usually with marked relief of distress, but other sensory modalities are unaffected. In acute haemodynamic studies beneficial changes have been shown, with reduced left ventricular end-diastolic pressure, reduced cardiac work and reduced myocardial oxygen consumption (Alderman et al. 1972) (Table 5.3). Hypotension may occur in patients who are tilted up after parenteral administration. The mechanism of hypotension may in part be due to histamine release. Vasodilation, however, is only partially blocked by H_1-receptor blockade and the depressant action on the vasomotor centre may be more important (Reynolds and Randall 1957). Hypotension may be pronounced in patients who are hypovolaemic secondary to prolonged diuretic therapy (Thomas et al. 1965). It may reduce coronary perfusion pressure, which may be deleterious in the early stage of acute myocardial infarction. Hypotension may be reversed by postural adjustment, fluid replacement, blood volume expansion or the use of pressor agents. Bradycardia may occur following high dose administration secondary to a central effect or direct stimulation of the vagal nucleus (Reynolds and Randall 1957). This can be easily reversed by atropine administration.

In patients with marked left ventricular impairment, morphine exhibits combined venous and arteriolar dilating actions. This leads to a beneficial reduction in the left ventricular filling pressure and to afterload reduction (Zelis et al. 1974).

In summary, the haemodynamic effects of morphine depend on the individual patient's haemodynamic status, and caution should be exercised if hypotension or evidence of hypovolaemia is present.

Respiratory Effects.   Morphine must be used with great caution in patients with chronic obstructive airways disease or cor pulmonale. Respiratory depression follows a direct effect on the brain stem respiratory centre, with reduced sensitivity of neurones in the brainstem to carbon dioxide. The respiratory rate, minute volume and tidal exchange are all reduced, and irregular or periodic breathing may occur. Respiratory depression may occur within 10 min of an intravenous injection and may last for up to 4–5 h. This may be reversed by administration of the opioid antagonist nalorphine. Additional side-effects include nausea and vomiting, which is the result of direct stimulation of the chemoreceptor trigger zone for emesis. This may be a major problem in patients with nausea in the early stage of acute myocardial infarction. The emetic effects may be blocked using phenothiazine derivatives and the combination of cyclizine and morphine may be used.

Gastrointestinal Effects.   There is a reduction in motility in the stomach, with reduced acid secretion, and gastric emptying may be delayed up to 12 h after the use of morphine. This may be of clinical importance in relation to concomitant administration of other cardioactive drugs given by the oral route in the early phase of myocardial infarction. Reduced absorption of mexilitene has been demonstrated and other agents may also be affected. Additional effects occur in the biliary tract, increased pressure within the ducts occurring within 5 min of intravenous administration and persisting for up to 2 h. Reduction in bowel motility may lead to troublesome constipation during the early clinical phase of acute myocardial infarction.

Problems of dependence do not occur in patients suffering from acute myocardial infarction as the pain is usually self-limiting and dosage requirements are usually limited to a period of several hours.

Diamorphine

Diacetyl morphine is in widespread clinical use in the United Kingdom; its dosage is 1–5 mg given intravenously, and its duration of action, 3–4 h. It is rapidly hydrolysed to monoacetyl morphine and to morphine. Its general haemodynamic effects are similar to those of morphine (Reynolds and Randall 1957). On the basis of comparison with previously published haemodynamic studies (Thomas et al. 1965), Macdonald et al. (1967) suggested that diamorphine is superior to morphine in providing analgesia, has less unpleasant or harmful side-effects and shows fewer haemodynamic effects. Scott and Orr (1969) compared the effects of several opioid analgesics and suggested that diamorphine (5 mg) provided earlier complete relief in a higher percentage of patients than morphine. There was no difference in side-effects of nausea or vomiting.

Pentazocine

Pentazocine is an opioid antagonist developed to have little abuse potential. Its clinical usefulness was suggested from early observations that it was associated with little hypotensive effect. Scott and Orr (1969) demonstrated a rise in arterial pressure in subjects with systolic blood pressure of less than 120 mmHg, and suggested it compared favourably with morphine and diamorphine. Other haemodynamic studies confirmed the rise in arterial pressure, but also showed a significant increase in cardiac work, left ventricular afterload and pulmonary vascular resistance (Jewitt et al. 1970; Alderman et al. 1972). In myocardial infarction, these haemodynamic changes are potentially hazardous in regard to extending myocardial infarct size. The rise in arterial pressure and heart rate may be associated with a rise in circulating adrenaline and noradrenaline. In the presence of hypotension, however, the rise in aortic pressure may help to perfuse the coronary arteries and pentazocine may therefore be of value in this subset of patients with acute myocardial infarction (Zola and McLeod 1983). As with other agonist/antagonists, there is a ceiling for respiratory depression, with a plateau and little further effect after 30 mg.

Buprenorphine

Buprenorphine is a semisynthetic highly lipophilic substance derived from thebaine; it has the same degree of analgesia as morphine but causes less dependence. Buprenorphine has mixed agonist/antagonist properties and is 25–50 times more potent than morphine. It produces analgesia and central nervous system effects qualitatively similar to those of morphine and can be given in a dose of 0.2–0.4 mg, this being comparative to 5–10 mg morphine (Mok et al. 1981). Buprenorphine is effective by the sublingual, oral or parenteral route. The sublingual route is attractive as it avoids the hepatic first pass effect.

Following sublingual administration, the plasma concentrations are similar after 80 min to those seen following the intravenous route. The systemic availability, however, is 30%, and the onset of analgesic activity is delayed, making this route unsuitable for use in acute myocardial infarction. The duration of analgesic activity by the intravenous route is longer than that of morphine.

Respiratory depression has been observed to be slower in onset but to last longer than with morphine. The maximum respiratory depression occurs at 3 h. It is unclear whether there is a ceiling effect as it appears that buprenorphine's respiratory effects are not readily reversed by the administration of naloxone (Steen et al. 1979). Its haemodynamic effects are similar to those of diamorphine, and there has been no difference in the reported incidence of side-effects compared with diamorphine in the treatment of acute myocardial infarction. Buprenorphine is an uncontrolled substance and may have obvious advantages in regard to storage and availability in the primary care setting.

In summary, the opioid analgesics are still the appropriate drugs of choice in acute myocardial infarction. Morphine and diamorphine remain those drugs with most widespread usage. However, careful subsetting of individual patients in regard to blood pressure measurements and potential respiratory complications may indicate that other compounds are more appropriate.

Bed Rest

Patients are usually rested for some 3–5 days, i.e. during treatment in the coronary care unit and immediately after transfer to a general medical ward or intermediate coronary care facility. Slower mobilisation should be considered in the presence of cardiac failure or continued cardiac arrhythmias. When in bed, active and passive leg movements should be encouraged and respiratory physiotherapy performed where indicated. Early gradual mobilisation should be undertaken and guidelines concerning progressive ambulation drawn up for each patient. Information leaflets may also be used to encourage rehabilitation.

Bowel function may be sluggish in the early period following myocardial infarction and may worry the patient. Use of a bed-commode should be encouraged and aperients given as required. The time of ultimate discharge from the hospital depends on the clinical status of the patient and the severity of myocardial damage. Up to 30% of hospital deaths occur more than 72 h after hospitalisation, and careful observation should be maintained in patients with (a) IV conduction defects, (b) continuing sinus tachycardia, (c) extensive anterior infarction or (d) a history of continuing arrhythmias. Patients may be kept under intermediate coronary care with appropriately trained staff (Resnekov 1977).

Oxygen Therapy

In the early stage of acute myocardial infarction, ventilation perfusion abnormalities have been noted which may lead to hypoxia. Early oxygen administration may protect ischaemic myocardium (Maroko et al. 1975). Unless contra-indicated, this should be given as 100% oxygen, 2–4 litres/min, via a close-fitting mask or nasal prongs. Hyperbaric oxygen has been advocated in the past; however, this is impractical and appears to confer no long-term benefit.

Treatment of Complications (Table 5.4)

Arrhythmias

The introduction of electrocardiographic monitoring in the early stages of acute myocardial infarction has identified a high incidence of arrhythmic events. All forms of cardiac arrhythmias occur, and indeed ventricular extrasystoles occur in virtually all patients who are monitored early in their clinical course. Treatment is required:

1. When there are haemodynamic sequelae with hypotension or cardiac decompensation.
2. When the arrhythmia leads to augmented myocardial oxygen consumption with a potential increase in infarct size.
3. When the existing arrhythmia predisposes to the development of malignant ventricular arrhythmias. In general terms the threshold and incidence of ventricular arrhythmias correlates with the extent of myocardial damage.

Table 5.4. Complications of acute myocardial infarction

1. Arrhythmias and conduction defects
2. Conditions secondary to myocardial damage
    Cardiac failure
    Cardiogenic shock
3. Thrombosis and thromboembolism

VENTRICULAR EXTRASYSTOLES

Routine monitoring confirms the presence of ventricular extrasystoles in virtually all patients during the early phase of myocardial infarction. During this time the threshold for induction of ventricular fibrillation is reduced, and observations during the early development of coronary care units suggested that the presence of ventricular extrasystoles is a warning arrhythmia and reflects electrical instability. Lown (1967) advanced his classification of the ventricular arrhythmias and emphasised the prophylactic use of anti-arrhythmic compounds to prevent the development of ventricular fibrillation. Further observations have shown that ventricular fibrillation is unheralded by warning arrhythmias in some 70% of patients and that warning arrhythmias may occur without resulting development of serious ventricular arrhythmias (Campbell and Murray 1980). Most authorities agree that several forms of ventricular extrasystoles still suggest a propensity to electrical instability, including R on T forms, multifocal extrasystoles and extrasystoles presenting in short salvoes. The use of standard class I anti-arrhythmics has been advocated in this setting. During the first hour of myocardial infarction, class I anti-arrhythmics may be less effective than during the later stages of development. The standard regimes used in myocardial infarction are as indicated in Chap. 8.

BRADYARRHYTHMIAS

Sinus Bradycardia. This arrhythmia is common in the early stage of myocardial infarction, possibly due to stimulation of cardiac afferent receptors, and occurs frequently in inferior or posterior myocardial infarction. If it occurs within the first 2–3 h of myocardial infarction, it may be associated with a significant incidence of ventricular tachycardia or ventricular fibrillation occurring by a re-entry mechanism or, alternatively, late enhanced automaticity. Atropine 0.6–1.2 mg i.v. should be administered, particularly if there is associated hypertension, and the dose should be repeated to maintain the heart rate and blood pressure at an adequate level. If ventricular extrasystoles are present in association with sinus bradycardia, the administration of atropine usually abolishes this arrhythmia (Adgey et al. 1968).

When seen in the period beyond 6 h after the onset of infarct, sinus bradycardia usually reflects atrial ischemia with sinus node dysfunction. At this time sinus bradycardia is usually not accompanied by hypotension and there is no apparent predisposition to ventricular arrhythmias. Treatment is not required unless there is secondary haemodynamic decompensation. If sinus bradycardia remains resistant to atropine therapy, then the use of ventricular electrical pacing may be required.

First Degree Heart Block. First degree heart block requires no specific therapy unless it is associated with sinus bradycardia and hypotension, in which case atropine should be used as indicated above.

Second Degree Heart Block. There are two types of second degree heart block:

1. *Wenckebach type.* No specific therapy is indicated when the ventricular rate is adequate. When associated with bradycardia, and particularly when ventricular irritability, cardiac failure or shock is present, pacemaker insertion is indicated.
2. *Mobitz Type II.* This form of second degree heart block is rare in acute myocardial infarction, but is a potentially serious conduction defect with the associated danger of sudden asystole. It usually requires the use of a pacemaker.

Complete Heart Block. Most patients with complete heart block will be those with inferior infarctions in whom ischaemia of the AV node artery leads to this major conduction defect. A pacemaker should be inserted to protect against the results of even transient haemodynamic disturbance. In general terms the conduction defect will become less marked during the next week of the clinical course and permanent pacing will seldom be required. Complete heart block in the presence of anterior myocardial infarction generally reflects severe damage to the intraventricular septum and although temporary pacing may stabilise the patient's condition, the long-term prognosis remains poor. Permanent pacing will usually be required, although it is uncertain whether or not this improves the long-term prognosis.

Tachyarrhythmias. Owing to increased myocardial oxygen demands, tachyarrhythmias tend to have a deleterious haemodynamic effect. In addition, when the heart rate is over 150 beats/min, the time available for ventricular filling during diastole is limited, as is the left ventricular ejection time, leading to a lowered ejection fraction and reduced cardiac output. These arrhythmias should be aggressively treated, particularly when the haemodynamic status is compromised (Maling and Moran 1957). Electrolyte and acid-base abnormalities should be treated and hypoxaemia corrected. Specific anti-arrhythmics with atrial or ventricular activity should be used as indicated.

Sinus Tachycardia. One-third of patients in the early stage of myocardial infarction will have sinus tachycardia with transient hyper- or hypotension. There is enhanced early sympathetic activity during myocardial infarction, resulting in both circulating and locally released cardiac catecholamines. When associated with cardiac failure, sinus tachycardia should be treated with diuretic therapy and cardiac glycosides. In the absence of cardiac failure, and particularly if sinus tachycardia is accompanied by ventricular extrasystoles, β-adrenoceptor blocking compounds may be helpful.

Supraventricular Tachycardia. The treatment of supraventricular tachycardia should be in accordance with its haemodynamic sequelae. In the presence of hypotension, cardiac failure or cardiac pain, electrical cardioversion may be required, although the use of standard anti-arrhythmic drugs may be preferred. Consideration should be given to the use of verapamil, disopyramide, procainamide or cardiac glycosides.

Ventricular Tachycardia. When ventricular tachycardia occurs at a rate greater than 150 beats/min, immediate control is mandatory. If intravenous class I anti-arrhythmic therapy is unsuccessful, then electrical cardioversion should be performed immediately.

Ventricular Fibrillation. This is the most serious arrhythmia complicating the early phase of acute myocardial infarction. Early sympathetic and parasympathetic overactivity leads to inhomogeneous depolarisation of adjacent ischaemic and non-ischaemic myocardium. The mechanism is probably due to re-entry in this early period (Han and Moe 1964).

Immediate defibrillation can usually be performed in the coronary care units together with cardiopulmonary resuscitation (see pp. 55–60).

Complications Which Result from Myocardial Damage

The mortality in the early stages of myocardia infarction is secondary to electrical instability and associated primary ventricular fibrillation. Thereafter the major determinant of prognosis is the mass of the damaged heart muscle (Page et al. 1971). The development of cardiogenic shock or cardiac failure is related to the amount of myocardial damage which occurs after coronary artery occlusion. Much interest has been shown in experimental models and subsequent clinical applications which might reduce the extent of acute myocardial damage, with resultant "salvage" of the myocardium (Maroko et al. 1971). Many studies have been performed in numerous animal models, including isolated heart preparations, open-chested anaesthetised animals and intact conscious animals, to investigate the functional effects of various interventions. Unfortunately the methods of study of the functional changes (measurement of ST segment elevation), the assessment of infarct size (creatinine phosphokinase release) and measurement of myocardial blood flow (using radioactive microspheres) have been difficult to translate to the clinical setting (Rude et al. 1981). The increasing use of haemodynamic monitoring in patients with acute myocardial infarction has allowed careful study of interventions which might alter the myocardial supply and demand ratio in a beneficial manner. The primary aim in these studies has been to affect the degree of ischaemic damage at the cellular level, to restore contractile function and to maintain stability of the myocardial cells until adequate perfusion is obtained via collateral channels. The major lines of research have been in the areas discussed below.

REDUCTION OF MYOCARDIAL OXYGEN CONSUMPTION

1. β-Adrenergic blocking compounds block the effects of high circulating catecholamines and their local myocardial effects. By reducing heart rate and

contractility, they affect two of the major determinants of myocardial oxygen consumption. Regional myocardial blood flow redistribution may be facilitated by enhancement of collateral flow to the ischaemic area of myocardium. Arrhythmias may also be reduced. These changes may be of particular value in patients in whom there is an inappropriate sympathetic response following acute myocardial infarction when sinus tachycardia and systolic hypertension are present in the absence of cardiac failure. In early myocardial infarction the parenteral use of metoprolol and atenolol has reduced indices reflecting myocardial oxygen consumption and indirect indices of infarct size. Unfortunately it is difficult to predetermine those patients who may react adversely to this therapy.

2. Mechanical methods of reducing ventricular afterload, including aortic balloon counter pulsation and external counter pulsation, have shown promising results in stabilising patients with severe ischaemic damage. Lack of availability and the need for trained staff to control this therapy make its widespread application impracticable.

3. Parenteral nitrate therapy may reduce left ventricular cavity size secondary to its effects on venous capacitance vessels. In addition it may enhance collateral blood supply by reducing the left ventricular volume and hence reducing compression or stretching forces on collateral vessels. Its use in clinical infarction may be complicated by the precipitation of bradycardia requiring supportive therapy.

4. Inhibition of lipolysis with reduction in free fatty acid production has been shown to reduce myocardial oxygen demand. Most compounds which reduce free fatty acid levels, however, have been limited in their clinical use owing to side-effects.

5. Reduction in left ventricular size by the use of cardiac glycosides or vasodilators in patients with myocardial infarction and cardiac failure has potential benefits when severe left ventricular dysfunction is present.

PROTECTION AGAINST LOCAL AUTOLYTIC DAMAGE

Administration of hydrocortisone has been shown to limit local cellular damage by stabilisation of lysosomal membranes. Clinical evaluation is awaited.

ENHANCED TRANSPORT OF ENERGY SUBSTRATE TO ISCHAEMIC MYOCARDIUM

Hyaluronidase has been used to facilitate transport of substrates from the circulation through the interstitium to myocardial cells. The mechanism is thought to be related to depolymerisation of hyaluronic acid or to enhanced capillary permeability (Maroko et al. 1977).

INCREASED PLASMA OSMOLALITY

Mannitol and hypertonic glucose have been used in experimental preparations. Their clinical benefits have been suggested by their peripheral effects in maintaining renal blood flow, and their primary cardiac effects are unclear.

ENHANCEMENT OF ANAEROBIC METABOLISM

Experimental effects on infarct size have been shown following administration of glucose–insulin–potassium and hypertonic glucose.

INCREASING MYOCARDIAL OXYGEN DELIVERY

1. Increased collateral flow from unobstructed coronary arteries can be demonstrated following administration of calcium antagonists, e.g. nifedipine or nitrates, or by increasing coronary perfusion pressure following α-adrenergic agonists. A similar effect may be demonstrated with intra-aortic balloon counter pulsation.

2. Increased arterial oxygen concentration may be achieved using high flow or hyperbaric oxygen. Clinical application has not shown a successful reduction in mortality.

3. Immediate surgical reperfusion by coronary artery bypass surgery has been successfully demonstrated in a few centres. Its widespread application is obviously limited by the resources required.

4. Thrombolysis using pharmacological methods has had much recent interest and is at present under widespread investigation (see following sections).

THROMBOLYTIC THERAPY

Coronary artery thrombus is found in 95% of patients dying from acute transmural myocardial infarction (Davies et al. 1976). A lesser incidence is found in those dying from subendocardial myocardial infarction or sustaining sudden cardiac death (Roberts and Buja 1972). Acute coronary arteriography conducted during the early hours of transmural myocardial infarction has confirmed total obstruction in some 85% during the first 4 h (DeWood et al. 1980). When studied between 12 and 24 h, a lesser incidence (65%) of total obstruction is evident. This suggests that spasm may play a role in the early stage of infarction and that subsequent recanalisation may occur following the evolution of the infarction.

Lysis of obstructing thrombus is an exciting therapeutic intervention with a potential for myocardial reperfusion and infarct size limitation. The ideal fibrinolytic agent has properties including:

1. Potent local fibrinolytic activity on obstructing thrombus
2. Little or no systemic effects, with a resulting low incidence of bleeding complications
3. Ease of administration by the intravenous route, allowing therapy by a primary care physician without recourse to specialised facilities

Early studies were performed using streptokinase administered by the intravenous route. The results were not wholly convincing, and the therapy had significant associated complications. This may have been due to (a) lack of an adequate placebo control base, (b) late entry of patients (up to 12 h after the onset of ischaemic symptoms, by which time myocardial damage may be irreversible), or (c) variation in dosage schedules and duration of therapy. A recent review has analysed the results of eight randomised trials which used the established intravenous regime of 250 000 units of streptokinase loading dose and then constant intravenous infusions administered within 24 h of acute myocardial infarction (Stampfer et al. 1982). A complicated statistical method was used to allow pooling of the data. These results suggested a reduction by some 20% in mortality at 40 days following acute myocardial infarction. Some of these studies were performed before the establishment of coronary care units and the wide-spread use of anti-arrhythmic compounds, including β-blockers and other pharmacological agents, which may be beneficial in reducing myocardial infarct size. Overall the results supported the possibility that fibrinolytic therapy was a promising approach. Further studies have now been carried out using high dose, brief duration intravenous infusions of streptokinase (Shroeder et al. 1983). Such a regime has been advocated to allow a high incidence of reperfusion without the protracted period of circulatory hyperplasminaemia so that there would be rapid recovery of the systemic effects with a reduced risk of bleeding complications. Using these regimes successful recanalisation, demonstrated by coronary arteriography, can be obtained in 45%–50% of patients.

Recently interest has centred on the use of regional fibrinolysis using semi-selective or subselective intracoronary infusion of streptokinase. The potential benefits of this route of administration include:

1. Specific visualisation of the infarct vessel, allowing both pharmacological and mechanical methods to be used to obtain reperfusion
2. Assurance of delivery of the thrombolytic agent to the intended site, with a resultant high concentration at the luminal–thrombus interface
3. Avoidance of a large loading dose, which may decrease bleeding complications and decrease the systemic effects

A number of major difficulties limit widespread use of the intracoronary route of administration.

1. The procedure is difficult and complex and requires coronary arteriography to be performed within a short time of the onset of ischaemic symptoms.
2. The number of hospitals admitting patients with acute myocardial infarction also having facilities and personnel available to perform coronary arteriography is limited.
3. Even those hospitals with catheter laboratories have difficulties in maintaining a service over the whole 24 h period. Cost implications are evident. The interruption of an existing investigational programme may also create major problems.
4. The necessity of transporting the patient to the catheter laboratory may delay the initiation of thrombolytic therapy. The success of reperfusion may be limited by such delays. Many of these problems may be solved, however, by performing coronary arteriography within coronary care units using

existing image intensifiers linked to relatively inexpensive video-tape recording facilities.

Although in the long-term preparations which are active by the intravenous route would be preferable, the studies published have shown a success rate of reperfusion of 40%–50% using the intravenous route, as against rates in excess of 75% with intracoronary administration. This suggests that where ideal conditions and facilities are available, the intracoronary route should be used.

Results.   In the initial reports Rentrop and his colleagues (1979) achieved reperfusion in some 76% of patients using conventional streptokinase. Ganz et al. (1983) have reported 95% successful reperfusion using thrombolysin (streptokinase/plasmin combinations). Many other centres have shown a similar incidence of success. Reperfusion rates with left anterior descending and right coronary artery occlusions are similar. Results with circumflex occlusions are less promising. Failure of reperfusion may be due to:

1. Absence of thrombus
2. Insufficient dosage of thrombolytic therapy
3. The presence of multiple occlusions, particularly in patients with a history of previous myocardial infarction
4. Antibody neutralisation following recent streptococcal infections
5. Inability to deliver high local concentrations of thrombolytic material due to distal site of occlusion

Early reocclusion is a variable occurrence and appears to be dependent on the extent of underlying vessel disease.

Assessment of Efficacy.   Although the early studies using intravenous streptokinase were promising, further information regarding the influence of successful reperfusion on mortality is awaited. Many controlled trials have been initiated and preliminary results suggest that at least in anterior infarcts, mortality may be influenced (Anderson et al. 1983; Kennedy et al. 1983). Ethical problems have limited the ability of many centres to enrol control subjects for such a trial.

Studies have been performed looking at other softer end-points to assess cardiac status, including clinical progress, electrocardiographic changes and measures of left ventricular function. The early comparative results were obtained using patients in whom reperfusion was not achieved and this may not be an adequate control group (Hugenholtz and Rentrop 1982).

1. Successful reperfusion is often accompanied by *relief of cardiac pain*, although analgesic has always been administered in the reported studies. In a small percentage of patients, reperfusion is associated with a return of cardiac pain, which may represent reversal of potential myocardial necrosis to a degree of myocardial ischaemia.

2. An accelerated pattern of sequential *electrocardiographic changes* is shown after reperfusion. ST elevation is usually dramatically reduced; however, Q wave

development usually occurs and appears early. The distribution of these changes may be less than that predicted from the admission electrocardiogram at the early stage of the ischaemic injury. In addition, experimental work suggests that there is dissociation between the extent of distribution of Q waves and the retention of regional contractile performance following reperfusion.

3. Reperfusion is associated with a *wash-out of cardiac enzymes* from previously ischaemic zones. There is an early peak in release of creatine phosphokinase and this appears to distort enzyme modelling estimates of infarct size. Animal studies suggest that established modelling techniques will grossly overestimate myocardial damage in reperfused patients (Blanke et al. 1984)

4. *Left ventricular function* is improved in those patients who reperfuse. This has been shown to occur in the region of reperfusion but also when global contraction is examined. Improved regional and global function has been demonstrated in comparison with control subjects and assessed by radionuclide, echocardiographic and invasive ventriculography.

The initial results of reperfusion therefore appear promising. This intervention appears to reduce myocardial infarct size with clinical evidence of salvage of the myocardium. Many questions concerning patient selection, time of intervention and specific dose regimes of thrombolytic compounds remain. Newer agents which may have properties of local thrombolysis without systemic effects have been developed and would appear to have the potential to play an increasing role in the treatment of the early phase of acute myocardial infarction.

Following reperfusion, patients are treated with conventional treatment; however, in addition they are anticoagulated with heparin, and then warfarin, and have anti-platelet therapy with aspirin and dipyridamole, usually with an additional calcium channel blocker. In due course the patients are reviewed with the intention of identifying the high-risk group who have been left with significant coronary artery obstruction after reperfusion. Exercise tests are performed at some 10–12 days post-infarct and further long-term therapy introduced. Early repeat coronary arteriography is indicated in those patients who have evidence of multivessel disease and due consideration will be given to their suitability for percutaneous transluminal balloon angioplasty or coronary artery bypass surgery.

Cardiogenic Shock

The clinical course of acute myocardial infarction may be complicated by shock if major myocardial damage has occurred or if mechanical complications intervene. The shock syndrome results from a reduction in blood flow to the vital organs secondary to (a) an inadequate cardiac output, (b) maldistribution of blood flow, or (c) both. It presents with arterial hypotension, restlessness, impaired cerebration, tachypnoea and oliguria or anuria. Cardiogenic shock usually results from acute myocardial infarction; however, it may also be a late clinical presentation in patients with diffuse myocardial disease, as in cardiomyopathy, or with end-stage valvular disease causing either major obstruction or regurgitation.

The development of cardiogenic shock accounts for 10%–15% of the hospital mortality following acute myocardial infarction. Most patients have three-vessel coronary artery disease, usually with left anterior descending artery occlusion, and pathological studies have confirmed extensive ventricular damage, more than 40% of the left ventricular muscle mass being affected. In the presence of lesser degrees of myocardial damage, shock may be precipitated by arrhythmias or conduction defects. Ventricular arrhythmias cause asynchronous ventricular contraction, while supraventricular tachycardia or atrial fibrillation provides inadequate diastolic filling and systolic ejection to maintain organ perfusion pressure.

Bradycardia in the presence of a fixed stroke volume may precipitate hypotension and shock. Loss of atrial transport in patients with idioventricular rhythm may also precipitate shock when the haemodynamic status is already compromised. Although the primary problem is left ventricular damage, cardiogenic shock may also be precipitated by right ventricular infarction or major pulmonary embolism. The mechanical complication of acute mitral regurgitation or ventricular septal defect may lead to cardiogenic shock without associated major left ventricular damage.

The availability of invasive methods of haemodynamic monitoring has allowed the early diagnosis of "pump failure". Subsetting of patients is made on the basis of the following measurements, which allow the introduction of rational pharmacological therapy:

1. Systemic arterial pressure
2. Left ventricular filling pressure
3. Cardiac output (Swan et al. 1970)

CLINICAL SIGNS

The patient is restless, often confused and may be semiconscious. The skin is cold and clammy and the body core temperature reduced. Cyanosis and tachypnoea are often present. The pulse is weak and thready with hypotension and reduced pulse pressure. Cardiac pain may be prolonged. Urine output is greatly reduced and arrhythmias are common. Hypovolaemia may occur, developing with fluid loss from sweating, vomiting, bleeding or prior diuretic administration (Loeb et al. 1968). Evidence of acute left ventricular failure may be present, with either bronchospasm or frank pulmonary oedema. Cheyne-Stokes respiration may develop, particularly if opioid analgesics have been used. If right ventricular infarction is present, concomitant signs of right heart failure will be evident. Auscultation confirms muffled heart sounds. Additional heart sounds may be evident or the murmurs of mitral regurgitation or ventricular septal defect may be present.

LABORATORY FINDINGS

1. Metabolic acidosis secondary to lactic acid accumulation
2. Arterial hypoxaemia with or without hypercapnia

3. Electrolyte disturbances, including hypo- or hyperkalaemia, may be present if the condition is maintained

4. Evidence of myocardial necrosis with grossly elevated cardiac enzymes and a marked leucocytosis may be present

HAEMODYNAMIC CHANGES

1. Cardiac output is low even in the presence of an increased left ventricular filling pressure.

2. Left ventricular filling pressure is elevated except in the present of hypovolaemia. Increased left ventricular filling pressure leads to increased left atrial, pulmonary venous and pulmonary arterial pressures and may precipitate right heart failure with elevated right atrial pressures and systemic venous engorgement. Functional tricuspid regurgitation may result. Coronary perfusion is reduced and subendocardial ischaemic injury may result in a reduction in the coronary perfusion gradient secondary to arterial hypotension and elevated left ventricular end-diastolic pressure. Further functional impairment results secondary to this ischaemia.

3. Increased total vascular resistance occurs secondary to the neurohumeral response to hypotension.

TREATMENT

When the shock state is secondary to extensive myocardial damage, the mortality approaches 100% no matter what pharmacological intervention is used. In view of this, haemodynamic assessment is advocated in all patients with evidence of early pump failure, including those with "normotensive shock" and heart failure. Theoretically, interventions which might lead to reduction of infarct size, i.e. salvage of the myocardium, should have potential benefit. However, despite attempts to improve oxygen delivery, interventions to reduce myocardial oxygen demand or facilitate the removal of metabolites accumulating in the myocardium, and pharmacological support of the circulation, the mortality from cardiogenic shock has not been significantly reduced. Early aggressive assessment and management is advocated to promote maximal collateral blood flow development in order to maintain function in initially ischaemic and threatened myocardium.

General measures to be taken include:

1. Relief of pain. Continued pain may induce a vasovagal contribution to the hypotension and associated profuse sweating may lead to hypovolaemia. Adrenergic stimulation leads to marked peripheral vasoconstriction. These factors may be reversed by the cautious introduction of opiate analgesics. Care must be used that the venous and arteriolar dilating activity of these compounds does not cause further hypotension. Small intravenous doses are used.

2. Relief of precipitating factors. Brady- and tachyarrhythmias are vigorously treated. Atropine should be used if sinus bradycardia persists. The

early introduction of a transvenous pacemaker should be considered. Anti-arrhythmics should be used cautiously in view of their negative inotropic action, and pre-treatment with β-blockers should be reversed using β-agonists.

3. High flow oxygen via a Ventimask. Occasionally ventilatory assistance may be required and a combined intensive care/coronary care approach undertaken.

4. Acidosis and electrolyte imbalance such as hypokalaemia are corrected, particularly since arrhythmias may be precipitated.

5. Mechanical factors must be sought and invasive investigations may be required to identify and quantify mitral regurgitation, acquired ventricular septal defect or early aneurysm formation so that surgical correction may be considered.

Haemodynamic monitoring with a Swan-Ganz catheter should be considered. In the presence of established cardiogenic shock, the haemodynamic findings are:

1. Increased peripheral resistance
2. Hypotension — systolic pressure less than 80 mmHg
3. Elevated left ventricular filling pressure — greater than 18 mmHg
4. Cardiac index < 1.8 litres/min/m^2

Pharmacological treatment should:

1. Obtain maximum left ventricular function by adjusting the left ventricular filling pressure to obtain optimal preload. If hypovolaemia is present, the filling pressure may be less than 15 mmHg. Cautious administration of a plasma expander, 5% albumin or dextran, in 50-ml aliquots should be carried out until the filling pressure is 18–20 mmHg. If the filling pressure is markedly elevated, then the powerful loop diuretics frusemide, bumetanide or ethacrynic acid should be given. Frusemide may be particularly useful as its venodilating activity may reduce preload before the diuresis is commenced. The osmotic diuretic mannitol (200 ml of 20% solution) may allow a diuresis to be established.

2. Enhance contractile function. Although cardiogenic shock may be accompanied by high circulating levels of catecholamines, inotropic support may be given using dopamine or dobutamine. Low dose dopamine (2–6 μg/kg/min) enhances contractile function and by direct activity on dopaminergic receptors enhances renal and mesenteric blood flow with resulting vasodilator activity. At higher doses α-activity may increase the arterial pressure due to α-adrenergic stimulation and an increased heart rate may also occur. Phentolamine has been advocated as adjunctive therapy to counteract these α-constrictor effects. Dobutamine may have an advantage in that it reduces total vascular resistance and leads to a modest increase in contractility. This synthetic sympathomimetic amine acts on adrenergic receptors and has a major inotropic action. Its pulmonary vascular effects are limited. Vasodilatation does occur due to withdrawal of sympathetic tone secondary to an increase in cardiac output (Loeb et al. 1977; Leir et al. 1978).

3. Adjust increased afterload. If the systolic blood pressure can be increased to 90 mmHg or more by inotropic support then the cautious introduction of vasodilator therapy may be helpful, provided continuous haemodynamic monitoring is available (since such patients are particularly sensitive to haemodynamic changes). As a consequence of the reduction in aortic impedence, enhanced forward ejection and improved organ perfusion should occur.

Phentolamine, nitroprusside and parenteral nitrate may be used. Experimental evidence suggests that problems of coronary artery "steal" may occur, with preferential blood flow to non-ischaemic areas (Kotter et al. 1977). The continued use of veno mixed or arteriolar dilators should depend on the haemodynamic profile and response to individual pharmacological intervention.

MECHANICAL TREATMENT

The use of intra-aortic balloon counter pulsation has been beneficial in offloading the systemic circulation and augmenting coronary artery perfusion. This treatment is not widely available, but it has been suggested as being helpful in maintaining haemodynamic stability before definitive cardiac surgical procedures are performed, such as repair of a ventricular septal defect or mitral valve replacement.

The counter pulsating balloon gives phase pulsation, synchronised with the electrocardiogram. Inflation is commenced at the time of closure of the aortic valve, and deflation prior to the onset of ventricular systole. This augments coronary perfusion pressure during early and mid diastole and increases coronary blood flow. Left ventricular ejections occur against a lower aortic impedence, leading to a 10%–20% enhancement of cardiac output with an associated reduction in left ventricular filling pressure. Associated beneficial haemodynamic changes include a reduced aortic systolic and an increased diastolic pressure, reduction in tachycardia and enhanced urinary output. The presence of uncontrolled tachycardia or arrhythmias with an irregular ventricular response are contra-indications to the use of aortic counter pulsation, as is the presence of aortic aneurysm or aortic valve regurgitation. Haemodynamic stability may be achieved and allow definitive investigation by means of left ventricular angiography and selective coronary arteriography.

Although haemodynamic improvement may be achieved, stability may be dependent on continued use of the balloon. Gradual "weaning" of the patient must be attempted by reducing the duration of the counter pulse and the ratio from 1:1 to 2:1 and gradually allowing the patient to become independent, though with continued use of maintenance pharmacological therapy.

In general, counter pulsation should only be considered when surgery is contemplated. Prolonged counter pulsation has unfortunately been disappointing in terms of recovery.

Although the prognosis of cardiogenic shock is poor, there is no reason for inactivity. Early adequate and appropriate treatment may prevent the development of an irreversibly deteriorating situation.

Cardiac Failure

The onset of cardiac failure may be a reflection of the degree of myocardial damage secondary to the coronary artery occlusion. Rarely it may be a reflection of a mechanical complication of the infarct, such as development of mitral regurgitation secondary to papillary muscle rupture or of a ventricular septal defect following rupture of the intraventricular septum. Although the early management will involve standard anti-failure measures, in these circumstances the long-term management will involve surgery, and appropriate haemodynamic investigations and angiography must be considered. Rupture of papillary muscle usually occurs in a transmural inferior infarct when the posteromedial papillary muscle has ruptured in part. The rapid onset of mitral regurgitation leads to a very marked increase in left atrial and pulmonary venous pressure and may lead to acute pulmonary oedema. Rupture of the intraventricular septum usually occurs as a single perforation; the resulting left-to-right shunt is determined by the size of the perforation.

Standard treatment of acute left ventricular failure is established as detailed in Chap. 9. If cardiac surgical facilities are not immediately available, patients should be stabilised and transfer arranged to an appropriate investigative centre.

Thrombosis and Thromboembolism

The introduction of anticoagulant drugs was followed by a wave of enthusiasm for their use in patients with acute myocardial infarction. The rationale for their use was the prevention of extension of coronary artery thrombus, to reduce infarct size or prevent reinfarction. In initial studies it was suggested that they reduce early mortality and that long-term treatment prevents late recurrence. These results have not been substantiated in further large detailed studies and there has been no apparent change in overall mortality (Goldman and Feinstein 1979).

The major indication for anticoagulants is now the prevention of thromboembolic complications, including systemic embolisation from mural thrombus and pulmonary embolism from venous thrombosis. Mural thrombus is frequently found in autopsy studies following fatal acute myocardial infarction. The incidence is 20%–60% and increases with age, large anterior infarct, congestive cardiac failure and left ventricular hypertrophy. Systemic embolisation is, however, relatively infrequent and mural thrombus may decrease in size or disappear even without anticoagulant therapy. Systemic embolisation occurs in 5% of patients with some 80% of events occurring in the cerebral circulation. Emboli may also occur to the limbs or the renal or mesenteric arteries. The use of anticoagulants has been shown to reduce significantly the incidence of systemic emboli from mural thrombus. In the Veterans' Administration Study, the endpoint was identifiable embolic episodes. All arterial emboli were reduced, including strokes (3.8% to 1%), by the use of full heparinisation followed by oral anticoagulants. The role of low dose heparin regimes has not yet been clearly defined. Full anticoagulation has been advocated for secondary prevention after clinical events representing systemic embolisation.

The frequency of deep venous thrombosis in patients with acute infarction is some 10%–35%, although few clinical episodes of pulmonary embolism result. Risk factors for development of venous thrombosis include age, congestive cardiac failure, shock, hypotension, obesity and a history of previous pulmonary embolism (Report of the Working Party on Anticoagulant Therapy in Coronary Thrombosis 1969; Anticoagulants in Acute Myocardial Infarction 1973). Both heparin and oral anticoagulants have been shown to be useful in reducing the incidence of venous thrombosis. Low dose heparin has also been applied with success. A low dose regime may have an advantage in reducing the risk of haemorrhagic complications, which occur in some 5%–10% of patients on full anticoagulation.

CLINICAL INDICATIONS FOR ANTICOAGULANTS

Some centres routinely administer anticoagulants in patients with acute myocardial infarction except in the presence of specific contraindications such as severe hypertension, extremely old age, active peptic ulceration or previous gastrointestinal bleeding and cerebrovascular disease. Such routine use of anticoagulants remains controversial. Our policy is to consider the use of anticoagulants in patients with transmural myocardial infarction during the acute phase of their illness. Heparin in moderate doses of 18 000 – 20 000 per 24 h will achieve prophylaxis for venous thrombosis and may give some cover against the development of mural thrombi. The presence of pericarditis is not an absolute contraindication to anticoagulation but close observation to exclude developing pericardial tamponade should be maintained. Full dose anticoagulation should be introduced in the presence of deep venous thrombosis, pulmonary embolism or systemic emboli. Following cerebral emboli, advantage may be gained by withholding anticoagulants for at least 2–3 days. Heparin should be given to prolong the PTT to $1\frac{1}{2}$–2 times normal control; oral anticoagulants should be introduced and should be continued for some 3 months (Genton and Turpie 1983).

References

Adgey AAJ, Geddes JS, Mulholland HC, Keegan DAJ, Pantridge JF (1968) Incidence, significance, and management of early bradyarrhythmia complicating acute myocardial infarction. Lancet II: 1097–1101

Alderman EL, Barry WH, Graham AF, Harrison DC (1972) Haemodynamic effects of morphine and pentazocine differ in cardiac patients. N Engl J Med 287: 13, 623–625

Anderson JL, Marshall HW, Bray BE (1983) A randomised trial of intracoronary streptokinase in the treatment of acute myocardial infarction. N Engl J Med 308: 1312–1318

Anticoagulants in acute myocardial infarction; results of co-operative clinical trial. (1973) JAMA 225: 724–729

Blanke H, Von Hardenberg D, Cohen M (1984) Patterns of creatine kinase release during acute myocardial infarction after non surgical reperfusion: comparison with conventional treatment and correlation with infarct size. J Am Coll Cardiol 3: 675–680

Campbell RWF, Murray A (1980) Significance of arrhythmias in the early and late phase of myocardial infarction. In: Lindgren A, Söner AB (eds) Acute and long-term management of myocardial ischaemia. Hjalmarson and Wilhelmson, Mölndal, Sweden, pp 130–136

Colling A, Dellipiani AW, Donaldson RJ, MacCormack P (1976) Teesside coronary survey: an epidemiological study of acute attacks of myocardial infarction. Br Med J II: 1169–1172

Davies MJ, Woolf N, Robertson WB (1976) Pathology of acute myocardial infarction with particular reference to occlusive coronary thrombi. Br Heart J 38: 659–664

Dellipiani AW, Colling WA, Donaldson RJ, McCormack P (1977) Teesside coronary survey: fatality and comparative severity of patients treated at home, in the hospital ward and in the coronary care unit after myocardial infarction. Br Heart J 39: 1172–1178

DeWood MA, Spores J, Notske R (1980) Prevalence of total coronary occlusion during the early hours of trasmural myocardial infarction. N Engl J Med 303: 897–902

Ganz W, Geft I, Maddahi J, Berman D, Charuzi Y, Shah PK, Swan HJ (1983) Nonsurgical reperfusion in evolving myocardial infarction. J Am Coll Cardiol I: 1247–1253

Genton MD, Turpie AGG (1983) Anticoagulant therapy following acute myocardial infarction. Part II antithrombotic therapy. Mod Conc Cardiovasc Dis 52: 10: 49–51

Goldman L, Feinstein AR (1979) Anticoagulants and myocardial infarction. Ann Intern Med 90: 92–94

Han J, Moe GK (1964) Nonuniform recovery of excitability in ventricular muscle. Circ Res 14: 44

Hill JD, Hampton JR, Mitchell JRA (1978) A randomised trial of home versus hospital management for patients with suspected myocardial infarction. Lancet I: 837

Hugenholtz PG, Rentrop P (1982) Thrombolytic therapy for acute myocardial infarction quo vadis? A review of the recent literature. Eur Heart J 2: 395–403

Jewitt DE, Maurer BJ, Hubner PJB (1970) Increased pulmonary arterial pressures after pentazocine in myocardial infarction. Br Med J I: 795–796

Kennedy JW, Ritchie JL, Davis KB, Fritz JK (1983) Western Washington Randomised Trial of intracoronary streptokinase in acute myocardial infarction. N Engl J Med 309: 1477–1482

Kotter V, Von Leatner ER, Wunderlich J, Schroder R (1977) Comparison of effects of phentolamine, sodium nitroprusside and glyceryl trinitrate in acute myocardial infarction. Br Heart J 39: 1196–1204

Leir CV, Heban PT, Huss P, Bush CA, Lewis RP (1978) Comparative systemic and regional haemodynamic effects of dopamine and dobutamine in patients with cardiomyopathic heart failure. Circulation 58: 466–475

Loeb HS, Pietras RJ, Tobin JR, Gunnar RM (1968) Hypovolaemia in shock due to acute myocardial infarction. Circulation 40: 653–659

Loeb HS, Bredakis J, Gunnar R (1977) Superiority of dobutamine over dopamine for augmentation of cardiac output in patients with chronic low output cardiac failure. Circulation 55: 375–381

Lown B, Fakhro AM, Hood WB Jr, Thorn GW (1967) The coronary care unit: new perspectives and directions. JAMA 199: 188

MacDonald HR, Rees HA, Muir AL, Lawrie DM, Burton JL, Donald KW (1967) Circulatory effects of heroin in patients with acute myocardial infarction. Lancet I: 1070–1074

Maling HM, Moran NC (1957) Ventricular arrhythmias induced by sympathomimetic amines in unanaesthetized dogs following coronary artery occlusion. Circ Res 5: 409

Maroko PR, Kjekshus JK, Sobel BE, Watanabe T, Covell JW, Ross J, Braunwald E (1971) Factors influencing infarct size following experimental coronary artery occlusion. Circulation 43: 67

Maroko PR, Radvany P, Braunwald E, Hale SL (1975) Reduction of infarct size of oxygen inhalation following acute coronary occlusion. Circulation 52: 360

Maroko PR, Hillis LD, Muller JE, Braunwald E (1977) Favorable effects of hyaluronidase on electrocardiographic evidence of necrosis in patients with acute myocardial infarction. N Engl J Med 296: 898

Maseri A, L'Abbate A, Baroldi G, Chierchia S, Marzilli M, Ballestra AM, Severi S, Parodi A, Distante A, Pesola A (1978) Coronary vasospasm as a possible cause of myocardial infarction. A conclusion derived from the study of "preinfarction" angina. N Engl J Med 299: 1271

Mather HG, Morgan DC, Pearson NG, Read KLO, Shaw DB, Steed GR, Thorne MG, Lawrence CJ, Riley IS (1976) Myocardial infarction: a comparison between home and hospital care for patients. Br Med J I: 925

Mok MS, Lippmann M, Steen SN (1981) Multidose/observational, comparative clinical analgetic evaluation of buprenorphine. J Clin Pharmacol 21: 323–329

Page DL, Caulfield JB, Kastor JA, Sanders CA (1971) Myocardial changes associated with cardiogenic shock. N Engl J Med 285: 133

Pantridge JF, Adgey AAJ (1969) Pre-hospital coronary care. The mobile coronary care unit. Am J Cardiol 24: 666

Rentrop KP, Blanke H, Karsch KR, Kreuzer H (1979) Initial experience with transluminal recanalisation of the recently occluded infarct-related coronary artery in acute myocardial infarction: comparison with conventionally treated patients. Clin Cardiol 2: 92–105

Report of the Working Party on Anticoagulant Therapy in Coronary Thrombosis to the Medical Research Council (1969) Assessment of short-term anticoagulant administration after cardiac infarction. Br Med J I: 335–342

Resnekov L (1977) Intermediate coronary care units. JAMA 237: 1697

Reynolds AK, Randall LI (1957) Morphine and allied drugs. University of Toronto Press, Toronto

Roberts WC, Buja LM (1972) The frequency and significance of coronary arterial thrombi and other observations in fatal acute myocardial infarction. Am J Med 52: 425

Rude RE, Muller JE, Braunwald E (1981) Efforts to limit the size of myocardial infarcts. Ann Intern Med 95: 736–761

Schroeder R, Biamino G, Enz-Rudiger VL (1983) Intravenous short term infusion of streptokinase in acute myocardial infarction. Circulation 67: 536–548

Scott ME, Orr R (1969) Effects of diamorphine, methadone, morphine and pentazocine in patients with suspected acute myocardial infarction. Lancet I: 1065–1067

Stampfer MJ, Goldhaber SZ, Yusuf S, Peto R, Hennekens J (1982) Effects of intravenous streptokinase on acute myocardial infarction. N Engl J Med 307: 19 1180–1182

Steen SN, Smith RL, Jeretin S (1979) Effect of i.v. buprenorphine in the human respiratory centre. I.R.C.S. Med Sci 7: 597–598

Swan HJC, Ganz W, Forrester J, Marcus H, Diamond G, Chonetti D (1970) Catheterisation of the heart in man with the use of a flow-directed balloon-tipped catheter. N Engl J Med 283: 447–451

Thomas M, Malcrona R, Fillmore S, Shillingford J (1965) Haemodynamic effects of morphine in patients with acute myocardial infarction. Br Heart J 27: 863–875

Valori C, Thomas M, Shillingford J (1969) Free noradrenaline and adrenaline excretion in relation to clinical syndromes following myocardial infarction. Am J Cardiol 20: 605–617

Zelis R, Mansour EJ, Capone RJ, Mason DT (1974) The cardiovascular effects of morphine. J Clin Invest 54: 1247–1258

Zola EM, McLeod DC (1983) Comparative effects and analgesic efficacy of the agonist–antagonist opioids. Drug Intell Clin Pharm 17: 411–417

6 Secondary Prevention Following Acute Myocardial Infarction

It is recognised that over 50% of deaths following acute myocardial infarction occur within 1 h as the result of the onset of electrical instability and the development of ventricular fibrillation. This observation has led to the development of community health care systems and the concept of coronary care units. There remains, however, an in-hospital mortality of some 12%–18% and a variable long-term mortality related to the extent of myocardial damage and severity of coronary artery atheroma. The prognosis following acute myocardial infarction may be influenced by:

1. Continued development of obstructive coronary artery disease with atheroma, spasm and platelet aggregation, with associated thrombosis leading to further acute myocardial infarction
2. Ventricular arrhythmias predisposing to sudden death
3. Cardiac failure secondary to major myocardial damage

Many secondary prevention trials have been performed in an attempt to reduce both the short- and long-term mortality. Extensive reviews have recently been published regarding both short-term acute phase and long-term trials (May et al. 1982, 1983). The general classes of therapeutic interventions are shown in Table 6.1. Some drugs may have more than one action and overlap may occur.

Secondary prevention therapy has been aimed at:

1. Prophylaxis of ventricular fibrillation
2. Reduction of myocardial damage
3. Slowing the progression and complications of coronary atheroma and prevention of coronary thrombosis

Secondary Prevention Trial Design

As secondary prevention trials have been developed, several general problems related to patient selection and trial design have been identified. Recent

Table 6.1. Secondary intervention following myocardial infarction

	Acute interventions	Chronic interventions
1. Anti-arrhythmics	Quinidine Lignocaine Procainamide Disopyramide β-blockers Glucose Insulin Potassium	Phenytoin Tocainide Mexilitene
2. Reduced progression of coronary atheroma		Diet Lipid-lowering drugs Cigarette cessation Bypass surgery Blood pressure reduction
3. Treatment of coronary thrombus	Thrombolytic agents Anticoagulants	Anticoagulants Platelet-active drugs β-blockers Exercise
4. Limitation of myocardial infarct size	a) By reducing oxygen requirements (β-blocking compounds) b) Increased myocardial blood flow Anticoagulants Platelet-active agents Fibrinolytics Hyaluronidase c) Enhanced anaerobic metabolism Glucose Insulin Potassium d) Reduced autolysis Corticosteroids	

interest has been focused on the use of β-adrenoreceptor blocking compounds in the treatment of survivors of acute myocardial infarction. Several extensive critical reviews have been written dwelling on the development of trial design and resulting interpretation of results (Hampton 1982; Shand 1982; Chamberlain 1983; Frishman et al. 1984). These reviews have promoted discussion, and several methods of presentation have been developed to allow comparison of results; these now provide a model to study the results of other secondary prevention trials.

It is worthwhile examining the particular problems faced when using β-blockers following myocardial infarction, as they can be borne in mind when setting up other secondary prevention studies.

1. The end-points in any specific trial may be difficult to define if limited to symptomatic relief or patient well-being. In general terms the end-point studied has been overall mortality, sudden cardiac death or further myocardial

infarction. Problems may remain in defining the mode of death in long-term out-of-hospital studies as many sudden deaths may occur in the presence of a further myocardial infarction.

2. The widespread use of β-blockers in the community for the treatment of hypertension and angina pectoris means that a significant proportion of patients admitted with acute myocardial infarction are excluded from a trial of β-blockers and the resulting trial results may not be applicable to the general population with coronary heart disease.

3. In the early hours following myocardial infarction, sympathetic or para-sympathetic imbalance may predominate. Considerable heart rate and blood pressure variation may occur, and a low percentage input of the total patient population may result.

4. If patients are treated in the early stages of myocardial infarction the control group mortality may be high. If major benefit results from a therapeutic intervention, then studies with relatively smaller numbers of patients may be adequate. As the mechanism of sudden death and reinfarction is ill-understood, the precise mode of action of any therapeutic intervention may be difficult to determine although it may be suggested by experimental observations. The scale of mortality reduction which might be achieved is accordingly difficult to predict, as are the numbers of a patient population to be studied.

5. After recovery from an acute myocardial infarction, the subsequent annual mortality is low and large patient numbers are necessary for study. Multicentre trials are therefore required to recruit adequate subjects. This may lead to logistic problems of uniformity of patient selection. Each centre should enlist an equivalent number and the total patient population must be known. If only a small proportion of the total population is entered, the results from the study may not be widely applicable.

6. Stratification or subdivision into subsets of patients according to age, sex, site of infarct or clinical examination prior to randomisation has been used to prove comparability of the control and intervention groups. This may be helpful in identifying particular groups who benefited by the therapeutic intervention and in addition may help to establish the potential mechanism of action. Subsetting the study population may increase the possibility that a positive result will arise by chance, and the application of conventional methods of statistical analysis may be inappropriate. Retrospective subsetting of the patient population should not be carried out.

7. When active drugs are used in large population studies, significant numbers of patients may be withdrawn following the development of side-effects. The subsequent analysis of such patients becomes difficult. The results should be analysed according to the original allocation on an "intention to treat" or pragmatic approach. Analysis of the results in patients who actually remain in the treatment or placebo group throughout may also be useful (explicative analysis). This is particularly so in trials of long duration, when many deaths may occur after the patients have been withdrawn from treatment.

Several studies have been reported which go a long way towards satisfying the early criticisms and which fulfil several important admission criteria, including (a) large enough numbers, with more than 20 deaths in the control group, (b) taking into account of additional risk factors, (c) acceptable randomisation procedures and (d) analysis on an "intention to treat" basis with withdrawal rates minimised. The methods of presentation are demonstrated in Figs. 6.1–6.3. The first method (Fig. 6.1) allows trials to be compared easily (Hampton 1982).

The results of the trials may also be usefully and conveniently compared using the method suggested by Baber and Lewis (1980) (Fig. 6.2). They divided the trials into early and late intervention groups with an arbitrary cut-off point of 72 h. The central line separates beneficial effects (on the right) and negative effects (on the left). The small vertical line within each study block shows the mean effect obtained within each trial. The width of the base indicates 95%

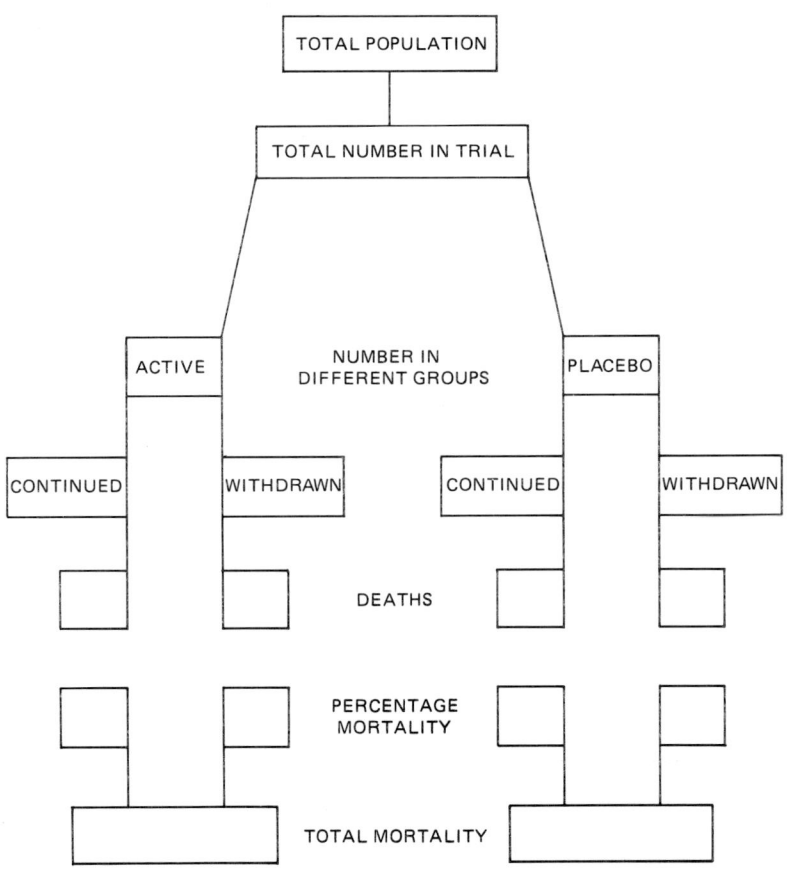

Fig. 6.1. Hampton's method of presenting trial results.

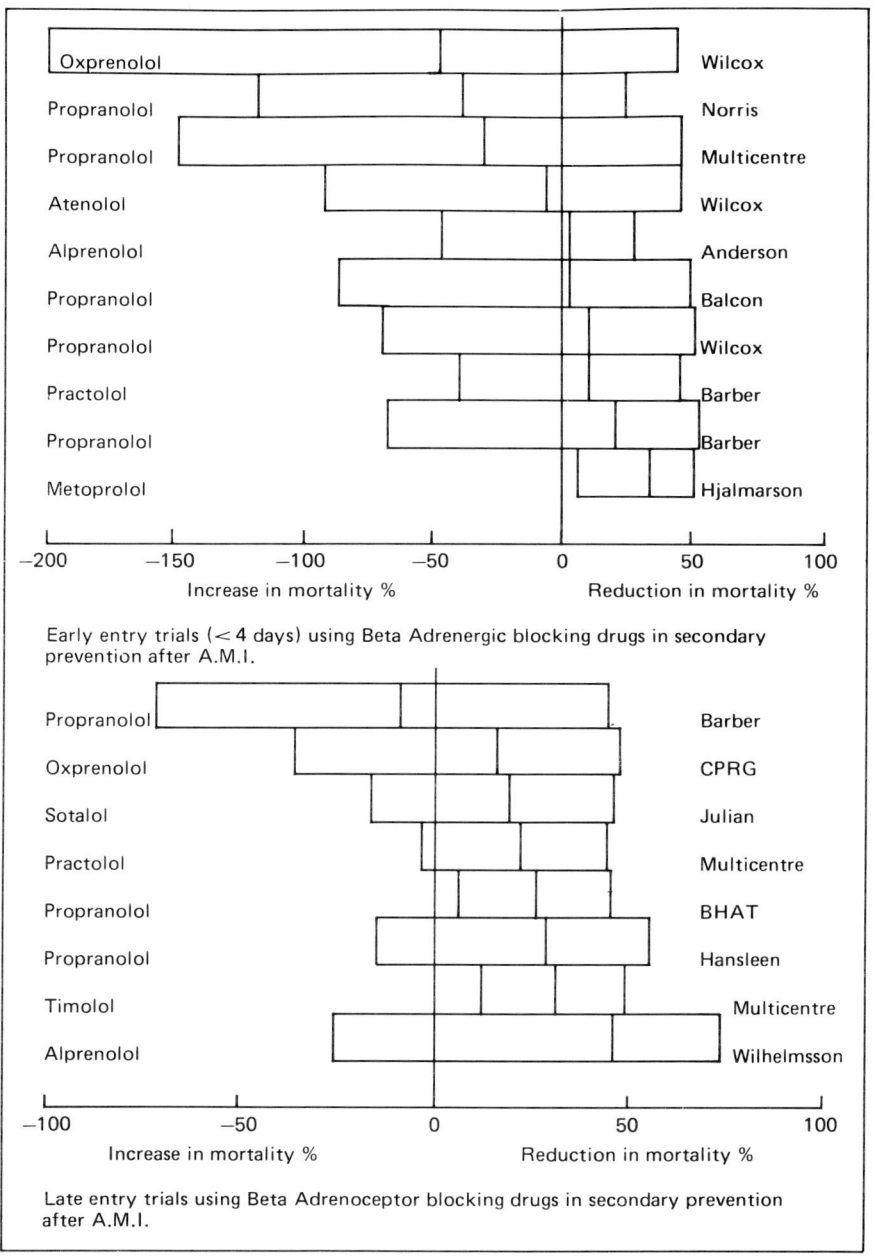

Early entry trials (< 4 days) using Beta Adrenergic blocking drugs in secondary prevention after A.M.I.

Late entry trials using Beta Adrenoceptor blocking drugs in secondary prevention after A.M.I.

Fig. 6.2. Baber and Lewis's method of presenting trial results.

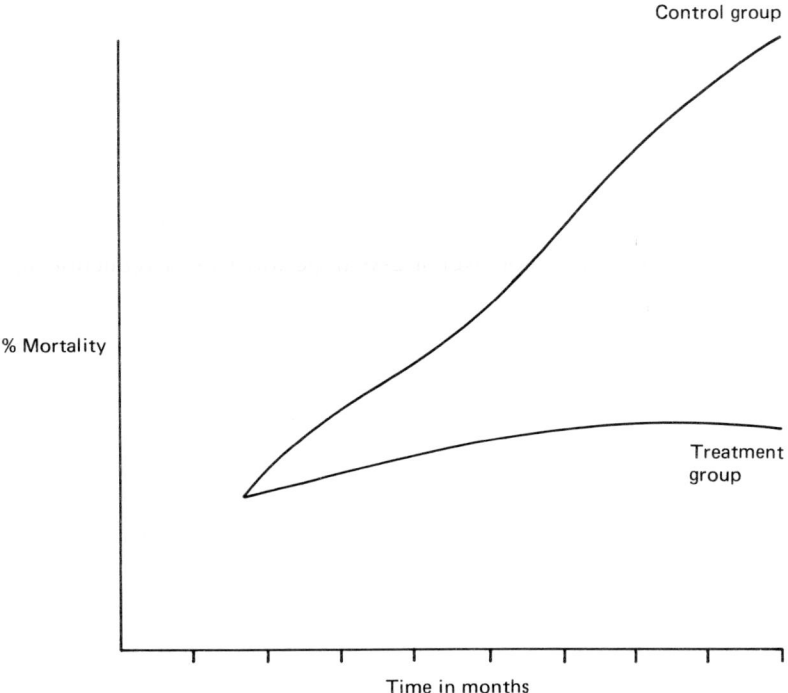

Fig. 6.3. A third possible method of presenting trial results.

confidence limits. Only trial results lying wholly on one side of the division have achieved conventional levels of significance, but a favourable trend may be reflected by the mean value.

The third method of display (Fig. 6.3) allows comparison of the mortality between active and control groups with time and gives evidence of serial observation. Divergent lines suggest differences, and statistical comparison can be made at different times. The duration of the beneficial effects may also be determined (Beta Blocker Heart Attack Research Group 1982).

Clinical Studies

β-Blockers

β-Adrenoceptor blocking compounds have had widespread use in the treatment of angina pectoris, arrhythmias and hypertension. Snow in 1965 first suggested that propranolol might reduce the mortality in patients with acute myocardial infarction. This study was not randomised nor double-blind. It raised the attractive possibility that by reducing sympathetic drive in the early phase of myocardial infarction, clinical benefit might accrue; however, several other studies were performed with negative results when using propranolol in a dose of 30–160 mg daily. These studies may have been flawed by the use of an inadequate dose, continued for an inadequate time. Several groups reported positive studies with other agents. Wilhelmsson et al. (1974) and Ahlmark et al. (1974) reported using alprenolol over a 2-year period with a reduction in mortality. Anderson et al. (1979) also suggested benefit by subsetting patients by age, showing advantage in patients younger than 65 years. A multicentre practolol trial (Multicentre International Study 1975) also showed benefit over placebo in patients with anterior myocardial infarction. Criticisms have been levelled at relatively small numbers of patients included in the alprenolol studies, and further analysis of the practolol study on an "intention to treat" basis has refuted the initial conclusions.

Recent studies have suggested that the introduction of β-blockade given parenterally in the early phase of acute myocardial infarction may reduce mortality (Hjalmarson et al. 1981) or myocardial infarct size (Yusef et al. 1980). Care must be taken during this phase, particularly in the presence of haemodynamic instability, and these agents are obviously contraindicated in patients with cardiac failure, bradycardia, hypotension or peripheral vascular disease.

Further studies have reported a reduction in mortality following the introduction of β-blocking compounds 1–3 weeks after the onset of symptoms. These studies, using both propranolol (BHAT 1981; Hansteen et al. 1982) and timolol (The Norwegian Multicentre Study Group 1981), have shown a significant reduction in mortality. It appears that these compounds have an increased role to play in long-term secondary prevention. Nevertheless, problems still remain concerning the best time of introduction of therapy, the duration of therapy and the particular agent to be used. Beneficial results have been obtained with β-adrenoceptor blocking compounds with different ancillary pharmacological properties. Metoprolol and atenolol are cardioselective. Propranolol, timolol and sotalol are non-selective. Propranolol has membrane-stabilising properties which none of the other compounds have, and alprenolol has intrinsic sympathomimetic activity. Most evidence suggests that sudden cardiac death and non-fatal myocardial reinfarction are reduced following β-blockade. It is difficult to ascribe the reduction in both these clinical events to a single mechanism.

β-Adrenergic blocking compounds are useful in patients with arrhythmias with associated high sympathetic drive; however, little effect has been demonstrated on non-fatal ventricular arrhythmias in the early weeks following acute myocardial infarction (Roland et al. 1979). Administration of β-blocking compounds has also been shown to increase the threshold for induction of ventricular fibrillation in experimental myocardial infarction (Verrier et al. 1974) and to suppress clinically overt ventricular arrhythmias (Lemberg et al. 1970).

β-Blockers have an influence on regional myocardial blood flow. Subendocardial myocardial blood flow may be enhanced during experimental acute myocardial infarction following β-blockade. Similar long-term effects may lessen arrhythmic events. Long-term metabolic effects may also occur, with enhancement of nutrient supply for metabolic requirements (Mueller et al. 1974), and altered lipolysis by non-selective β-blockade may also modify myocardial metabolism (Newman 1977). Additional potential beneficial properties of individual β-blockers include reduction in platelet aggregation and effects on thromboxane synthesis (Weksler et al. 1977; Campbell et al. 1981). The overall mechanism remains uncertain.

Anti-arrhythmic Drugs

Continuous monitoring in the early stage of myocardial infarction has identified a high incidence of ventricular arrhythmias. Treatment has been introduced either before the onset of ventricular arrhythmias using a prophylactic regime or alternatively when arrhythmias have developed. In addition to mortality, the incidence of ventricular arrhythmias has usually been monitored as a marker of electrical instability.

Quinidine

Quinidine, a standard class I anti-arrhythmic, is orally active and is effective in treating both atrial and ventricular arrhythmias (Chap. 8). Two double-blind studies have been performed using quinidine and are detailed in Table 6.2. These were started within 24 h of admission to hospital and mortality was reviewed within the first 2 weeks. Although the incidence of ventricular arrhythmias was reduced in the quinidine group, there was no difference in mortality between the treated and control groups.

Procainamide

Procainamide can be given both parenterally and orally. It has class I anti-arrhythmic activity and is effective in both atrial and ventricular arrhythmias. Slow release preparations are now available (Chap. 8). In the open study of Reynell (1961) there was no reduction in ventricular arrhythmias nor was there any difference in mortality (Table 6.2). Koch-Weser et al. (1969) showed a reduction in ventricular arrhythmias, but again there was no difference in mortality between the two groups. In these two studies varying dosage schedules were used.

Disopyramide (Chap. 8)

Although an early report suggested that disopyramide was effective in preventing arrhythmias in patients following acute myocardial infarction (Zainal et al. 1977), criticism was levelled regarding the control group mortality and conclusions drawn. Three further studies examined the mortality following the introduction of disopyramide within 48 h of myocardial infarction with a follow-up period of up to 6 weeks. Jennings et al. (1980) reported that twice as many patients in the placebo group required other anti-arrhythmic therapy as compared with the active intervention group. At the time of hospital discharge, five patients in the placebo group and two in the intervention group had died. This reduction in mortality was not statistically significant.

Lignocaine

Lignocaine, a standard class I anti-arrhythmic agent, is used during the coronary care phase of treatment of acute myocardial infarction (Chap. 8). The clinical studies performed using lignocaine are summarised in Table 6.2. The loading dose administered and infusion rates used in these studies have varied. The success in suppressing ventricular arrhythmias in general reflects the infusion rates and resulting plasma levels. High infusion rates are most effective. Primary ventricular fibrillation was suppressed when infusions of 2.5 mg/min or greater were used. The resulting high plasma levels were associated with unwarranted effects in up to 15% of patients. Overall the total mortality has been uninfluenced by lignocaine.

Lignocaine has also been assessed in the prehospital phase of coronary care in two studies in which the drug was administered by the intramuscular route by primary care physicians. When analysed according to the "intention to treat" principle, neither study showed a significant reduction in mortality. In the study of Lie et al. (1974) it was demonstrated that unsatisfactory plasma levels of lignocaine were achieved using this route. This may have been a reflection of the poor haemodynamic status and absorption from the intramuscular site of injection. A high intramuscular dose has therefore been advocated.

Others

Six controlled studies have been performed using other anti-arrhythmics in an attempt to reduce mortality on a long-term basis. Table 6.2 shows the agents used, the trial designs and the results. Chamberlain et al. (1980) selected a high-risk group of patients on the basis of clinical and electrocardiographic findings and the Ghent/Rotterdam (Van Durme et al. 1977) group were selected on the basis of the presence of ventricular arrhythmias. The other studies have recruited low-risk subject groups using anti-arrhythmic therapy on a prophylactic basis. Arrhythmia suppression as measured by 24-h ECG tape monitoring and mortality have been evaluated.

Four of the studies suggested that the anti-arrhythmic agents used might be detrimental, whereas in the Ghent/Rotterdam study, in which the patients selected had arrhythmias, the trend favoured the intervention therapy. Side-effects were fairly common, particularly involving the central nervous system, and caused 25% of patients to be withdrawn from the phenytoin study reported by Peter et al. (1979).

Table 6.2. Secondary prevention after acute myocardial infarction by means of anti-arrhythmic drugs (after Mav et al. 1982, 1983)

Trial	Time of entry	Intervention(s)	Length of follow-up	Control			Intervention		
				No. random-ised	No. of deaths	Per cent mortality	No. random-ised	No. of deaths	Per cent mortality
Quinidine									
Holmberg and Bergman (1967)	<24 h	Quinidine p.o. 1200 mg/day	14 days	55	4	7.3	49	9	18.4
Jones et al. (1974)	<24 h	Quinidine p.o. 1200 mg/day for 3 days	14 days	58	6	10.3	45	4	8.9
Procainamide									
Reynell (1961)	<96 h	Procainamide 2–4 g/day for 2–3 wk	Hospital discharge	55	5	9.1	51	5	9.8
Koch-Weser et al. (1969)	<72 h	Procainamide 1 g stat. + 2–4 g/day	7 days	33	3	9.1	37	3	8.1
Disopyramide									
Jennings et al. (1976)	<48 h	Disopyramide 100 mg stat. + 400 mg/day for time in CCU	Hospital discharge	49	5	10.2	46	2	4.0
Nicholls et al. (1980)	<24 h	Disopyramide 100 mg i.v. stat. + 400 mg/day p.o.	Hospital discharge	99	12	12.1	100	10	10.0
Wilcox et al. (1980)	<24 h	Disopyramide 450 mg/day	42 days	158	10	6.3	158	14	8.9
Lignocaine									
Bennett et al. (1970)	<48 h	Lignocaine 50 mg i.v. stat. + 0.5–1.0 mg/min for 48 h	Hospital discharge	125	8	6.4	249	25	10.0
Pitt et al. (1971)	<24 h	Lignocaine 75–100 mg i.v. stat. + 2.5 mg/min for 48 h	Hospital discharge	114	16	14.0	108	9	8.3

SECONDARY PREVENTION FOLLOWING ACUTE MYOCARDIAL INFARCTION

Table 6.2. (cont.)

Darby et al. (1972)	<48 h	Lignocaine 200 mg i.m. stat. + 2 mg/min i.v. for 48 h	Hospital discharge	100	11	11.0	103	12	11.7
O'Brien et al. (1973)	On hospital adm.	Lignocaine 75 mg i.v. stat. + 2.5 mg/min for 48 h	2 days	146	4	2.7	154	11	7.1
Lie et al. (1974)	<6 h	Lignocaine 100 mg i.v. stat. + 3 mg/min for 48 h	CCU discharge	105	10	9.5	107	8	7.5
Valentine et al. (1974)	<12 h	Lignocaine 300 mg i.m. stat.	30 days	157	18	11.5	207	26	12.6
Lie et al. (1978)	<6 h	Lignocaine 300 mg i.m. stat.	Hospital discharge	153	6	3.9	157	5	3.2
Others									
Collaborative Group Australia/Britain (1971)	At hospital discharge	Phenytoin (300–400 mg/day)	12 mo	285	23	8.1	283	26	9.2
Peter et al. (1978)	Before CCU discharge	Phenytoin (variable to maintain serum levels of 40–80 mol/litre)	24 mo	76	14	18.4	74	18	24.3
Ryden et al. (1980)	<2 days	Tocainide (750 mg i.v. stat. + 1200 mg/day)	6 mo	56	5	8.9	56	5	8.9
Bastian et al. (1980)	7–10 days	Tocainide (1200 mg/day)	6 mo	74	3	4.1	72	4	5.6
Chamberlain et al. (1980)	6–14 days	Mexiletine (600–750 mg/day)	4 mo 3 mo intervention	163	19	11.7	181	24	13.3
Ghent–Rotterdam Study (to be published)	<14 days	Aprindine (100–200 mg/day)	12 mo	152	19	12.5	153	12	7.8

Those studies using 24-h tape monitoring showed that the drugs tested reduced the incidence of ventricular arrhythmias but did not affect the total mortality.

Anticoagulant Drugs

Following observation of a high incidence of occluding coronary arterial thrombus in patients dying from acute myocardial infarction, trials of anti-coagulant therapy were performed on both a short- and a long-term basis. The early studies had many problems related to trial design and conduct, with inadequate controls, small sample size and open design.

The rationale for the use of anticoagulants in the acute phase of myocardial infarction was:

1. To prevent extension of occluding thrombus in the affected coronary vessel
2. To reduce the risk of systemic arterial embolism from left ventricular mural thrombus and pulmonary embolism from deep venous thrombosis

It was also suggested that the long-term use of anticoagulants prevents subsequent coronary thrombosis and reinfarction.

Four short-term trials were conducted using anticoagulants following acute myocardial infarction (Table 6.3). The numbers of patients randomised, the time of entry and the duration of follow-up are shown. The active therapy was either continuous heparin or initial heparin followed by either phenindione or warfarin. Two of the studies were placebo controlled. The Medical Research Council control group were given low dose phenindione (Second Report of the Working Party on Anticoagulant Therapy in Coronary Thrombosis 1964).

The studies of Drapkin and Merskey (1972) showed a statistically significant reduction in overall mortality between the intervention and control groups. This benefit was confined, however, to females, who made up only one-third of the study population. It should be noted that the control group mortality in females (31%) was much higher than that in males (16.4%). These positive results were not confirmed in the other studies. The trials in general failed to demonstrate that anticoagulants reduce mortality, although there was a reduction in systemic and pulmonary thromboembolic events.

Five long-term studies continued intervention after hospital discharge. Again they are summarised in Table 6.2. There were variable times of randomisation, durations and follow-ups. The active intervention was either coumarin or phenindione derivatives prescribed either alone or following initial heparinisation. Dosage was adjusted to maintain "effective" anti-coagulation. Varying standards of control were used and the adequacy of control is doubtful in some of the studies. None of the studies found a statistically significant difference in mortality between the intervention and control groups. Although The Sixty Plus Reinfarction Study Research Group (1980) reported a significant reduction in mortality, when the figures are analysed on

Table 6.3. Secondary prevention after acute myocardial infarction by means of anticoagulant drugs (after May et al. 1982, 1983)

Trial	Time of entry	Intervention(s)	Length of follow-up	Control			Intervention		
				No. random-ised	No. of deaths	Per cent mortality	No. random-ised	No. of deaths	Percent mortality
Carleton et al. (1960)	< 48 h	i.v. heparin	29 days	65	13	20.0	60	18	30.0
Medical Research Council Short-Term (1969)	< 14 days	Phenindione	28 days	715	129	18.0	712	115	16.2
Drapkin and Merskey (1972)	< 24 h	Phenindione	21 days approx.	452	88	19.5	822	111	13.5
Veterans' Administration Cooperative (1973)	< 72 h	Warfarin	28 days	513	58	11.3	513	49	9.6
Medical Research Council Long-Term (1959, 1965)	29–43 days	Phenindione	25 mo	188	40	21.3	195	29	14.9
Wasserman et al. (1966)	< 7 days	Warfarin	< 36 mo	70	15	21.4	77	12	15.6
Seaman et al. (1969)	2–80 mo	Phenindione	72 mo (6-wk inter-vention)	87 81	31 33	35.6 40.7	88	36	40.9
German–Austrian Multicenter Prospective Clinical Trial (Breddin 1977; Breddin et al. 1979)	28–42 days	Phenprocoumon	24 mo	309	22	7.1	320	26	8.1
The Sixty Plus Reinfarction Study (1980)	6 mo – 6+ yr	Acenocoumarin/phenprocoumon	24 mo	456	70	15.4	456	53	11.6

the "intention to treat" principle, the reduction in mortality unfortunately is no longer statistically significant.

Three of the five studies showed a trend in favour of the anticoagulant group. There was a highly significant reduction in the incidence of recurrent myocardial infarction at 2 years in the Sixty Plus Reinfarction Trial. A similar reduction was shown in the Medical Research Council trial, although it appeared to be restricted to men (Report of Working Party on Anticoagulant Therapy in Coronary Thrombosis 1969). In these long-term trials thromboembolic incidents were reduced. Haemorrhagic complications, however, were more frequent in the group given anticoagulants.

When the results of all reported randomised controlled trials are pooled, there is an overall reduction of some 21% in mortality. This suggests that the small sample size in individual studies was inadequate to detect such a reduction in fatality rate. A further two prospective surveys also suggested a large difference in mortality favouring anticoagulant-treated groups (Chalmers et al. 1977; Modan et al. 1975). Their control groups, however, were not recruited by generally accepted methods.

From these studies it appears that although thromboembolism may be reduced, the case for long-term anticoagulants following acute myocardial infarction is not fully proved. Further studies using more stringent trial design are indicated.

Platelet-Active Drugs

Pathological studies suggest that platelets play a major role in the initiation of thrombus formation in atherosclerotic arteries and may play a role in atherogenesis. A decreased platelet survival time has been shown in some two-thirds of patients with coronary artery disease (Steele et al. 1978). In addition, increased platelet aggregation has been demonstrated in patients with angina and abnormal exercise tests (Frishman et al. 1974). Acetylsalicylic acid (aspirin) has been shown to have a potent inhibitory effect on platelet adhesion and aggregation. Other drugs with anti-platelet properties include dipyridamole and sulfinpyrazone. In addition clofibrate has been shown to increase platelet survival time.

Two short-term trials of platelet-active drugs have been reported and are summarised in Table 6.4. In neither of the two trials was benefit conferred with regard to survival.

Aspirin

Seven long-term studies have been reported and are summarised in Table 6.4. It can be seen that the dose of aspirin used in these studies varied greatly, involving subgroups on relatively low doses and others on conventional regimes. None of the seven studies demonstrated a statistically significant difference between the intervention and control groups in terms of total

Table 6.4. Secondary prevention after acute myocardial infarction by means of platelet-active drugs (after May et al. 1982, 1983)

Trial	Time of entry	Intervention(s)	Length of follow-up	Control			Intervention		
				No. random-ised	No. of deaths	Per cent mortality	No. random-ised	No. of deaths	Per cent mortality
Gent et al. (1968)	< 14 days	Dipyridamole (400 mg/day)	28 days	52	3	5.8	51	8	15.7
Elwood and Williams (1979)	h–days	Aspirin (300 mg stat)	28 days	1281	172	13.4	1249	159	12.7
Elwood et al. (1974)	< 6 mo	Aspirin (300 mg/day)	12 mo	624	61	9.8 (18.5)	615	47	7.6 (12.2)
Coronary Drug Project Aspirin Study (CDPA) (1976)	wk–yr	Aspirin (972 mg/day)	22 mo	771	64	8.3	758	44	5.8
German–Austrian Multicenter Prospective Clinical Trial (Breddin 1977, Breddin et al. 1979)	28–42 days	Aspirin (1500 mg/day)	24 mo	309	22	7.1	317	13	4.1
Elwood and Sweetnam (1979)	Days–wk	Aspirin (900 mg/day)	12 mo	878	127	14.5	847	103	12.2
Aspirin Myocardial Infarction Study (AMIS) (1980)	2–60 mo	Aspirin (1000 mg/day)	40 mo	2257	219	9.7	2267	246	10.8
Persantin Aspirin Reinfarction Study (PARIS) (1980)	2–60 mo	Aspirin (972 mg/day)	41 mo	406	52	12.8	810	85	10.5
		Aspirin (972 mg/day) + dipyridamole (225 mg/day)					810	87	10.7
The Anturan Reinfarction Trial (ART) (1978); Boelaert (1980)	25–35 days	Sulfinpyrazone (800 mg/day)	16 mo	816	89	10.9	813	74	9.1

mortality. However, in all of the studies a trend was reported in favour of the active intervention.

Platelet-suppressing drugs also affect prostaglandin synthesis and through this mechanism may affect the balance of vasoactivity and platelet aggregation in local circulations. Thromboxane A_2 produced by platelets stimulates platelet aggregation and is a potent vasoconstrictor. It has been postulated that endothelial damage in the coronary circulation may release thromboxane A_2. This leads to increased coronary artery tone, may induce spasm and promotes further platelet aggregation. Vascular endothelium produces prostacyclin (PGI_2), which inhibits platelet aggregation and is a potent vasodilator. The ideal prostaglandin synthetase inhibitor for use in the therapy of ischaemic heart disease would be one which reduces thromboxane A_2 production but which maintains prostacyclin output. In this regard observations concerning the action of aspirin have been directed towards both the dose and the dosing interval used. It has been suggested that very low doses of aspirin, i.e. half an aspirin tablet or even less daily, may selectively block thromboxane synthesis without affecting prostacyclin production (Burch et al. 1978). More recent studies, however, have suggested that both cyclo-oxygenase systems are affected equally, but that regeneration may occur within 36 h by endothelial cells whereas platelets are incapable of such enzyme regeneration. It may be that by extending the intervals between dosing, thromboxane A_2 may be inhibited without affecting prostacyclin production. The negative results obtained in previous clinical studies may be a reflection of the dosage used, with the resultant mixed action of aspirin.

Sulfinpyrazone (Anturan)

Sulfinpyrazone was introduced as a uricosuric agent in 1959. It has several actions on platelet function that appear to be due to reversible competitive inhibition of prostaglandin synthesis, which leads to an increased platelet survival time in patients with coronary artery disease (Steele et al. 1978). It also inhibits platelet adhesion and aggregation, while experimental evidence has suggested that it inhibits re-entry ventricular arrhythmias arising from acutely ischaemic myocardium. In addition it may reduce coronary vascular tone and enhance collateral flow to marginal zones of infarcted myocardium. In experimental models pretreatment with sulfinpyrazone has reduced the incidence of ventricular fibrillation (Moschos et al. 1982). Unfortunately, this anti-arrhythmic potential has not been shown following acute myocardial infarction in man.

The Anturan Reinfarction Trial Research Group (1978) showed results that apparently demonstrated a significant reduction in cardiac mortality in the early stages following acute myocardial infarction. A major benefit was noted between the 2nd and 7th month. The reduction in the incidence of sudden death continued through to 24 months, with 43% fewer cases in the active treatment group. By 24 months, however, the total mortality showed no significant difference. Unfortunately there appear to have been major problems with this study. On the basis of "intention to treat" analysis there was no significant difference in mortality. Further criticisms have been levelled at the definitions used in regard to both analysable deaths and sudden death. In addition, there was a higher pre-entry incidence of arrhythmias in the control than in the active intervention group. A further Italian study (Anturan Reinfarction, Italian Study 1982) using sulfinpyrazone showed a reduction in nonfatal myocardial infarctions, but there was no difference in the total mortality or in sudden deaths between the groups.

Dipyridamole

Dipyridamole acts as a phosphodiesterase inhibitor and by this mechanism raises the intracellular concentration of cyclic AMP. This enhanced level of cyclic AMP prevents platelet aggregation and tends to favour vasodilation. In addition the vessel wall is more sensitive to the vasodilating activities of adenosine (Kalsner 1975). Dipyridamole also potentiates the effects of prostacyclin and again this increases cyclic AMP with associated stimulation of adenyl cyclase (Moncada and Korbut 1978). In in vitro studies it appears that dipyridamole and aspirin have different and additive mechanisms as far as platelet function is concerned, and this led to their combined use in the "Paris" study (The Persantin–Aspirin Reinfarction Study Research Group 1980). In this study the results showed a trend in favour of both aspirin and combined aspirin and Persantin groups, although the total mortality was not significantly reduced.

Physical Exercise

The influence of physical exercise training has been studied in both North America and in Europe. The studies are detailed in Table 6.5. Supervised submaximal exercise training sessions were designed. Each programme was determined by performance during a baseline exercise test or by age-predicted pulse rate responses. Additional home exercise periods were undertaken in the study by Palatsi (1976) and the National Exercise and Heart Disease Project (Naughton 1979). In the study by Kallio et al. (1979) emphasis was placed not only on exercise but also on modification of other risk factors.

In general the studies were accompanied by poor compliance, with 40%–60% of subjects discontinuing the training schedule. An additional group of patients were withdrawn for medical reasons. The results show a trend towards reduction in mortality, although statistical significance was not reached, probably because of the small number of patients.

Risk Factor Modification

Lipid-Lowering Agents

There has been a long recognised association between hyperlipoproteinaemia and the risk of development of coronary heart disease, though it is less certain

Table 6.5. Secondary prevention after acute myocardial infarction by means of physical exercise (after May et al. 1982, 1983)

Trial	Time of entry	Intervention(s)	Length of follow-up	Control			Intervention		
				No. randomised	No. of deaths	Per cent mortality	No. randomised	No. of deaths	Per cent mortality
Sanne et al. (1973)	3 mo	Individualised supervised training 3×/wk	48 mo	157	35	22.3	158	28	17.7
Kentala (1972)	6–8 wk	Individualised supervised training 2–3×/wk	12 mo	146 (81)	32 (8)	21.9 (9.9)	152 (77)	26 (5)	17.1 (6.5)
Palatsi (1976)	2.5 mo	Daily home exercise	29 mo (12 mo intervention)	200	28	14.0	180	18	10.0
Kallio et al. (1979)	On hospital	Physical exercise and health education	36 mo	187	56	29.9	188	41	21.8
National Exercise and Heart Disease Project (NEHDP) (Naughton 1979)	2–12 mo	Individualised supervised training 3×/wk	30–54 mo	328	24	7.3	323	15	4.6
Southern Ontario Multicenter Exercise Heart Trial (to be published)	< 12 mo	Individualised partially supervised training 2–4×/wk	48 mo	354	26	7.3	379	36	9.5

whether hyperlipidaemia remains a risk factor for myocardial reinfarction in patients surviving their first attack (The Coronary Drug Project Research Group 1976). Several controlled trials have assessed the effect of either lipid-lowering agents or diet on morbidity and mortality in patients with established coronary heart disease. The details of these trials are shown in Table 6.6. It can be seen that the Coronary Drug Project was by far the largest study group. Several drug regimes have been developed using agents either singly or in combination. The times of entry and duration of follow-up varied greatly.

Oestrogen Therapy.   In general the trials using oestrogen therapy have been associated with problems of compliance caused by the development of side-effects including breast tenderness, gynaecomastia and decreased libido. Adverse cardiovascular events resulted in the termination of the oestrogen regimes in the Coronary Drug Project. An excess of non-fatal myocardial infarction, pulmonary embolism and thrombophlebitis was recorded in the 5-mg oestrogen group, and there was also a trend towards an excess total mortality as well as venous thrombosis and possible malignant disease in the group taking 2.5 mg daily. Stamler et al. (1963) reported a beneficial effect from low-dose therapy, although the overall group mortality was not reduced.

Dextrothyroxine.   The effect of this drug in long-term usage was assessed as part of the Coronary Drug Project and also in the Veterans' Administration Drug Lipid Cooperative study. In neither study was mortality reduced, and indeed in the Coronary Drug Project, where a high dose (0.6 mg/day) was used, there was a trend towards a higher mortality not only in the subset of patients with a high incidence of ventricular extrasystoles recorded on routine electrocardiograms but also in those with no apparent ectopic activity. This portion of the study was terminated at an earlier stage than had been intended.

Clofibrate.   Clofibrate has been widely used to treat hyperlipoproteinaemia and has been assessed in secondary prevention studies following acute myocardial infarction. The Coronary Drug Project showed that the results in total mortality in the treated and non-treated groups were identical, and no beneficial subgroups were identified on clinical grounds. There appeared to be a trend towards a reduction in coronary deaths and definite non-fatal myocardial infarction; however, this was not significant. There was a higher incidence of morbidity in the active intervention group, including angina pectoris, intermittent claudication and arrhythmias. In addition, gallstone development was twice as common among patients in the clofibrate treatment group. No significant difference was noted in cardiac mortality in the Newcastle study (Five-year study. . . 1971) when looking at the subset of patients who had sustained a previous myocardial infection, although there was a trend towards a reduction in the intervention group. In the overall patient group, including patients with coronary heart disease but no previous myocardial infarction, a statistically significant reduction in mortality was reported. It has been suggested, however, that these figures should be adjusted using continuity correction for small number studies, and that with such an adjustment statistical significance is lost

Table 6.6. Secondary prevention after acute myocardial infarction by means of lipid-lowering agents or diet (after May et al. 1982, 1983)

Trial	Time of entry	Intervention(s)	Length of follow-up	Control			Intervention		
				No. random-ised	No. of deaths	Per cent mortality	No. random-ised	No. of deaths	Per cent mortality
Oliver and Boyd (1961)	3–4 mo	Oestradiol (0.2 mg/day)	60 mo	50	12	24.0	50	17	34.0
Stamler et al. (1963)	< 2 mo	Oestrogen (10 mg/day)	58 mo	119	–	33.8	156	–	23.6
Oslo Diet Heart Study (Leren 1970)	1–2 yr	Diet	60 mo	206	55	26.7	206	41	19.9
Medical Research Council (Gent et al. 1968)	2–13 wk	Diet	11 yr 2–81 mo	206 207	108 31	52.4 15.0	206 214	101 28	49.0 13.1
The Coronary Drug Project (CDP) (1970)	< 3 mo	Oestrogen (2.5 mg/day)	56 mo	2789	525	18.8	1101	219	19.9
		Oestrogen (5.0 mg/day)	21 mo	2789	230	8.2	1119	108	9.7
		Dextrothyroxine (6.0 mg/day)	36 mo	2715	339	12.5	1083	160	14.8
		Clofibrate (1800 mg/day)	74 mo	2789	709	25.4	1103	281	25.5
		Nicotinic acid (3000 mg/day)	74 mo	2789	709	25.4	1119	273	24.4

Table 6.6. *(cont.)*

Trial	Time of entry	Intervention(s)	Length of follow-up	Control			Intervention		
				No. randomised	No. of deaths	Per cent mortality	No. randomised	No. of deaths	Per cent mortality
Veterans' Administration Drug Lipid Cooperative Study (Detre and Shaw 1974)	1–16 mo	Oestrogen (1.25 mg/day)		143	41	28.7	141	40	28.4
		Nicotinic acid (4000 mg/day)					77	24	31.2
		Nicotinic acid (4000 mg/day) + oestrogen (1.25 mg/day)					68	21	30.9
		Dextrothyroxine (4 mg/day)					74	17	23.0
		Dextrothyroxine (4 mg/day) + oestrogen (1.25 mg/day)					67	20	29.9
Physicians of the Newcastle upon Tyne Region (1971)	< 6 wk	Clofibrate (1500–2000 mg/day)	43 mo	253	48	19.0	244	27	11.1
Scottish Society of Physicians (1971)	8–16 wk	Clofibrate (1600–2000 mg/day)	40 mo	263	29	11.0	260	29	11.2
Carlson et al. (1977)	4 mo	Clofibrate 2000 mg/day + nicotinic acid (3000 mg/day) + diet	9–48 mo	279	26	9.3	279	24	8.6

(Armitage 1971). Although no reduction in overall mortality was noted in the Scottish Society of Physicians Trial (Report by a Research Committee of the Scottish Society of Physicians 1971), both cardiac mortality and non-fatal infarcts were reduced in those patients with existing angina. It is difficult to explain this trial result on the basis of any specific factor related to the patient's clinical condition or the action of clofibrate itself.

In the study performed by Carlson et al. (1977) fixed doses of both clofibrate and niacin were given. No difference in total mortality was observed between the intervention and control groups. However, there was a statistically significant reduction in the incidence of non-fatal myocardial infarction in the clofibrate/niacin group.

Nicotinic Acid (Niacin).   In two studies nicotinic acid alone was used as an intervention. In the Coronary Drug Project there was no statistically significant reduction in total mortality (Coronary Drug Project Research Group 1975). The incidence of non-fatal myocardial infarction was significantly lower in the group treated with nicotinic acid; however, atrial fibrillation, other cardiac rhythm disturbances, other side-effects (including gastrointestinal problems) and abnormal liver function tests were more common. In the Veterans' Administration Drug Lipid Cooperative study, too, there was no reduction in mortality in the group treated with nicotinic acid.

Dietary Intervention

The Oslo Diet Heart Study (Leren 1970) (Table 6.6), performed in patients who had sustained an acute infarct, involved an attempt to reduce serum cholesterol by dietary intervention. A mean reduction in serum cholesterol levels of 17.6% was obtained in the diet group, as compared with only 3.7% in the control group. There was a 25% lower total mortality in the intervention group at the end of 5 years; however, this was not statistically significant. The combined incidence of both fatal and non-fatal infarcts and of major cardiovascular incidents appeared to be significantly reduced in the diet group. After 11 years of follow-up there was a statistically significant reduction in fatal myocardial infarction in the diet group, but the difference in total mortality between the intervention and control groups was only 6%.

The Medical Research Council trial (Research Committee to the Medical Research Council 1968) again altered diet by replacing saturated fats by polyunsaturated fats in an attempt to reduce the reinfarction rate in patients under 60 who had survived a first attack. There was no reduction in the reinfarction incidence, and the total mortality was also approximately the same in both groups. The serum cholesterol was reduced by 12% in those on the test diet and by 6% in those in the control group.

In general terms it appears that attempts to reduce plasma lipids in patients following acute myocardial infarction do not reduce overall mortality. These studies nevertheless demonstrate that therapeutic intervention can reduce the serum cholesterol by between 6.5 and 20%. The reduction is usually evident within 6 months of commencing therapy and may be the result of either dietary intervention or drug administration. It must be emphasised, however, that the patients studied were not selected on the basis of an elevated serum cholesterol level and that in those with normal baseline lipids little therapeutic efficacy was achieved. It is also unclear whether any reduction in other cardiovascular events is related to the lipid-lowering activity of the agents used. A considerable incidence of adverse effects occurs, suggesting that this therapy should only be introduced in those patients who have been confirmed to have a specific hyperlipoproteinaemia.

References

Ahlmark G, Saetre H, Korsgren M (1974) Reduction of sudden deaths after myocardial infarction. Lancet II: 1563

Andersson MP, Bechsgaard P, Frederiksen J et al. (1979) Effect of alprenolol on mortality among patients with definite or suspected acute myocardial infarction. Lancet II: 865–867

Anturan Reinfarction, Italian Study (1982) Sulfinpyrazone in post-myocardial infarction. Lancet I: 237–242

Armitage P (1971) Statistical methods in medical research. Blackwell Scientific, Oxford, p 134

Aspirin Myocardial Infarction Study Research Group (1980) A randomised controlled trial of persons recovered from myocardial infarction. JAMA 243: 661–668

Baber NS, Lewis JA (1980) Betablockers in the treatment of myocardial infarction. Br Med J 281: 59

Bastian BC, McFarland PW, McLauchlan JH et al. (1980) A prospective randomized trial of tocainide in patients following myocardial infarction. Am Heart J 100: 1017–1022

Bennett MA, Wilner JM, Pentecost BL (1970) Controlled trial of lignocaine in prophylaxis of ventricular arrhythmias complicating myocardial infarction. Lancet II: 909–911

Beta Blocker Heart Attack Research Group (1982) A randomised trial of propranolol in patients with acute myocardial infarction. JAMA 247: 1707–1714

Boelaert J, Van Eeghem P, Daneels R (1980) The Anturan Reinfarction Trial. N Engl J Med 303: 49

Breddin K (1977) Multicenter two-year prospective study on the prevention of secondary myocardial infarction by ASA in comparison with phenprocoumon and placebo. In: Boissel P, Klimt CR (eds) Multicenter controlled trials: principles and problems. INSERM, Paris, p 79

Breddin K, Loew D, Lechner K, Uberta K, Walter E (1979) Secondary prevention of myocardial infarction. Comparison of acetylsalicylic acid, phenprocoumon and placebo. A multicenter two-year prospective study. Thromb Haemost 4: 225–236

Burch JW, Stanford N, Majerus PW (1978) Inhibition of platelet prostaglandin synthetase by oral aspirin. J Clin Invest 61: 314–319

Campbell WB, Johnson AR, Callahan KS, Graham RM (1981) Anti-platelet activity of beta-adrenergic antagonists: inhibition of thromboxane synthesis and platelet aggregation in patients receiving long-term propranolol treatment. Lancet II: 1382–1384

Carleton RA, Sanders CA, Burack WR (1960) Heparin administration after acute myocardial infarction. N Engl J Med 263: 1002–1005

Carlson LA, Danielson M, Ekbert I et al. (1977) Reduction of myocardial infarction by the combination treatment with clofibrate and nicotinic acid. Atherosclerosis 28: 81–86

Chalmers TC, Matta RJ, Smith H Jr et al. (1977) Evidence favoring the use of anticoagulants in the hospital phase of acute myocardial infarction. N Engl J Med 297: 1091–1096

Chamberlain DA, Jewitt DE, Julian DG et al. (1980) Oral mexiletine in high-risk patients after myocardial infarction. Lancet II: 1324

Chamberlain DA (1983) Beta-adrenoceptor antagonists after myocardial infarction — where are we now? Br Heart J 49: 105–110

Coronary Drug Project Research Group (1975) Clofibrate and niacin in coronary heart disease. JAMA 231: 360–381

Darby S, Bennett MA, Cruickshank JC et al. (1972) Trial of combined intramuscular and intravenous lignocaine in prophylaxis of ventricular tachyarrhythmias. Lancet I: 817–819

Detre KM, Shaw L (1974) Long-term changes of serum cholesterol with cholesterol-altering drugs in patients with coronary heart disease: Veterans' Administration Drug-Lipid Cooperative Study. Circulation 50: 998–1005

Drapkin A, Merskey C (1972) Anticoagulant therapy after acute myocardial infarction: relation of therapeutic benefit of patient's age, sex, and severity of infarction. JAMA 222: 541–548

Elwood PC, Cochrane AL, Burr ML et al. (1974) A randomized controlled trial of acetylsalicylic acid in the secondary prevention of mortality from myocardial infarction. Br Med J I: 436–440

Elwood PC, Sweetnam PM (1979) Aspirin and secondary mortality after myocardial infarction. Lancet II: 1313–1315

Elwood PC, Williams WO (1979) A randomized controlled trial of aspirin in the prevention of early mortality in myocardial infarction. J R Coll Gen Pract 29: 413–416

Five-year study by a group of Physicians of the Newcastle upon Tyne region (1971) Trial of clofibrate in the treatment of ischaemic heart disease. Br Med J 4: 767–775

Frishman WA, Weksler B, Cristal Doulou P et al. (1974) Reversal of abnormal platelet aggregability and change in exercise tolerance in patients with angina pectoris following oral propranolol. Circulation 50: 887–896

Frishman WH, Furberg CD, Friedewald WT (1984) Beta adrenergic blockade for survivors of acute myocardial infarction. N Engl J Med 310: 830–837

Gent AE, Brook OGD, Foley TH (1968) Dipyridamole; a controlled trial of its effect in acute myocardial infarction. Br Med J 4: 366–368

Hampton JR (1982) Should every survivor of a heart attack be given a betablocker? Part I. Evidence from clinical trials. Br Med J 285: 33–36

Hansteen V, Moinichen E, Lorensteen E et al. (1982) One year's treatment with propranolol after myocardial infarction: preliminary report of Norwegian Multicentre trial. Br Med J 284: 155–160

Hjalmarson A, Herlitz J, Malek I et al. (1981) Effect on mortality of metroprolol in acute myocardial infarction. A double-blind randomised trial. Lancet II: 823–827

Holmberg S, Bergman H (1967) Prophylactic quinidine treatment in myocardial infarction: A double-blind study. Acta Med Scand 181: 296–304

Jennings G, Model DG, Jones MBS et al. (1980) Oral disopyramide in prophylaxis of arrhythmias following myocardial infarction. Lancet II: 934–936

Jones DT, Kostuk, WJ, Gunton RW (1974) Prophylactic quinidine for the prevention of arrhythmias after acute myocardial infarction. Am J Cardiol 33: 655–660

Kallio V, Hamalainen H, Hakkila J et al. (1979) Reduction in sudden death by a multifactorial intervention programme after acute myocardial infarction. Lancet II: 1091–1094

Kalsner S (1975) Adenosine and dipyridamole actions and interactions on isolated coronary artery strips of cattle. Br J Pharmacol 55: 439–445

Kentala E (1972) Physical fitness and feasibility of physical rehabilitation after myocardial infarction in men of working age. Ann Clin Res 4 [Suppl 9] 1–84

Koch-Weser J, Klein SW, Foo-Canto LL et al. (1969) Antiarrhythmic prophylaxis with procainamide in acute myocardial infarction. N Engl J Med 281:1253–1260

Lemberg L, Castellanos A, Arcebal AG (1970) The use of propranolol in arrhythmias complicating acute myocardial infarction. Am Heart J 80: 479–487

Leren P (1970) The Oslo Diet Heart Study: Eleven year report. Circulation 42: 935–942

Lie KI, Wellens HJ, Van Capelle FJ et al. (1974) Lidocaine in the prevention of primary ventricular fibrillation; A double-blind randomised study of 212 consecutive patients. N Engl J Med 291: 1324–1326

Lie KI, Liem KL, Louridtz WJ (1978) Efficacy of lidocaine in preventing primary ventricular fibrillation within 1 hour after a 300 mg intramuscular injection. A double blind, randomised study of 300 hospitalized patients with acute myocardial infarction. Am J Cardiol 42: 486–488

May GS, Eberlein KA, Furberg CD, Passamani ER, Demets DL (1982) Secondary prevention after myocardial infarction: A review of long-term trials. Prog Cardiovasc Dis 24: 331–352

May GS, Furberg CD, Eberlain KA, Geraci BJ (1983) Secondary prevention after myocardial infarction: A review of short-term acute phase trials. Prog Cardiovasc Dis 1983: 24: 335–359

Modan B, Shani M, Schor S. et al. (1975) Reduction of hospital mortality from acute myocardial infarction by anticoagulant therapy. N Engl J Med 292: 1359–1362

Moncada S, Korbut R (1978) Dipyridamole and other phosphodiesterase inhibitors act as anti-thrombotic agents by potentiating prostacyclin. Lancet I: 1286–1289

Moschos CB, Escobinas AJ, Jorgensen OB et al. (1981) Effect of sulfinpyrazone on ventricular fibrillation during acute myocardial ischemia. Circulation 64: 13–18

Mueller HS, Ayres SM, Religa A, Evans RG (1974) Propranolol in the treatment of acute myocardial infarction. Effect on myocardial oxygenation and haemodynamics. Circulation 49: 1078–1087

Multicentre International Study (1975) Improvement in prognosis of myocardial infarction by long-term beta adrenoreceptor blockade using practolol. Br Med J 3: 735–740

Naughton J (1979) Exercise and myocardial infarction: The National Exercise and Heart Disease Project: an overview. Proceedings of the Workshop on Physical Conditioning and Rehabilitation. US DHSS, PHS, NIH

Newman RJ (1977) Comparison of the antilipolytic effects of metoprolol, acebutolol and propranolol in man. Br Med J II: 601–603

Nicholls DP, Haybyrne T, Barnes PC (1980) Intravenous and oral disopyramide after myocardial infarction. Lancet II: 936–938

O'Brien KP, Taylor PM, Croxson RS (1973) Prophylactic lidocaine in hospitalized patients with acute myocardial infarction. Med J Aust II [Suppl]: 36–37

Oliver MF, Boyd GS (1961) Influence of reduction of serum lipids on prognosis of coronary heart disease: Five-year study using oestrogen. Lancet II: 499–505

Palatsi I (1976) Feasibility of physical training after myocardial infarction and its effect on return to work morbidity and mortality. Acta Med Scand [Suppl] 599: 1–84

Peter T, Ross O, Duffield A et al. (1979) Effect on survival after myocardial infarction of long-term treatment with phenytoin. Br Heart J 40: 1356–1360

Pitt S, Lipp H, Anderson ST (1971) Lignocaine given prophylactically to patients with acute myocardial infarction. Lancet I: 612–615

Report by a Research Committee of the Scottish Society of Physicians (1971) Ischaemic heart disease: a secondary prevention trial using clofibrate. Br Med J 4: 775–784

Report of the Working Party on Anticoagulant Therapy in Coronary Thrombosis to the Medical Research Council (1959) An assessment of long-term anticoagulation administration after cardiac infarction. Br Med J I: 803–810

Report of Working Party on Anticoagulant Therapy in Coronary Thrombosis to the Medical Research Council (1969) Assessment of short-term anticoagulant administration after cardiac infarction. Br Med J I: 335–342

Research Committee to the Medical Research Council (1968) Controlled trial of soyabean oil in myocardial infarction. Lancet II: 693–700

Reynell PC (1961) Prophylactic procainamide in myocardial infarction. Br Heart J 23: 421–424

Roland JM, Wilcox RG, Banks DC, Edwards B, Fentem PH, Hampton JR (1979) Effect of betablockers on arrhythmias during six weeks after suspected myocardial infarction. Br Med J II: 518–521

Ryden L, Arnman K, Conradson TB et al. (1980) Prophylaxis of ventricular tachyarrhythmias with intravenous and oral tocainide in patients with and recovering from acute myocardial infarction. Am Heart J 100: 1006–1012

Sanne H (1973) Exercise tolerance and physical training of non-selected patients after myocardial infarction. Acta Med Scand [Suppl] 551: 1–112

Seaman AJ, Griswold HE, Beaume RB et al. (1969) Long-term anticoagulant prophylaxis after myocardial infarction. N Engl J Med 281: 115–119

Second Report of the Working Party on Anticoagulant Therapy in Coronary Thrombosis to the Medical Research Council (1964) An assessment of long-term anticoagulant administration after cardiac infarction: Br Med J II: 837–843

Shand DG (1982) Beta adrenergic blocking drugs after acute myocardial infarction. Mod Concs Cariovasc Dis 51: 103–106

Snow PJD (1965) Effect of propranolol in myocardial infarction. Lancet II: 551–553

Stamler J, Pick R, Katz LN et al. (1963) Effectiveness of estrogens for therapy of myocardial infarction in middle-aged men. JAMA 240: 228–231

Steele P, Rainwater J, Vogel R et al. (1978) Platelet-suppressant therapy in patients with coronary artery disease. JAMA 240: 228–231

The Anturan Reinfarction Trial Research Group (1978) Sulfinpyrazone in the prevention of cardiac death after myocardial infarction. N Engl J Med 298: 289–295

The Coronary Drug Project Research Group (1970) Initial findings leading to modifications of its research protocol. JAMA 214: 1303–1313

The Coronary Drug Project Research Group (1976) Aspirin in coronary heart disease. J Chron Dis 29: 625

The Norwegian Multicentre Study Group (1981) Timolol induced reduction in mortality and reinfarction in patients surviving acute myocardial infarction. N Engl J Med 304: 801–807

The Persantin–Aspirin Reinfarction Study Research Group (1980) Persantin and aspirin in coronary heart disease. Circulation 62: 449–461

The Sixty Plus Reinfarction Study Research Group (1980) A double-blind trial to assess longterm oral anticoagulant therapy in elderly patients after myocardial infarction. Lancet II: 989–993

Valentine PA, Frew JL, Mashford ML et al. (1974) Lidocaine in the prevention of sudden death in the pre-hospital phase of acute infarction: A double-blind study. N Engl J Med 291: 1327–1331

Van Durme JP, Hagemeijer F, Bogaert M et al. (1977) Chronic anti-dysrhythmic treatment after myocardial infarction. Design of the Gent-Rotterdam Aprindine Study. In: Boissel JP, Klimt CR (eds) Multicenter controlled trials: principles and problems. INSERM, Paris, p 43

Verrier RL, Thompson PL, Lown B (1974) Ventricular vulnerability during sympathetic stimulation: role of heart rate and blood pressure. Cardiovasc Res 8: 602–610

Veterans' Administration Cooperative (1973) Anticoagulants in acute myocardial infarction. Results of a cooperative clinical trial. JAMA 225: 724–729

Wasserman AJ, Gutterman LA, Yoe KB et al. (1966) Anticoagulants in acute myocardial infarction: The failure of anticoagulants to alter mortality in randomized series. Am Heart J 81: 43–49

Weksler BB, Gillick M, Pink J (1977) Effect of propranolol on platelet function. Blood 49: 185–196

Wilcox RG, Rowley JM, Hampton JR et al. (1980) Randomized placebo-controlled trial comparing oxprenolol with disopyramide phosphate in immediate treatment of suspected myocardial infarction. Lancet II: 764–766

Wilhelmsson C, Vedin JA, Wilhelmsen L et al. (1974) Reduction of sudden deaths after myocardial infarction by treatment with alprenolol. Lancet II: 1157–1160

Yusuf S, Ramsdale D, Peto R et al. (1980) Early intravenous atenolol in suspected acute myocardial infarction. Preliminary report of a randomised trial. Lancet II: 273–276

Zainal N, Carmichael DJS, Griffiths JW et al. (1977) Oral disopyramide for the prevention of arrhythmias in patients with acute myocardial infarction admitted to open wards. Lancet II: 887–889

7 Indications for Surgery in Coronary Heart Disease

Cardiologists and cardiac surgeons work closely together in the selection of patients for surgery, in postoperative management and in long-term follow-up. In terms of coronary heart disease, surgery may be required as an emergency, urgently within a few days or as an elective procedure (Table 7.1).

Table 7.1 Surgery of CHD

A. *Emergency or urgent*
   1. Mechanical complication following acute myocardial infarction
     a) Ventricular septal defect
     b) Mitral incompetence
   2. Unstable angina not controlled by medical therapy
   3. Left main coronary artery disease

B. *Elective*
   1. Stable angina not adequately controlled by medical therapy
   2. Repair of ventricular aneurysm

Emergency or Urgent Surgery

Ventricular Septal Defects

Postinfarction ventricular septal defect (VSD) is uncommon but not rare. A pansystolic murmur often associated with a thrill develops at the left sternal edge 24–96 h after infarction. The clinical picture subsequently varies considerably. Haemodynamic changes may be slight or left and right heart failure may occur insidiously or rapidly. If haemodynamics are stable, early investigation is not necessary. However, in the presence of clinical deterioration intensive management and early investigation become appropriate. Treatment is by:

1. Diuretic — usually intravenous frusemide 40–80 mg
2. Off-loading — consideration should be given to nitroprusside or nitrate as a veno-arteriolar or venous dilator.

3. In specialised cardiac centres it may be feasible to provide circulatory assistance by an aortic balloon pump to augment coronary and cerebral blood flow.

The investigations required are right and left heart catheterisation and selective coronary angiography. The right heart catheterisation data required are both pressure and oxygen saturation. These allow an assessment of the size and site of the left to right flow and the effects on the pulmonary circulation. Pulmonary to systemic flow rates of more than 2:1 usually merit closure (Table 7.2). Left ventricular angiography delineates the site of the VSD (anterior or posterior) and whether it is single or multiple. Selective coronary angiography is also done to assess all potentially diseased vessels and to indicate the scope of the surgery required.

Early cardiac surgery may be needed in life-threatening situations but the mortality remains high (approximately 50%). Surgery 3–4 weeks later carries a much better prognosis. By this time the margins of the VSD have become firmer and more suitable for surgical repair.

Table 7.2. Data consistent with significant postinfarction VSD

Site	Pressure (mmHg)	O$_2$ saturation (%)
Superior vena cava	Mean 6	70
Right atrium	Mean 6	70
Right ventricle	70/8	86
Pulmonary artery	70/35[a]	86
Pulmonary capillary wedge	Mean 24[a]	96
Aorta	96/70	96

$$\text{Pulmonary : systemic flow} = \frac{\text{Aortic} - \text{mixed venous (RA) saturation}}{\text{Aortic} - \text{pulmonary arterial saturation}}$$

$$= \frac{96-70}{96-86}$$

$$= 2.6 : 1$$

[a] There is pulmonary hypertension and the pulmonary wedge pressure is raised, reflecting left heart failure due to the infarction.

Mitral Incompetence

Papillary muscle rupture or severe dysfunction can occur following myocardial infarction. The subsequent mitral incompetence can be slight, moderate or torrential. It is commoner after inferior but can also occur with anterior infarction. The clinical feature is the development of a long apical systolic murmur. The haemodynamic consequences vary considerably. There can be little upset or varying degrees of left heart failure.

Many patients will respond to treatment with oral or intravenous diuretics or by off-loading if need be. An inadequate response is the indication for further investigation with a view to mitral valve replacement although this will only seldom be required (Table 7.3).

Table 7.3. Data consistent with postinfarction mitral incompetence

Site	Pressure (mmHg)	O$_2$ saturation (%)
Superior vena cava	Mean 6	84
Right atrium	Mean 6	84
Right ventricle	60/8	84
Pulmonary artery	60/40[a]	84
Pulmonary capillary wedge	Mean 24 v = 40[a]	98
Aorta	100.70	98

[a] There is pulmonary hypertension with a raised pulmonary wedge pressure. The high 'v' wave reflects the mitral incompetence.

Unstable Angina Not Controlled by Medical Treatment

Unstable angina can be defined as episodes of chest pain at rest or minimal exertion, ST or T wave changes on the ECG and normal cardiac enzymes. Such patients should be initially treated medically by oral or intravenous nitrates and a calcium channel blocker. If they fail to settle in 24–48 h then coronary angiography may be needed. These patients suffer from a variety of coronary problems ranging from "pure" vasoconstriction, through a mixture of vasoconstriction and coronary atherosclerosis, to severe coronary artery stenosis due to atherosclerosis and with no contribution from vasoconstriction.

A management plan is outlined in Fig. 7.1. The subsequent clinical course is unpredictable. A proportion of cases, especially those with predominant coronary vasoconstriction, will settle. Of patients who have done well at 4–8 weeks, around 30% will require investigation and probable surgery within the next year.

Left Main Coronary Disease

Left main coronary disease is associated with an increased risk of coronary events (Mock et al. 1982), including the risk of sudden death. It should be suspected when symptoms are severe and when formal exercise testing is associated with the early onset of symptoms and a failure of the systolic blood pressure to rise. Left main disease can at times also be unexpectedly revealed at angiography when symptoms have been relatively mild.

Because of the increased risk of sudden death, many centres will not allow patients with a diagnosis of left main coronary obstruction of more than 50% to go home but will keep them in hospital for early surgery. There are also those who advocate emergency coronary bypass surgery within hours. Our own policy is to keep the patient in hospital, operate as soon as possible but not to consider emergency surgery unless the clinical situation becomes unstable.

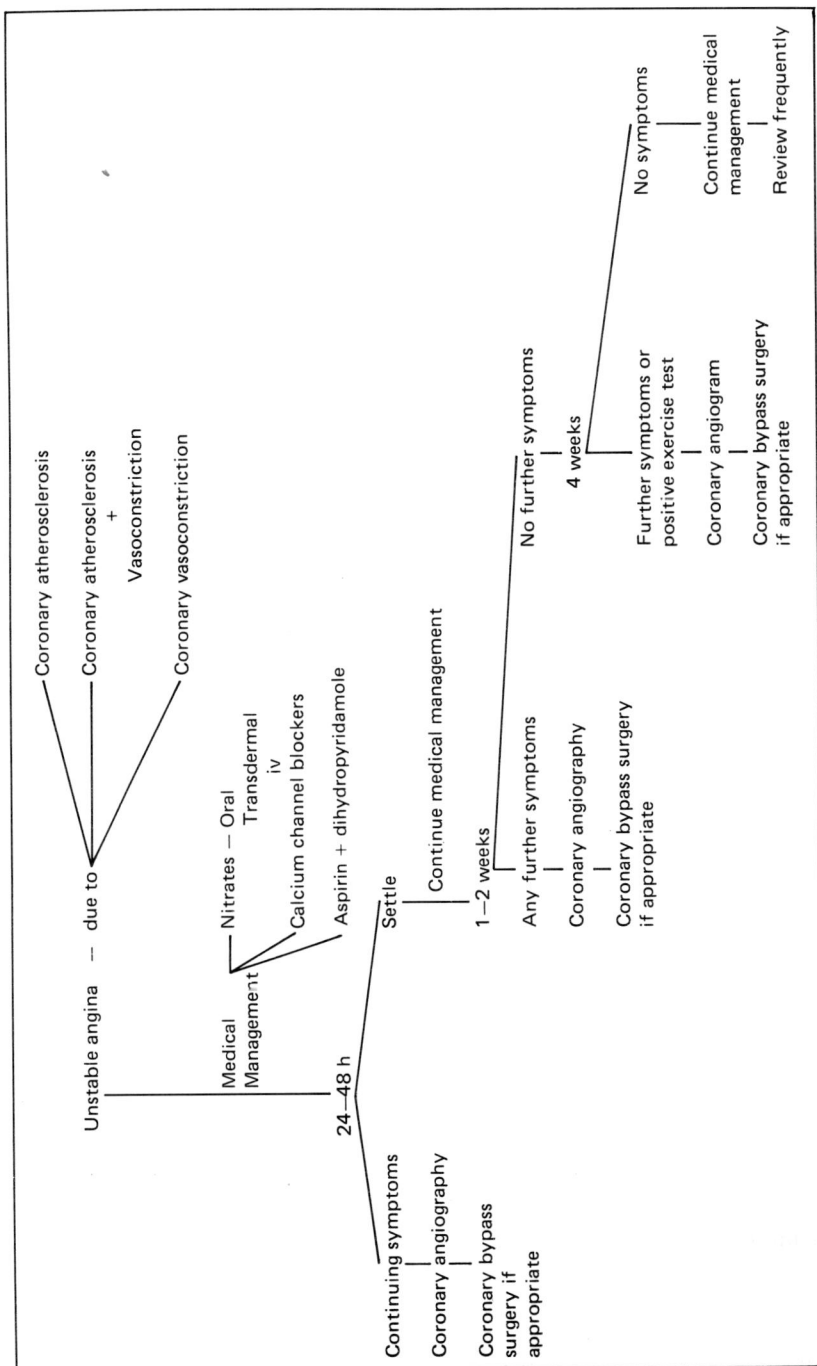

Fig. 7.1. Management plan for unstable angina.

Elective Coronary Surgery

There has been an explosive increase in coronary artery bypass surgery. It was quickly shown to relieve symptoms of angina and it was anticipated that it would improve prognosis. Recent studies have clarified the position in this regard (CASS 1983; European Coronary Surgery Study Group 1980).

At present there seems general agreement that coronary bypass surgery should be offered to those with (a) left main coronary disease, (b) angina despite intensive medical management, (c) angina and intolerance of the medical regime. In general terms such patients will have around a 70%–80% chance of significant improvement, with an operative mortality of 2%–3% and an average stay in hospital of 9 days. The role of the relatively new procedure of coronary angioplasty by means of balloon catheter remains uncertain but is promising. Initially used for patients with proximal single vessel obstruction, the indications now seem to be expanding; however, it remains a procedure only for the highly skilled investigative cardiologist or radiologist.

In terms of prognosis it has been shown that the outlook for those treated medically is better than previously thought — an annual mortality of around 1.6%. Both the European and CASS reports have shown an improved survival in those with left main coronary disease. The European study indicates an improved prognosis in those with triple vessel disease — around a 6% improvement at 5 years — while no statistical differences were found by the CASS group. Both trials agree that the prognosis is not improved in those with angina and underlying single or double vessel disease. At present it would seem logical to treat medically those presenting with angina, going forward to coronary angiography in those whose quality of life remains impaired in terms of work or leisure. There is no doubt that coronary bypass surgery has meant a dramatic improvement in symptoms without necessarily considering an additional improvement in prognosis.

Surgery of Ventricular Aneurysm

After myocardial infarction the damaged left ventricle is usually akinetic, i.e. does not contract; alternatively it may be dyskinetic, which implies paradoxical movement, i.e. outward movement during ventricular systole. The presence of a dyskinetic segment is not in itself an indication for surgery. Surgery may need to be considered, however, if there is evidence that the segment is expanding or that symptoms are developing. Patients with a ventricular aneurysm who develop significant angina may be considered for resection of aneurysm and grafting of any other diseased vessels. There is no point in grafting the vessels supplying the dyskinetic segment. It is essentially an avascular scar whose function cannot be improved by an increase in blood supply. Results of

resection of aneurysm for symptoms of breathlessness or recurrent dys-
rhythmia have in general been disappointing. The decision on each patient has
to be made after a full haemodynamic assessment in a specialised unit.

References

CASS Principal Investigations and Their Associates (1983) Coronary artery surgery study (CASS):
    a randomised trial of coronary artery bypass surgery. Circulation 68: 939–950
European Coronary Surgery Study Group (1980) Prospective randomised study of coronary artery
    bypass surgery in stable angina pectoris. Lancet II: 491–495
Mock M, Ringqvist I, Fisher L, Davis K, Chaitman BR, Kouchoukos N, Kaiser G, Alderman E,
    Ryan T, Russell R, Mullen S, Fray D, Killip T (1982) The survival of medically treated
    patients in the coronary artery surgery study (CASS) registry. Circulation 66: 562–568

8 Arrhythmias

The term "cardiac arrhythmia" encompasses disturbances of the normal rhythmic activity of the heart, including both the initiation and the conduction of the impulse. Recent methods of investigation have shown that arrhythmias are common in apparently normal individuals as well as in those with cardiac disease. Understanding arrhythmias and their treatment requires knowledge of the anatomy and electrophysiological properties of the specialised conducting system. Likewise, the selection of an anti-arrhythmic agent demands knowledge of its pharmacological properties, its site of action and its range of anti-arrhythmic activity. Rational therapy depends on establishing the correct diagnosis, which is often difficult since arrhythmias may be paroxysmal rather than sustained and infrequent rather than constant. The diagnosis of an arrhythmia in itself does not necessarily indicate a need for treatment. The decision to treat is influenced by the nature of the arrhythmia, the potential complications and the level of accompanying symptoms.

Mechanisms

The two major mechanisms of arrhythmia production are enhanced automaticity and re-entrant or circus movements.

Enhanced Automaticity

The use of glass capillary micro-electrodes has allowed measurement of intra- and extracellular differences in electrolyte distribution and electrical potential. In a non-automatic cardiac fibre in diastole the resting potential is stable until excited by a propagated action potential (Fig. 8.1). Following excitation, an increased permeability to sodium occurs, with a rapid phase of depolarisation (phase zero). The potential gradually reverts towards normal during repolarisation. As the inward sodium current subsides, potassium ions move out across the membranes. Automatic cells from specialised areas in the myocardium have the property of slow diastolic depolarisation (phase 4).

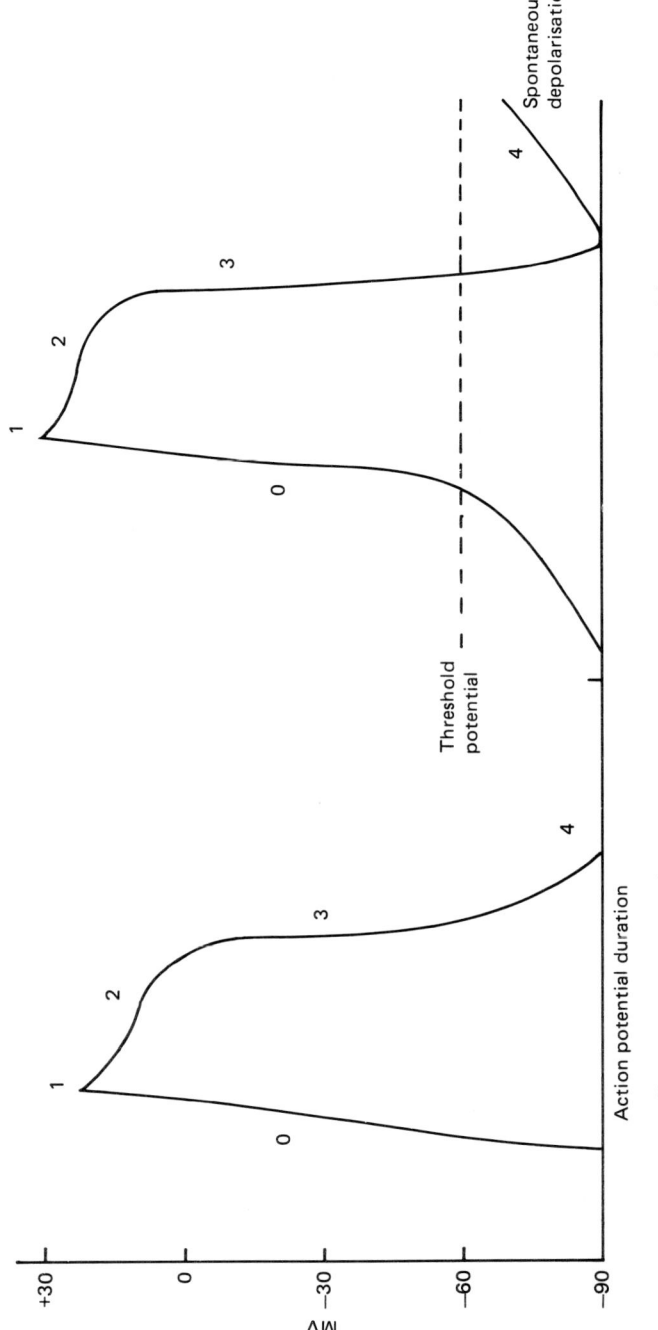

Fig. 8.1. Schematic representation of action potential in non-automatic cardiac fibre and cell with automatic activity.

When slow diastolic depolarisation reaches a critical point, the threshold potential, an action potential develops. Two inward calcium currents also contribute to the transmembrane potential in automatic cells. The intrinsic rate of automatic discharge is determined by the slope of phase 4 depolarisation, the value of the resting potential and the threshold potential. Enhanced or developed automaticity may occur by more rapid spontaneous phase 4 diastolic depolarisation in an established automatic or pacemaker cell or by transformation of an ordinary myocardial fibre by some pathological process such as ischaemia. Repetitive discharges may be precipitated by local myocardial hypokalaemia, anoxia, acidosis or local release of catecholamines.

Re-entrant Mechanism

Re-entrant or circus movement arrhythmias occur when a single excitatory wave is continuously propagated within a closed circuit. The circuit acts as a physiological or functional electrical pathway. It may have an anatomical structure involving specialised conducting tissue or be associated with an accessory bypass tract. The mechanism of re-entry is demonstrated (Fig. 8.2). The circuit requires two interconnected pathways which are functionally disassociated, having different conduction properties and refractory periods when stimulated. (a) A common distal pathway must link the two proximal pathways. In response to an appropriately timed impulse, one pathway (the retrograde limb) must block and fail to conduct. (b) The other limb (anterograde) conducts to the distal tissue. (c) The block in the retrograde limb is unidirectional and the impulse conducts in retrograde direction. If this conducted impulse is sufficiently slow, the anterograde limb regains excitability and again conducts the propagated impulse. (d) Continued repetition of the sequence results in a sustained re-entrant arrhythmia.

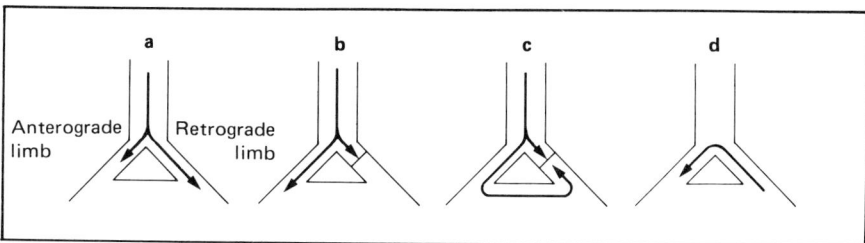

Fig. 8.2. Schematic representation of re-entrant mechanism of arrhythmia.

Anti-arrhythmic Drugs

Although recent advances in pacing techniques and surgical intervention are promising, most patients with cardiac arrhythmias require treatment with anti-arrhythmic drugs. The ideal anti-arrhythmic compound should have:

1. Parenteral and oral formulations to allow rapid onset of action and simple dosage schedules
2. A wide spectrum of therapeutic activity in both atrial and ventricular arrhythmias
3. Lack of significant cardiac depressant activity or non-cardiac side-effects
4. Pharmacokinetic properties which allow long-term prophylactic therapy

The ideal agent has not yet been found, although at present most patient's symptoms can be controlled. There is a continued search for drugs with anti-fibrillatory activity which might reduce the incidence of sudden death.

Therapeutic drug monitoring is important. Rapid analytical methods to measure concentrations of most anti-arrhythmics are now available. Many patients with arrhythmias are seriously ill and this may lead to considerable inter- and intrasubject differences in pharmacokinetics. Variations in absorption, clearance and volumes of distribution may lead to marked differences in concentration-effect relationships. Logical anti-arrhythmic therapy involves attaining an effective plasma concentration. The safe and effective plasma concentration of most agents is now known, though in most cases it has a narrow range, necessitating careful dose titration. Dosage is determined by the combination of measurement of concentration and clinical observation. Efficacy may be difficult to determine if an arrhythmia occurs infrequently, no matter what its clinical importance may be. Treatment should only be regarded as ineffective if the arrhythmia is not controlled after the therapeutic plasma concentrations have been achieved.

Classification of Anti-arrhythmic Drugs

The chemical structures of drugs with anti-arrhythmic activity show great variation. Several classifications have been used according to:

1. The clinical spectrum of activity
2. The anatomical site of action (Table 8.1)
3. Electrophysiological action on isolated cardiac fibres (Vaughan Williams 1970) (Table 8.2).

This latter classification was developed following observations on electrical activity of isolated cardiac fibres. It allows drugs to be characterised at the pre-clinical phase of development, although it has practical clinical limitations and unfortunately excludes some agents with anti-arrhythmic activity such as the cardiac glycosides. Four types of basic activity are recognised, although present developmental agents may require at least one further class recognition. Many

Table 8.1. Site of action of anti-arrhythmic compounds

Site	Anti-arrhythmic
Sinus node ⎫ Atrium ⎬	β-Adrenoceptor blocking agents Digoxin Verapamil Procainamide Disopyramide Amiodarone Quinidine
A-V node	Digoxin Verapamil β-Blockers
Anomalous pathway	Disopyramide Amiodarone Procainamide Quinidine
Ventricle	Lignocaine Disopyramide Tocainide Mexiletine Phenytoin Procainamide Quinidine Amiodarone

Table 8.2. Classification (Vaughan-Williams) of anti-arrhythmic drugs

	Class I	Class II	Class III	Class IV
A	Quinidine Procainamide Disopyramide	β-Adrenoceptor blocking compounds Bretylium	Amiodarone Disopyramide Sotalol	Verapamil
B	Lignocaine Mexiletine Aprindine Phenytoin Tocainide			
C	Lorcainide Flecainide			

drugs have more than one action as defined in this classification; however, their therapeutic activity is usually associated with a dominant action.

Class I. These agents have membrane-stabilising activity and interfere with depolarisation of the cardiac cell membrane by restricting the entry of the depolarising fast sodium current. The maximum rate of rise of phase zero action potential is reduced, and the rate of phase 4 diastolic depolarisation is depressed. These effects reduce spontaneous automaticity. Class I compounds can be further subdivided according to their influence on the duration of the action potential, which may be lengthened (group IA), shortened (group IB) or unaffected (group IC).

Class II. Increased catecholamine discharge can induce cardiac arrhythmias. Agents with class II activity reduce the potential for such arrhythmias. β-Adrenoceptor blocking compounds act as competitive antagonists and block the possible arrhythmogenic effect of cyclic AMP. Bretylium blocks the release of sympathetic transmitter with a similar anti-arrhythmic effect.

Class III. Agents with class III activity prolong the total duration of the action potential. Amiodarone has marked class III activity, while sotalol and bretylium have weak class III activity.

Class IV. These drugs inhibit the slow inward calcium-mediated current and depress phase II and phase III of the action potential. These actions are of particular importance in the upper and middle parts of the A-V node and are useful in blocking one limb of a re-entry circuit.

Class I Anti-arrhythmics

Quinidine

This dextroisomer of quinine is the parent compound of the class I anti-arrhythmics. It reduces the maximum rate of depolarisation, depresses spontaneous phase 4 diastolic depolarisation in automatic cells and slows conduction and prolongs the effective refractory period of atrial, ventricular and Purkinje fibres.

Clinical Use

No adequate parenteral formulation is available and this restricts the use of quinidine to prophylaxis of atrial arrhythmias after cardioversion or as oral therapy in suppression of ventricular arrhythmias after the parenteral administration of an alternative agent. It has activity against both atrial and ventricular arrhythmias, has a vagolytic action which increases A-V conduction, and may lead to rapid conduction from atria to ventricles. This may occur in the presence of atrial flutter and atrial tachycardia. Prior therapy with cardiac glycosides should be given. Quinidine is administered orally 200–600 mg 6 hourly after an initial test dose. Sustained release formulations are now available.

Pharmacokinetics

About 70% of an oral dose is absorbed from the gut. Measurable drug levels are obtained within 15 min, with the peak effect at 1–3 h and a half-life of 7 h.

Sustained release preparations are also in use, though their bio-availability may be lower than that of standard quinidine (Ueda 1976). Anti-arrhythmic effects are seen with drug levels of 2–8 µg/ml (2.5–5 µg/ml with a specific assay being used). Standard assay methods may also measure inactive metabolites. Quinidine is highly protein bound (89%) and metabolised by hydroxylation, the inactive metabolites being excreted in the urine. These metabolites are polar and the excretion depends on urinary pH. The clearance is reduced in liver disease, with an increase in the half-life; protein binding is reduced and lower total plasma levels may be effective. The half-life is unaffected by congestive heart failure. Quinidine interacts with digoxin and higher plasma digoxin levels may result. Accordingly, the dose of cardiac glycoside may require reduction.

Adverse Effects

1. *Cardiac.*   Vasodilatation and hypotension may occur with a high plasma concentration, resulting in myocardial depression. The effects on specialised conducting tissue may lead to sinus node arrest, sino-atrial block, A-V dissociation or progressive QRS and QT prolongation. This latter effect may facilitate the development of re-entry arrhythmias, including paroxysmal ventricular tachycardia (Selzer and Wray 1964).

2. *Extracardiac.*   Gastrointestinal side-effects (nausea, vomiting and diarrhoea) may occur. Cinchonism and hypersensitivity reactions with fever, purpura, thrombocytopenia and hepatic dysfunction may also occur.

Procainamide

Procainamide exhibits similar electrophysiological properties to those described for quinidine. Experimentally, the threshold for induction of ventricular fibrillation is increased.

Clinical Use

Procainamide is available for parenteral and oral use and is effective in the treatment of atrial, junctional and ventricular arrhythmias. It is administered intravenously in a dose of 100 mg every 2 min, to a total of 1000 mg over the first hour (Giardina et al. 1973). It is useful in the treatment of lignocaine-resistant ventricular arrhythmias. Its oral dose is 250–500 mg 3 hourly. Slow release preparations are now available.

Pharmacokinetics

Procainamide can be administered orally, being 85% bio-available. Peak action occurs at 45–90 min, and the mean half-life is some 3.5 h. It is metabolised to an active metabolite, *N*-acetyl-procainamide (NAPA). Ninety per cent of procainamide and NAPA is excreted in the urine. High plasma levels of procainamide and NAPA may be obtained in renal impairment and cardiac failure. The rate of metabolism in the population has a bimodal distribution, patients being classified as fast or slow acetylators. Slow acetylators require smaller doses during long-term administration (Reidenberg et al. 1975). Anti-arrhythmic activity has been shown at plasma levels of 4–8 µg/ml. Toxic effects are concentration related (Koch-Weser and Klein 1971), commencing at blood levels of 8–10 µg/ml and being marked at blood levels of > 16 µg/ml.

Adverse Effects

1. *Cardiac.*   Hypotension and vasodilatation may result from rapid intra-venous administration. There may also be electrocardiographic changes, i.e. P-R prolongation proceeding to heart block, and QRS and QT prolongation.

2. *Extracardiac.*   With chronic oral therapy involving high dosage, many patients develop a systemic lupus erythematosus-like syndrome with a positive antinuclear factor (ANF). Renal involvement is, however, usually absent, and the systemic effects are potentially reversible (Blomgren et al. 1972).

Disopyramide

Disopyramide has electrophysiological properties similar to those of quinidine; however, its different formulations allow a more versatile role.

Clinical Use

Both parenteral and oral preparations of disopyramide are available. Atrial and ventricular arrhythmias may be treated, including those resistant to ligno-caine (Härtel et al. 1974).

Pharmacokinetics

Disopyramide is available both as the base compound and as the phosphate salt. The bio-availability of the phosphate is 80%–90% while that of the free base is slightly less. The half-life is 6–8 h and slow release preparations are now available. There is non-linearity of protein binding, although the plasma concentration of the non-protein-bound drug is proportional to the admin-istered dose. Clearance is dependent on the free drug, with 50% being excreted unchanged in the urine and the remainder being metabolised to *N*-disopropyl-disopyramide. The dose should be reduced in severe renal failure. The therapeutic range is 2–7 µg/ml (total drug concentration) (Bryson et al. 1978).

Adverse Effects

1. *Cardiac.* Myocardial depression is clinically significant and is related both to the plasma level and to the rate of administration of the compound. Disopyramide should be used cautiously in patients with cardiac failure or severe left ventricular dysfunction. Sinus node depression may occur in patients with sick sinus syndrome. Concentration-related QT prolongation may also occur which may predispose to re-entry arrhythmias.

2. *Extracardiac.* Disopyramide has anticholinergic activity. Dry mouth and blurred vision occur commonly and urinary retention may be a problem, particularly in elderly male patients. Glaucoma may rarely be precipitated.

Lignocaine

Lignocaine has typical class I electrophysiological effects and also exhibits local anaesthetic activity. The conduction velocity of Purkinje fibres and ventricular muscles is only slightly slowed (Harrison and Alderman 1972).

Clinical Use

Lignocaine remains the standard compound used in the coronary care unit phase of acute myocardial infarction and following cardiac surgery. It is administered by bolus injection (1–2 mg/kg body weight), with a constant infusion thereafter (2–4 mg/min), and long-term treatment, if indicated, requires an alternative orally active class I anti-arrhythmic. After intramuscular injection, absorption may be somewhat erratic and the blood levels achieved vary widely according to the haemodynamic state of the patient.

Pharmacokinetics

When given orally, lignocaine is hydrolysed in the gastrointestinal tract and there is extensive first pass metabolism in the liver. Following intravenous administration, the elimination half-life is approximately 2 h (Rowland et al. 1971). Therapeutic efficacy is associated with blood levels in the range of 1.5–5 μg/ml. The two main metabolites are monoethyl glycine xylidide (MEGX) and glycine xylidide (GX). The hepatic clearance is flow limited and a smaller dosage may be adequate in the presence of reduced hepatic blood flow, e.g. in cardiac failure and in the presence of hepatic disease (Thomson et al. 1973). Clearance is also prolonged in the elderly, and infusion rates require appropriate adjustment. Toxicity can occur at a wide range of total blood concentration and may show considerable overlap with the therapeutic range. This may be particularly troublesome after bolus injection, and the rate of administration is important. Toxic effects, however, correlate better with free drug levels than with the total plasma concentrations. The free drug fraction in plasma varies from 20%–40% and is determined largely by the concentration of the acute phase proteins, notably α_1 acid glycoprotein. Long-term infusion following myocardial infarction leads to a progressively increasing plasma concentration, and a true steady state may not be achieved. This may be related to diminished plasma clearance, but may also reflect increasing levels of α_1 acid glycoprotein. The relationship between the total and free levels of lignocaine and their anti-arrhythmic activity during prolonged infusions remains to be clarified.

Adverse Effects

1. *Cardiac.* Lignocaine has little haemodynamic effect when given in therapeutic doses. High levels may be associated with bradycardia, hypotension and even asystole (Gupta et al. 1974).
2. *Extracardiac.* Nausea and vomiting may follow intravenous administration at levels higher than 5 μg/ml. Central nervous system side-effects predominate, with twitching, paraesthesia and convulsions.

Mexiletine

Mexiletine, a primary amine, has similar electrophysiological actions to lignocaine (Chew et al. 1979).

Clinical Use

Mexiletine is effective after intravenous and oral administration. It has no atrial activity and has been advocated mainly for the acute and chronic control of ventricular arrhythmias following myocardial infarction.

Pharmacokinetics

Following oral administration, peak plasma levels are obtained within 2–4 h. Mexiletine is extensively metabolised to parahydroxy- and hydroxymethymexiletine and to their corresponding deaminated alcohols by hepatic metabolism. The half-life of mexiletine is 9–12 h in normal subjects, but may be prolonged following acute myocardial infarction (to up to 24 h). The concomitant administration of analgesics, particularly the opiates, may be associated with reduced absorption (Campbell et al. 1975). Ten to 20 per cent of the administered dose is excreted unchanged in the urine at normal urinary pH, but this may be reduced when the urine is alkalinised by antacids. There is a narrow therapeutic range since the effective plasma levels are 0.75–2 μg/ml.

Adverse Effects

1. *Cardiac.* Hypotension, bradycardia and transient atrioventricular block may occur with high dosage.
2. *Extracardiac.* Neurological side-effects are common. These include

tremor, nystagmus, diplopia, dizziness, dysarthria, paraesthesia, ataxia and confusion. Gastrointestinal side-effects may also be prominent in some patients.

Tocainide

Tocainide, another primary amine, is an analogue of lignocaine and has similar electrophysiological and anti-arrhythmic properties.

Clinical Use

Tocainide is active after both intravenous and oral administration. Its potential use is in the acute and chronic treatment of ventricular arrhythmias as an alternative to lignocaine following acute myocardial infarction.

Pharmacokinetics

Tocainide is virtually totally absorbed following oral administration (Lalka et al. 1976). Peak plasma levels are achieved within 60–90 min. Protein binding is in the order of 50%. Forty per cent of the drug is excreted unchanged in the urine and the remainder is metabolised in the liver. The elimination half-life is in the range of 11–15 h. There is a low degree of hepatic clearance, suggesting that a substantial first pass effect is unlikely. Twenty-five per cent is excreted as N-carboxy-tocainide. Other metabolites include the glucuronide and lactoxy-lidide salts, which are inactive. Anti-arrhythmic activity occurs within the plasma concentration range of 6–12 µg/ml (Winkle et al. 1976).

Adverse Effects

1. *Cardiac.* Haemodynamic effects are slight when plasma concentration is within the therapeutic range.
2. *Extracardiac.* The central nervous system effects are similar to those associated with lignocaine and mexiletine and appear to be related to peak plasma drug concentration. Gastrointestinal side-effects include anorexia, nausea, vomiting, constipation and abdominal pain. Morbilliform rashes and occasional interstitial pulmonary alveolitis have necessitated drug withdrawal.

Flecainide

Flecainide has typical class I activity with slow depolarisation of specialised cardiac cells. The duration of the action potential is unaffected. Conduction is slowed through the His-Purkinje system, with retrograde conduction through accessory pathways also being affected.

Clinical Use

Flecainide has been advocated for the chronic prophylaxis of ventricular tachyarrhythmias and has shown particular value in the treatment of A-V nodal re-entry tachyarrhythmias, with especially good effects in the treatment of Wolff-Parkinson-White syndrome (Anderson et al. 1981).

Pharmacokinetics

Flecainide is available for both intravenous and oral use. It has a half-life of some 20 h, which allows twice daily therapy (Conard et al. 1976, 1979). Although metabolised in the liver, there is no first pass effect. Excretion is in the urine as both unchanged flecainide and its metabolites meta-*O*-dealkylated flecainide and its lactam. The former metabolite has anti-arrhythmic activity. Flecainide is a basic drug and is bound to plasma proteins (37%–58%). Protein binding is unaltered following acute myocardial infarction. Flecainide elimination may be reduced in elderly patients.

Adverse Effects

1. *Cardiac.* QRS duration and QT interval may be prolonged and the A-V node effects may lead to the development of complete heart block. Sinus node activity is also affected in patients with sick sinus syndrome, and caution should be exercised in this condition. Negative inotropic activity is present and may precipitate cardiac failure in patients with marked left ventricular dysfunction. Pro-arrhythmic effects have been demonstrated in some 5% of patients treated with endocardial pacemakers. Flecainide should therefore be used with caution when treating concomitant arrhythmias in such patients (Bexton et al. 1983).

2. *Extracardiac.* Nausea and dizziness may occur, although they often decrease with continued therapy. Central nervous system effects have also been reported.

Class II Anti-arrhythmics

β-Adrenoceptor Compounds

Many compounds with β-blocking activity are available. Their differing pharmacokinetic properties are detailed elsewhere. The anti-arrhythmic activity of this group of compounds is similar, despite different ancillary properties. Cardioselectivity, partial agonist activity and membrane-stabilising activity appear to be unimportant (Coltart et al. 1971).

Mechanism of Action

Catecholamines augment phase 4 depolarisation. β-Blockers, by acting as competitive antagonists, reduce the slope of depolarisation. The action potential is shortened and the functional refractory period of the A-V node is prolonged.

Clinical Use

β-Adrenoceptor blocking drugs are useful for controlling inappropriate sinus tachycardia or supraventricular arrhythmias provoked by conditions of high catecholamine secretion, including emotion, exercise and anaesthesia. Their long-term use in secondary prevention trials following acute myocardial infarction is reviewed in Chap. 6. For intravenous use practolol has been generally administered as first-line treatment, particularly in the control of supraventricular arrhythmias, including atrial flutter and atrial fibrillation, or to cardiovert paroxysmal atrial tachycardia. Metoprolol and atenolol are now being increasingly used. Propranolol has been used most often in the treatment of arrhythmias associated with thyrotoxicosis. Sotalol has additional class III activity and may demonstrate a wider spectrum of anti-arrhythmic efficacy (Singh et al. 1980).

Other clinical situations in which β-blockers may be of value in arrhythmia control include mitral valve prolapse, hypertrophic obstructive cardiomyopathy, hereditary prolonged QT syndrome and the arrhythmias associated with phaeochromocytoma.

Adverse Effects

1. *Cardiac.* Myocardial depression with hypotension or cardiac failure in patients with left ventricular dysfunction may occur after intravenous or occasionally after oral use. Haemodynamic effects are less pronounced following the use of compounds with partial agonist activity.

2. *Extracardiac.* Increased airways obstruction occurs in patients with asthma or chronic obstructive airways disease. Peripheral limb blood flow may also be reduced in patients with peripheral vascular disease, and caution should be exercised even with selective agents in this clinical setting.

Bretylium Tosylate

Bretylium tosylate has adrenergic neurone blocking activity which suppresses noradrenaline release. It is administered intravenously or intramuscularly (5–10 mg/kg). There is little hepatic metabolism. The elimination half-life is 7.5 h, excretion being via the kidney. Bretylium has class III action on Purkinje fibres and is effective in ventricular dysrhythmias, especially in resistant ventricular fibrillation (Holder et al. 1977). It should be used cautiously in the presence of hypotension.

Class III Anti-arrythmics

Amiodarone

Mechanism of Action

Amiodarone prolongs the action potential duration and increases the effective refractive period of atria and ventricles. Additional anti-arrhythmic properties may be present following intravenous usage and it may have β-receptor inhibitory activity and quinidine-like effects (Zipes and Troup 1978).

Clinical Use

Amiodarone has been shown to be of great value in the treatment of a wide range of ventricular and supraventricular arrhythmias, especially re-entrant arrhythmias associated with accessory pathways in the Wolff-Parkinson-White syndrome. It acts on both the anomalous and normal pathways of conduction. Usage has increased in patients with complex arrhythmias refractory to other anti-arrhythmic compounds, and amiodarone is useful in control of arrhythmias associated with hypertrophic or congestive cardiomyopathy (McKenna et al. 1983).

Pharmacokinetics

Anti-arrhythmic activity may be quickly evident following intravenous use. However, following oral therapy activity is maximal only after some 4–6 days. The elimination half-life is very long (30–45 days) and anti-arrhythmic activity may continue for many months after stopping treatment. When given intravenously, the anti-arrhythmic efficacy of amiodarone does not bear a simple relationship to plasma concentration.

The amiodarone molecule is deiodinated, blocks the peripheral conversion of thyroxine to tri-iodothyronine (T_3) and leads to a rise in serum reverse T_3 (rT_3). Early studies suggest that serum T_3 levels may reflect amiodarone efficacy and toxicity (Nademanee et al. 1981). Plasma levels may or may not reflect tissue concentration and the effect on the QT interval may be a better guide to myocardial concentration and effect.

Adverse Effects

1. *Cardiac.* Vasodilatation after intravenous usage may occasionally occur and be associated with hypotension. Haemodynamic effects, however, are usually unimportant.
2. *Extracardiac.* These are common and include:
   a) Corneal deposits. Yellow-brown deposits are evident in almost all patients. They usually do not interfere with visual acuity and may reverse following cessation of therapy. Slit-lamp observation can be helpful when amiodarone is being used as chronic therapy.
   b) Photosensitisation may require the use of barrier creams if the patients are exposed to ultraviolet light.
   c) Skin discolouration with grey or bluish pigmentation.
   d) Hypo- or hyperthyroidism (2%–3% of patients).
   e) Elevation of hepatic enzymes.
   f) Interstitial pulmonary infiltration may occur. Caution must be exercised in patients with pre-existing lung disease, and serial chest X-rays may be required during follow-up.
   g) Proximal muscle weakness.

These adverse effects are usually reversible and seldom require cessation of therapy. The benefits of drug efficacy usually greatly outweigh these adverse effects.

Class IV Anti-arrythmics

Verapamil

Mechanism of Action

Verapamil inhibits slow inward calcium mediating current. The other calcium channel blockers presently available have little anti-arrhythmic effect in man.

Clinical Use

The major action of verapamil is exerted on conduction through the A-V node (Braunwald 1982). As supraventricular tachycardia has a re-entry mechanism in some 70% of cases, verapamil has become the drug of choice (Rinkenberger et al. 1980). The ventricular response in atrial fibrillation and flutter is controlled and verapamil may be used in conjunction with cardiac glycosides in this situation.

Pharmacokinetics

Verapamil can be given both intravenously and orally. The elimination half-life is 3–7 h, and although absorption is good, bio-availability is < 25%, which is consistent with a high first pass hepatic metabolism. The active metabolite norverapamil is formed. The elimination half-life is prolonged in patients with liver disease when the volume of distribution is increased and clearance is diminished. Excretion is essentially renal (70%) (Singh et al. 1978).

Adverse Effects

1. *Cardiac.*   Myocardial depression may occur in patients with cardiac failure and caution is necessary in patients with left ventricular dysfunction. Drug interactions may occur with β-adrenoceptor blocking drugs, leading to profound bradycardia, and parenteral usage of both agents is contra-indicated (Packer et al. 1982). Rapid intravenous administration should be avoided in patients with A-V conduction problems or glycoside toxicity since complete heart block may develop.

2. *Extracardiac.*   Nausea, dizziness and facial flushing occur rarely.

Diagnosis

The patient's description of symptoms and assessment of the rate (fast or slow) and rhythm (regular or irregular) should always be obtained. Specific questions should be directed towards identifying precipitating factors, including exercise, emotion, alcohol, excessive caffeine and tobacco. A description of the onset and cessation, whether abrupt or gradual, and the identification of physical manoeuvres which abolish the abnormal rhythm is important information. In addition to the general description of "palpitation", the patient should be questioned concerning other symptoms, including dyspnoea, ischaemic chest pain, dizziness or syncope, which may suggest significant haemodynamic sequelae.

General clinical examination may be helpful in the recognition of cardiac or extracardiac disease associated with arrhythmia. Valvular disease, hypertension, coronary heart disease and cardiomyopathy may all present with arrhythmia. Extracardiac disorders include pulmonary disease, especially thromboembolism and infection, thyroid disease and possible anaemia.

Clinical examination of the patient during the arrhythmia may allow a provisional diagnosis, e.g. atrial fibrillation, and allow an assessment of the haemodynamic consequences, e.g. cardiac failure or hypotension. Definitive diagnosis depends on electrocardiographic confirmation. In the case of paroxysmal disorders, the primary care physician is often best placed to make the diagnosis. Standard electrocardiography, especially a long lead II or right precordial lead (V_1), is especially helpful in demonstrating atrial activity. Casual electrocardiography is often unhelpful as it is recorded over a limited period.

In many situations prolonged continuous ambulatory monitoring electrocardiography is of value. Direct electromagnetic recording using small light-weight tape recorders allows patient monitoring during normal, daily, free-ranging activities. Clinical events can be noted on the tape and used with appropriately detailed diary cards to make clinical/electrocardiographic associations. Tape analysis is conducted using high-speed scanning systems, and "event markers" allow rapid scanning to be performed.

Real time tracings of arrhythmic events can be obtained. The usefulness of 24-h tape monitoring systems is limited if the arrhythmia is infrequent. The useful monitoring period may be extended using event recording monitoring activated by the patient at the time of symptoms. This simplifies tape analysis and is much less time consuming. Trans-telephone monitoring systems may also be used for transmission of rhythmic events.

In the case of complex arrhythmias, the surface electrocardiogram may not be fully diagnostic and intracardiac electrocardiograms may be helpful. Using multipolar catheter electrodes, electrocardiograms may be obtained from the atria, ventricles and His bundle. The additional use of programmed stimulation with timed extra stimuli may provide additional information on both the diagnosis and mechanism.

Treatment

The aim of treatment of cardiac arrhythmias is to improve the mechanical function of the heart by electrical or pharmacological methods. This may be done by control of the ventricular rate or restoration of sinus rhythm. The treatment depends on the site of origin of the arrhythmia, which may be sinus, atrial, junctional or ventricular.

Sinus Tachycardia

Sinus tachycardia is defined as a heart rate of more than 100 beats/minute due to a rapidly discharging S-A node. Clinical diagnostic points include:

1. Rate seldom over 130/minute except in response to exercise
2. Rhythm usually regular but perhaps varying with respiration and posture
3. Onset and resolution usually gradual
4. Carotid sinus massage or eyeball pressure leading to gradual rather than abrupt slowing of the heart rate

Sinus tachycardia may be associated with infection and toxaemia, heart failure or myocarditis, emotion or other medical conditions with an increased metabolic rate, including anaemia, thyrotoxicosis, A-V shunt, cor pulmonale or pregnancy.

Treatment is aimed at diagnosis and management of the underlying condition. No therapy is required in most cases. When seen as a manifestation of cardiac failure, treatment should be with diuretics, and digoxin is to be considered in the presence of cardiomegaly. With thyrotoxicosis, β-adrenoceptor blocking compounds are useful in controlling the tachycardia, the associated palpitation and peripheral symptoms such as tremor. β-Adrenergic receptor blocking compounds are also helpful in controlling ventricular extrasystoles associated with sinus tachycardia in subjects with stress- or exercise-related arrhythmias.

Sinus Bradycardia

Sinus bradycardia is defined as a heart rate of less than 60 beats/minute. This may occur secondary to enhanced vagal activity influencing the S-A node and may be seen in association with first degree heart block. It is associated with athletic training, vagotonic manoeuvres such as retching or pathological conditions such as obstructive jaundice, hypothyroidism or hypopituitarism, and raised intracranial pressure. It may be secondary to drug effects, including those of the cardiac glycosides or β-adrenoceptor blocking compounds.

Treatment is not usually required unless there is associated hypotension or cardiac failure. Atropine 0.6 mg intravenously is indicated and repeated according to the chronotropic and haemodynamic response. Isoprenaline by infusion may also be of value in the acute treatment, and in resistant cases a transvenous atrial or ventricular pacemaker may be required. Ventricular extrasystoles in the presence of sinus bradycardia may also be abolished by increasing the heart rate.

Atrial Extrasystoles

Atrial extrasystoles occur when an ectopic focus discharges prematurely before the next expected S-A nodal impulse. Diagnosis is made on the basis of the following electrocardiographic criteria:

1. A P wave configuration different from sinus beats, with a variable PR interval.
2. A fixed coupling interval to the preceding sinus beat.
3. An incomplete compensatory pause following the extrasystole. The P-P interval is only slightly longer than the sinus P-P interval.

Atrial extrasystoles may occur in normal hearts; however, they may be associated with pathological conditions, including rheumatic heart disease, hyperthyroidism and myocarditis.

Atrial extrasystoles are usually symptomless and do not require therapy unless indicative of underlying cardiac disease. Therapy may be required if the extrasystoles are (a) frequent and persistent, (b) multifocal or (c) bi- or trigeminal, or if the frequency is increased by exercise. These features may indicate early cardiac decompensation and may be followed by the onset of atrial fibrillation.

Pharmacological agents should be considered which have suppressive activity on the atria, i.e.

1. β-Adrenoceptor blocking compounds
2. Disopyramide
3. Quinidine
4. Procainamide

Atrial Fibrillation

The atria generate irregular deflections seen as f waves at the rate of 400–600/min in untreated patients. Haemodynamic disturbances occur following the onset of fibrillation secondary to:

1. Loss of the atrial transport component of ventricular filling.
2. Rapid irregular uncontrolled rates leading to inadequate ventricular filling and emptying.
3. A reduction in stroke volume and cardiac output, with forward and backward manifestations of cardiac failure. This is of particular importance in patients with mitral stenosis.

Atrial fibrillation may be heralded by prodromal atrial arrhythmias, including extrasystoles, tachycardia or atrial flutter.

Atrial fibrillation is especially common when associated with rheumatic valvular disease, particularly that involving the mitral or tricuspid valve. It is often seen secondary to congestive cardiomyopathy and may precipitate the onset of congestive cardiac failure. Common associations are coronary artery disease, pulmonary thromboembolic disease, hyperthyroidism, hypertension and uncorrected atrial septal defect presenting in middle age. Occasionally it may occur in apparently healthy individuals as lone fibrillation, while rarely it is associated with anomalous bypass tracts such as in the Wolff-Parkinson-White and related syndromes.

The long-term treatment includes the management of any underlying conditions predisposing to the development of the acute arrhythmia. The initial aim, however, is to reduce the ventricular response by blocking the number of impulses conducted through the A-V node or by cardioversion to sinus rhythm. If the onset is associated with an uncontrolled ventricular response leading to acute cardiac failure, then early electrical cardioversion may be indicated. When the clinical condition allows, early treatment should be with cardiac glycosides to slow the ventricular response. The route of administration of the loading dose will depend on the clinical condition.

Appropriate diuretic therapy will also be required in the presence of cardiac decompensation. When the ventricular response is difficult to control (which is especially the case during exercise), β-adrenoceptor blocking compounds may be added. Verapamil may also be used as an alternative or in addition to glycoside therapy. Cardiac glycosides are contra-indicated when atrial fibrillation is associated with the Wolff-Parkinson-White or related syndromes. In these conditions glycosides increase the block in the normal A-V conducting tissue and facilitate conduction in the faster conducting anomalous pathway, leading to a faster ventricular response. In these conditions agents should be used which have blocking activity on anomalous pathways such as verapamil, β-blockers or amiodarone. Direct current cardioversion may be used in those cases in which there has been reversal of a precipitating or associated cause. This includes:

1. Following corrective mitral valve surgery.
2. After therapy for thyrotoxicosis.
3. Following dissolution of an intercurrent illness, including respiratory infection or pulmonary embolism. Successful cardioversion and maintenance of sinus rhythm is unlikely if the fibrillation has been present for more than 6 months.

Direct Current Cardioversion.   This abolishes arrhythmias using an external direct current electrical shock. Energy is stored in a capacitor and the discharge is triggered by a monitored tracing by the QRS complex to ensure discharge delivery outside of the ventricular vulnerable period. The electrical discharge transiently depolarises the entire heart, allowing the sinus node, as the fastest intrinsic pacemaker, to reinstitute normal rhythmic function. Direct current cardioversion is unpleasant and the patient should be pretreated with a short-acting anaesthetic, a powerful analgesic or a tranquilliser with amnesic properties. The presence of an anaesthetist is indicated as respiratory depression may occur following the procedure. For atrial arrhythmias, a discharge of some 25–50 joules or watt seconds may be used, increasing this incrementally to 100, 200 and 400 watt seconds. Ventricular arrhythmias generally require this higher level of discharge. Occasional complications may occur following cardioversion. These include the onset of profound bradyarrhythmias or escape tachyarrhythmias. Cardioversion is indicated in the presence of tachyarrhythmias with major haemodynamic sequelae including hypotension or cardiac failure. It is contra-indicated if the tachyarrhythmia is intermittent. Caution must be exercised in the presence of digoxin, as potentially fatal tachyarrhythmias have been reported when there is digoxin toxicity.

Atrial Flutter

Rapid regular atrial activation occurs with a rate of 220–300 beats/minute and is seen as regular repetitive wide deflections of identical shape, size and timing. The rate of atrial discharge may be related to atrial size, slow rates being associated with large atria. Atrioventricular conduction shows variable degrees of block according to the atrial rate. One-to-one conduction may occur with slow flutter rates; however, increased degrees of block are more common (two-to-one or four-to-one). The degree of block may be increased following vagotonic manoeuvres which will not tend to abolish the underlying flutter.

Atrial flutter is associated with the same conditions as atrial fibrillation.

Direct current cardioversion should be performed when the rhythm has serious haemodynamic consequences.

Pharmacological choices include:

1. Cardiac glycosides. Digoxin increases the refractory period of the A-V node and reduces the refractory period of the atrial myocardium, increasing atrial automaticity. These effects may convert atrial flutter to atrial fibrillation. If digoxin is then withdrawn, the resulting increased atrial refractoriness facilitates a return to sinus rhythm.

2. Agents which depress atrial automaticity and block A-V conduction.
    a) β-Adrenoceptor blocking compounds normally slow the ventricular response.
    b) Verapamil may cardiovert or also slow the ventricular response.
    c) Amiodarone may be of particular value in the presence of anomalous pathways.
    d) Quinidine and disopyramide depress conduction in the A-V node, but vagolytic activity may facilitate conduction, converting atrial flutter with block to a lesser degree of block, e.g. two-to-one to one-to-one, and leading to an excessive tachycardia. Cardiac glycosides should be introduced prior to the introduction of these agents so that depression of A-V node conduction will predominate.

Atrial Tachycardia

Atrial tachycardia occurs when there is a rapid succession of three or more consecutive atrial impulses. Its features are as follows:

1. Sudden onset and termination
2. Rapid succession of abnormal P waves, the first and succeeding beats being premature
3. Rate of 160–220 beats/minute
4. Variable duration, from a few seconds to many hours
5. A-V conduction usually one-to-one when atrial rate is less than 200 beats/min. A-V block may occur with faster rates
6. Possible anomalous intraventricular conduction (RBBB, LBBB)

Table 8.3. Choice of drugs used in treatment of supraventricular arrhythmia

Drug (proprietary name)	Dose
1. Verapamil (Cordilox)	5–10 mg i.v. bolus over 30 s. Intravenous infusion 5–10 mg/h — total dose 25–100 mg daily. Oral dose 40–120 mg three times daily
2. *β-Blockers* Practolol (Eraldin)	5 mg i.v. bolus, which may be repeated until 20–25 mg is given
Propranolol (Inderal)	1 mg i.v. bolus, which may be repeated until 5 mg is given
Metoprolol (Betaloc, Lopresor)	5 mg i.v. bolus over 2 min, repeated at 5-min intervals up to a total of 15 mg. Oral dose 50–100 mg three times a day
3. *Others* Digoxin (Lanoxin)	0.5–0.75 mg i.v., then maintenance oral dose of 0.25 mg daily. Avoid in Wolff-Parkinson-White syndrome
Disopyramide (Rhythmodan, Norpace; slow release — Rhythmodan Retard, Dirythmin SA)	2 mg/kg up to 150 mg over 5 min. Repeat if necessary. Maintenance infusion 20–30 mg/h up to 800 mg daily. Oral dose 300–800 mg daily
Amiodarone (Cordarone X)	3.5 mg/kg i.v. over 5 min. Oral dose 200 mg three times daily for first week, then 200 mg daily
Procainamide (Pronestyl; Slow release — Procainamide durules)	100 mg i.v. bolus repeated up to 1 g in 1 h; maintenance 2–6 mg/min. Oral dose 250 mg every 4–6 h or durules 1.0–1.5 g every 8 h
Quinidine (Quinicardine; slow release — Kiditard, Kinidin Durules)	Oral dose 200–400 mg 3–4 times daily or slow release 500 mg every 12 h

The patient may be unaware of the arrhythmia or may have major associated symptoms, including dyspnoea, anginal chest pain and syncope.

Response to physical manoeuvres and standard anti-arrhythmic agents will depend on the mechanism of the arrhythmia. Most supraventricular tachycardias are secondary to re-entrant or circus movement. Vagal manoeuvres may terminate the tachycardia if the A-V node or S-A node is involved in the re-entry circuit. When the sinus or A-V node is not involved in a re-entry circuit, increased vagal tone may transiently decrease ventricular response. Pharmacological treatment is aimed at slowing or blocking conduction at some point within the re-entry circuit.

Pharmacological approaches include:

1. Cardiac glycosides or β-adrenoceptor blocking agents. These depress A-V conduction and prolong the refractory period. They act predominantly on the anterograde slow pathway in cases of A-V nodal re-entrant tachycardia.
2. Verapamil, which exerts a depressant activity in both the slow and fast A-V nodal pathways.
3. Procainamide, quinidine and disopyramide, which prolong the refractory period in the retrograde fast pathway.

4. Amiodarone, which is very effective both in terminating and in preventing episodes of A-V node re-entrant tachycardia.

Therapy can therefore involve compounds with actions on the A-V node, the bypass tract, the atrium, the ventricles or the His-Purkinje system (Table 8.3).

Pacing Techniques for Cardioversion

Cardioversion may be attempted using pacing techniques by inserting a catheter into the atrium. Overdrive pacing at fast rates to capture the S-A node may allow "capture" from the ectopic atrial focus. The patients may remain in sinus rhythm as the pacing rate is sequentially reduced. Underdrive pacing at slow rates may interrupt tachyarrhythmias by rendering one limb of the circuit refractory. Re-entry tachyarrhythmias may also be abolished using programmed stimulation with extra stimuli being introduced either to the atrium or to the ventricles. Varying coupling intervals can be used and the circuit interrupted. Re-entry arrhythmias may also be abolished using high frequency pacing discharges, so-called burst activity.

Ventricular Extrasystoles

Ventricular extrasystoles occur when an ectopic ventricular focus discharges prematurely. The ECG features include:

1. Extrasystole at any time in diastole.
2. A fixed coupling interval (variation less than 0.08) in most cases in which an extrasystole occurs singly.
3. A widened QRS complex, the configuration depending on the site of origin. Secondary ST/T wave changes usually occur.
4. A full compensatory pause, since the S-A node is not usually penetrated by retrograde activity.

Ventricular extrasystoles often occur without symptoms and frequently do not require therapy. The enhanced post-extrasystolic potentiation of the stroke volume may be noticed by the patient or detected in the peripheral pulse. The need for therapy depends on the clinical condition. If ventricular extrasystoles are found in the absence of cardiac disease, therapy is not indicated unless the patient is symptomatic. However, if they are associated with cardiac disease or ECG abnormalities, including ischaemic changes or left ventricular hypertrophy, then a more specific indication is present.

Treatment is usually indicated in these circumstances when ventricular extrasystoles show the following features:

1. Multifocal origin
2. Interspersion with other ventricular arrhythmias
3. Short coupling intervals (R on T)
4. Occurrence as bigemini or in groups
   (See section on acute myocardial infarction)

The various aspects of treatment are outlined below:

1. Avoid precipitating factors, including alcohol, caffeine and tobacco.
2. If the extrasystoles are induced by stress or exercise and are associated with a fast intrinsic sinus rate, β-adrenoceptor blocking compounds may be indicated.
3. If the extrasystoles are associated with sinus bradycardia, atropine may be used acutely while an underlying cause is sought.
4. In most clinical conditions the standard class I anti-arrhythmic agents with ventricular activity should be used (Table 8.4). Lignocaine is the standard drug for intravenous use. For chronic use, quinidine, disopyramide, mexiletine, tocainide and procainamide may all be of value.
5. In the presence of digoxin toxicity, the glycoside should be stopped, hypokalaemia corrected (if present) and an appropriate class I anti-arrhythmic administered.

Table 8.4. Choice of anti-arrhythmic drugs for ventricular arrhythmias

Drug (proprietary name)	Dose
Lignocaine (Xylocard, Lidothesin)	50–100 mg i.v. bolus; infusion 1–4 mg/min. Half dose in hepatic and cardiac failure (see text)
Mexiletine (Mexitil)	100–250 mg over 5–10 min followed by infusion of 250 mg over 1 h, 250 mg over 2 h, then 0.5 mg/min. Oral dose 200–300 mg 8 hourly
Disopyramide	See Table 8.3
Tocainide (Tonocard)	0.5–0.75 mg/kg/min for 15 min. Oral dose 400–800 mg, then 400 mg 8 hourly
Procainamide	See Table 8.3
Phenytoin (Epanutin)	50–100 mg i.v. over 5 min; repeat to 1 g. Oral dose 1 g then 500 mg for 2 days, then 400 mg daily
Quinidine	See Table 8.3
Bretylium tosylate (Bretylate)	5 mg/kg i.m. repeated 6–8 hourly at varying sites to avoid minor necrosis
Flecainide	2 mg/kg slow i.v. injection, maximum 150 mg. Infusion 1.5 mg/kg/h for 1 h, then 250 μg/kg/h

Ventricular Tachycardia

Ventricular tachycardia is defined as three or more consecutive ventricular extrasystoles and is usually a reflection of significant cardiac disease. ECG features include:

1. Widening of QRS complexes; they show bundle branch block configuration with associated ST/T wave changes
2. A heart rate of 140–180 beats/minute
3. A regular rhythm in most cases

Ventricular tachycardia may be of unifocal origin with uniform complexes or, alternatively, may have a varying QRS configuration, suggesting a multifocal origin. Ventricular tachycardia often has severe haemodynamic consequences; it may lead to hypotension, cardiac failure, cardiac pain or even syncope.

Direct current cardioversion is used in the presence of cardiac failure, hypotension or syncope. Parenteral administration of class I anti-arrhythmics may successfully cardiovert the tachycardia and standard prophylactic therapy should then be continued. Class I anti-arrhythmics should initially be administered by the intravenous route, with chronic oral therapy being given as required.

References

Anderson JL, Stewart JR, Perry BA et al. (1981) Oral flecainide acetate for the treatment of ventricular arrhythmias. N Engl J Med 305: 473–477

Bexton RS, Hellestrand KJ, Nathan AW, Spurrell RAJ, Camm AJ (1983) A comparison of the anti-arrhythmic effects on A-V junctional re-entrant tachycardia of oral and intravenous flecainide acetate. Eur Heart J 4 [2]: 92–102

Blomgren SE, Condemi JJ, Vaughan JH (1972) Procainamide-induced lupus erythematosus. Clinical and laboratory observations. Am J Med 53: 338–348

Braunwald E (1982) Mechanisms of action of calcium channel-blocking agents. N Engl J Med 307: 1618–1627

Bryson SM, Whiting B, Lawrence JR (1978) Disopyramide serum and pharmacologic effect kinetics applied to the assessment of bioavailability. Br J Clin Pharmacol 6: 409–419

Campbell RWF, Dolder MA, Prescott LF et al (1975) Comparison of procainamide and mexiletine in prevention of ventricular arrhythmias after acute myocardial infarction. Lancet II: 1257–1264

Chew CYC, Collett J, Singh BN (1979) Mexiletine: a review of its pharmacological properties and therapeutic efficacy in arrhythmias. Drugs 17: 161–181

Coltart DJ, Gibson DG, Shand DG (1971) Plasma propranolol levels associated with suppression of ventricular ectopic beats. Br Med J I: 490–495

Conard GJ, Carlson GL, Frost JW, Ober RE, Leon AS, Hunninghake DB (1976) Human plasma elimination kinetics of R818, a new anti-arrhythmic. Proc A Ph A Acad Pharmaceut Sci. Orlando: 106

Conard GJ, Carlson GL, Frost JW, Ober RE (1979) Human plasma pharmacokinetics of flecainide (R818) a new anti-arrhythmic following single oral and intravenous doses. Clin Pharmacol Ther 25: 218

Giardina EV, Heissenbuttel RH, Bigger JT Jr (1973) Intermittent intravenous procainamide to treat ventricular arrhythmias. Ann Intern Med 78: 183–193

Gupta PK, Lichstein E, Chadda KD (1974) Lidocaine-induced heart block in patients with bundle branch block. Am J Cardiol 33: 487–492

Harrison DC, Alderman EL (1972) The pharmacology and clinical use of Lidocaine as an antiarrhythmic drug — 1972. Harper and Row, Hagerstown, M.D. (Modern Treatment vol 9)

Härtel G, Louhija A, Konttinen A (1974) Disopyramide in the prevention of recurrence of atrial fibrillation after electroversion. Clin Pharmacol Ther 15: 551–555

Holder DA, Sniderman AD, Fraser G, Fallen EL (1977) Experience with bretylium tosylate by a hospital cardiac arrest team. Circulation 55: 541–544

Kessler KM, Lowenthal DT, Warner H et al. (1974) Quinidine elimination in patients with congestive heart failure on poor renal function. N Engl J Med 290: 706–709

Koch-Weser J, Klein SW (1971) Procainamide dosage schedules, plasma concentrations and clinical effects. JAMA 215: 1454–1460

Lalka D et al. (1976) Kinetics of the oral antiarrhythmic Lidocaine congener, tocainide. Clin Pharmacol Ther 19: 757–766

McKenna WJ, Rowland E, Krikler DM (1983) Amiodarone — the experience of the last decade. Br Med J 287: 1654–1656

Nademanee K, Melmed S, Hendrickson JA (1981) Role of serum T_4 and reverse T_3 in monitoring antiarrhythmic efficacy and toxicity of Amiodarone in resistant arrhythmias. Am J Cardiol 47: 482

Packer M, Meller J, Medina N (1982) Haemodynamic consequences of combined beta-adrenergic and slow calcium channel blockade in man. Circulation 65: 660–668

Reidenberg MM, Drayer DE, Levy M et al. (1975) Polymorphic acetylation of procainamide in man. Clin Pharmacol Ther 17: 722–730

Rinkenberger RL, Prystowsky EW, Heger JJ et al. (1980) Effect of intravenous and chronic oral verapamil administration in patients with supraventricular tachyarrhythmias. Circulation 62: 996–1010

Rowland M, Thomson PD, Guichard A et al. (1971) Disposition kinetics of Lidocaine in normal subjects. Ann NY Acad Sci 179: 383–397

Selzer A, Wray HW (1964) Quinidine syncope: paroxysmal ventricular fibrillation occurring during treatment of chronic atrial arrhythmias. Circulation 30: 17–26

Singh BN, Ellrodt G, Peter CT (1978) Verapamil: A review of its pharmacological properties and therapeutic uses. Drugs 15: 169–203

Singh BN, Collett JT, Chew CYC (1980) New perspectives in the pharmacologic therapy of cardiac arrhythmias. Prog Cardovasc Dis 22: 243–301

Thomson PD, Melmon KL, Richardson JA et al. (1973) Lidocaine pharmacokinetics in advanced heart failure, liver disease and renal failure in humans. Ann Intern Med 78: 499–508

Ueda CT, Williamson BJ, Bzindzio BS (1976) Absolute quinidine bioavailability. Clin Pharmacol Ther 20: 260–265

Vaughan Williams EM (1970) Classification of antiarrhythmic drugs. In: Sandboe E, Flensted-Jensen KH, Olesen AB (eds) Symposium on cardiac arrhythmias. Astra, Sodertalje, Sweden, pp 449–472

Winkle RA et al. (1976) Clinical efficacy and pharmacokinetics of a new orally effective anti-arrhythmic Tocainide. Circulation 54: 884–889

Zipes DP, Troup PJ (1978) New antiarrhythmic agents Amiodarone, Aprindine, disopyramide, Ethmozin, mexiletine, tocainide, verapamil. Am J Cardiol 41: 1005–1024

9 **Cardiac Failure**

The clinical syndrome of cardiac failure has long been recognised, but its management remains one of the major problems in clinical cardiology. About one-quarter of patients with cardiovascular disease have heart failure and the long-term prognosis is determined by the degree to which cardiac performance is impaired (Klainer et al. 1965). Recent innovations in the investigation of cardiac patients have increased our understanding of the mechanism of cardiac failure and aided the development of a logical approach to its long-term management.

Definition

Cardiac failure is defined as a "clinical state resulting from the inability of the heart to provide sufficient blood for tissue metabolic needs". Although the absolute value of the cardiac output is usually reduced, cardiac failure may occur with a normal or even high cardiac output, according to the underlying cause. Cardiac failure may affect the left ventricle alone, the right ventricle alone or both. Right ventricular failure may occur secondary to failure of the left ventricle or be the result of primary pulmonary disease involving the lung tissue or vessels, when it is termed cor pulmonale or pulmonary heart disease. The signs and symptoms of cardiac failure depend on the predominantly affected ventricle. They are due to poor organ and tissue perfusion associated with inadequate cardiac output (forward failure) and the effects of increased back pressure due to inadequate ventricular emptying.

Regulation of Cardiac Function

In the intact heart there are three principal determinants of the stroke volume: preload, contractility and afterload. (Fig. 9.1)

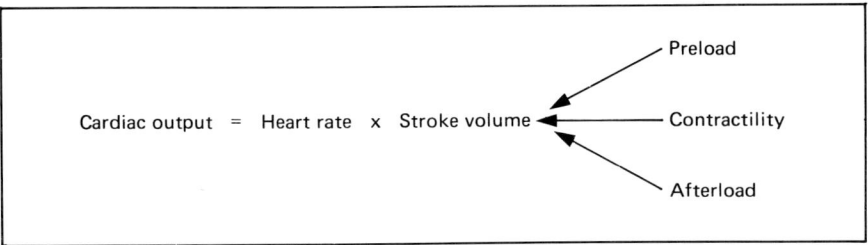

Fig. 9.1. Factors involved in the regulation of cardiac function.

Preload

The concept of preload arises from studies of contraction of isolated muscle strips (Sonnenblick et al. 1964). The force generated following stimulation is enhanced by increasing the resting fibre length. In the intact heart preload is determined by the volume of blood in the ventricle at the end of diastole. An increased end-diastolic volume increases the stroke volume ejected. Increased stretching of myocardial muscle fibres augments their contractile power. The left ventricular end-diastolic volume can be measured by contrast angiography, gated radionuclide ventriculography or echocardiography.

The left ventricular end-diastolic pressure (left atrial or left ventricular filling pressure) is closely related to the left ventricular end-diastolic volume and is often used as an expression of preload. It may be measured directly via left heart catheterisation or indirectly from a peripheral pulmonary artery (pulmonary wedge pressure).

Contractility

Contractility is the force of ventricular contraction and is independent of loading. Contractility depends on the interaction of the contractile proteins myosin and actin, which are found in the thick and thin filaments of the myocardial sarcomere. Energy is derived from ATP, which is rapidly hydrolysed by actomyosin ATPase, which transduces its chemical energy to mechanical work. The rate of contraction is proportional to the intrinsic ATPase of the myosin molecule. The amount of force generated depends on the number of actin and myosin interactions. Ca^{2+} initiates activation and determines the maximum force generated by controlling the number of active interactions between the thick and thin filaments (Fabiato and Fabiato 1979).

Afterload

Afterload is an expression of the resistance which a ventricle must overcome to eject the stroke volume. The total vascular resistance is the sum of the proximal resistance in the aorta (impedance) and the peripheral vascular resistance, which is a reflection of the cross-sectional area of the systemic vascular beds (Mason 1967). This distal resistance is controlled by several neurohumoral mechanisms.

The total vascular resistance may be derived from simultaneous measurements of the mean arterial pressure and cardiac output (Mills et al. 1970). If the vascular resistance is reduced, ventricular ejection is facilitated and the cardiac output raised (Miller et al. 1976). Conversely, increased peripheral vascular resistance increases ventricular systolic pressure, wall stress and ventricular radius. Myocardial oxygen consumption is increased and the ejection fraction reduced (Mason 1967).

Pathophysiology

The pathophysiological changes which result in cardiac failure in an individual depend on the mechanism and the resulting effects on the factors regulating cardiac function (Table 9.1). These factors include:

1. Pressure overload on a ventricle, leading to increased afterload.
2. Volume overload leading to ventricular dilatation and increased preload.
3. Myocardial disease, which affects contractility. It may be diffuse, as in cardiomyopathy, or segmental, as in coronary artery disease.

Cardiac failure may occur despite the maintenance of a high cardiac output in the presence of high metabolic or circulatory demands.

Compensatory Mechanisms

In cardiac failure several compensatory or adaptive mechanism are stimulated to maintain cardiac output and organ perfusion pressure (mean arterial pressure). These are both cardiac and extracardiac in origin.

Cardiac Mechanisms

1. *Heart rate*:   Tachycardia may occur when the stroke volume is reduced.

Table 9.1 Causes of cardiac failure

Pressure load		Volume overload		Myocardial disease	High output cardiac failure
Left ventricle	Right ventricle	Left ventricle	Right ventricle		
Aortic stenosis	Pulmonary stenosis	Aortic valve regurgitation	Atrial septal defect	Coronary artery disease	Hyperthyroidism
Hypertrophic obstructive cardiomyopathy	Pulmonary hypertension	Mitral valve regurgitation	Ventricular septal defect	Congestive cardiomyopathy	Beri beri
Hypertension		Arteriovenous fistula	Pulmonary valve regurgitation	Secondary cardiomyopathy	Paget's disease
			Tricuspid valve regurgitation	Myocarditis	Pulmonary emphysema

2. *Ventricular dilatation*:   The Frank-Starling mechanism is invoked. As the ventricular volume increases (preload), the cardiac output is increased. This response is progressively limited, however, with increasing ventricular dilatation. The beneficial effects are lost when volume is greater than twice normal (Sonnenblick et al. 1964). Further dilatation is accompanied by an increase in ventricular wall stress and an increase in left ventricular end-diastolic pressure.

3. *Ventricular hypertrophy*:   If an increased systolic load is sustained, compensatory left ventricular hypertrophy occurs to maintain pump function. This is also stimulated by loss of myocytes. When hypertrophy is associated with normal myosin ATPase activity, this increase in wall thickness is physiological. As cellular hypertrophy advances, increase in muscle mass is limited to the extent to which coronary vasodilatation may occur (Spann et al. 1967). An increase in connective tissue occurs, with interstitial fibrosis and a reduction in myofibril content with respect to the muscle cell volume (Wikman-Coffelt et al. 1979). These developments interfere with normal contractile function and eventually cardiac ejection is impaired.

Extracardiac Mechanisms (Fig. 9.2)

1. *Increased sympathetic nervous activity*:   Following the reduction in cardiac output, arterial pressure falls. This leads to stimulation of afferent impulses from baroreceptors in the aortic arch and carotid sinus. Inadequate emptying of the ventricle leads to an increase in the left ventricular end-diastolic pressure, and increased pressure in the left atrium and pulmonary veins. Mechanoreceptors are stimulated, giving an afferent input to the central motor cortex in the mid-brain. This leads to stimulation of sympathetic nervous activity and withdrawal of vagal tone (Malliani 1982). Sympathetic activity has an advantageous effect by increasing the heart rate and contractility. Subsequent depletion of cardiac catecholamine stores makes the heart less responsive (Zelis and Flaim 1982). Venoconstriction increases venous return and increases preload.

Arterial vasoconstriction occurs, with regional redistribution of the peripheral blood flow to maintain the supply to skeletal muscle and heart while that to the liver, gastrointestinal tract and kidneys is decreased (Nellis et al. 1980). Although this is a useful short-term change, in the long term it leads to a sustained rise in systemic vascular resistance and aortic impedance, with a secondary reduction in cardiac output.

2. *Renin-angiotensin-aldosterone system* (Fig. 9.3):   Stimulation of β-adrenoceptors in the juxtaglomerular apparatus of the kidney results in renin release (Watkins et al. 1976). Increased plasma renin activity stimulates production of angiotensin I, which in the presence of angiotensin converting enzyme is converted to the active vasoconstrictor substance angiotensin II. This further vasoconstriction has a beneficial effect in maintaining arterial pressure but again leads to a reduced cardiac output by increasing afterload

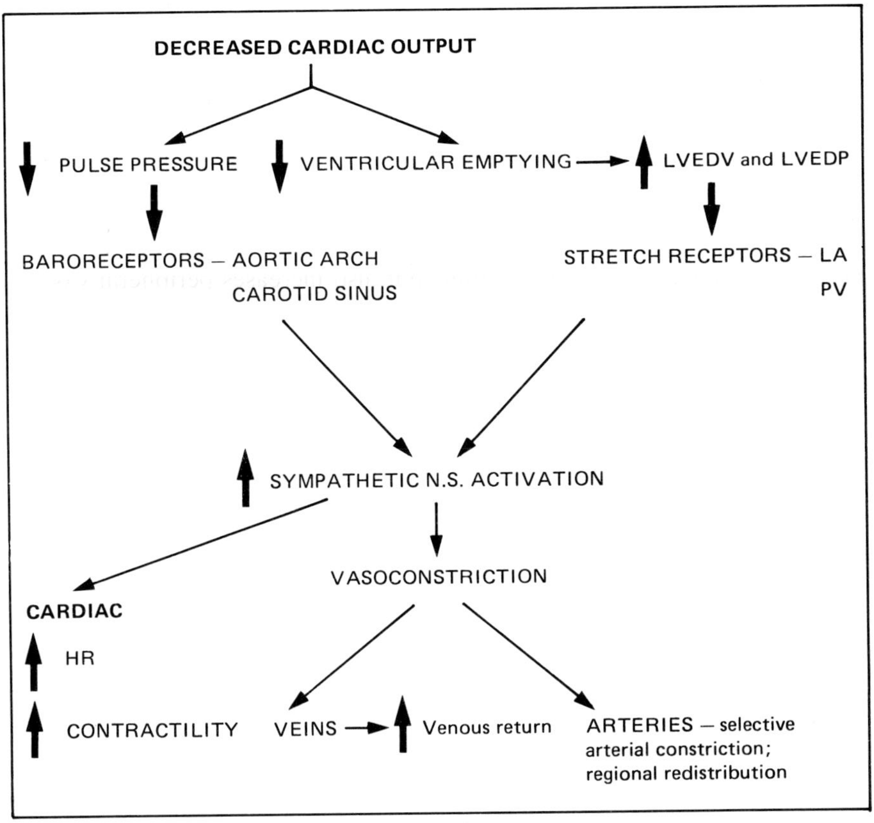

DECREASED CARDIAC OUTPUT

↓ PULSE PRESSURE   ↓ VENTRICULAR EMPTYING ⟶ ↑ LVEDV and LVEDP

↓ BARORECEPTORS – AORTIC ARCH
CAROTID SINUS

STRETCH RECEPTORS – LA
PV

↑ SYMPATHETIC N.S. ACTIVATION

VASOCONSTRICTION

CARDIAC

↑ HR

↑ CONTRACTILITY   VEINS ⟶ ↑ Venous return   ARTERIES – selective
arterial constriction;
regional redistribution

Fig. 9.2. Extracardiac compensatory mechanisms in cardiac failure.

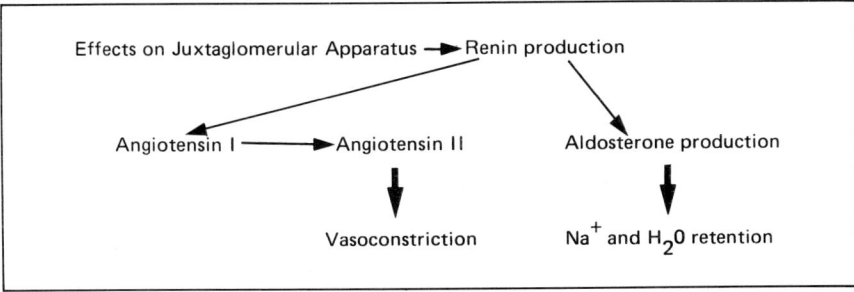

Effects on Juxtaglomerular Apparatus ⟶ Renin production

Angiotensin I ⟶ Angiotensin II   Aldosterone production

↓ Vasoconstriction   ↓ Na^+ and H_2O retention

Fig. 9.3. The renin-angiotensin-aldosterone system as an extracardiac compensatory mechanism.

(Davis and Freeman 1976). Within the kidney blood flow is reduced selectively to the outer cortical glomeruli, with the inner cortical glomeruli and loops of Henle being preferentially perfused. Adrenal aldosterone production is stimulated by renin and acts on the distal convoluted tubule with resultant sodium and water retention and plasma volume expansion (Nicholls et al. 1974). This maintains cardiac preload but eventually leads to the development of oedema (Watkins et al. 1976). In addition, renal retention of sodium leads to an increased vascular sodium content which causes an increased stiffness along the arterial tree (Zelis et al. 1970). This serves to maintain blood pressure in the face of an inadequate cardiac output, but also increases peripheral vascular resistance by impeding vascular relaxation.

Symptoms and Signs of Left Heart Failure

Dyspnoea

An increased awareness of respiration is the usual presenting symptom. Exertional dyspnoea is caused by increasing pulmonary vascular engorgement with decreased compliance secondary to inadequate emptying of the left ventricle. This leads to increased pressure in the left atrium and pulmonary veins. The New York Heart Association classification is useful in assessing the patient's symptomatic awareness (Table 9.2). There is not, however, always a close correlation with objective testing of exercise capacity.

Table 9.2. Functional status according to the N.Y.H.A.

Class I	Patients with cardiac disease but without limitation during ordinary physical activity.
Class II	Cardiac disease associated with slight limitations. Ordinary physical activity such as walking causes dyspnoea.
Class III	Marked limitation in physical activity. Unable to walk even on a level without disability. Less than ordinary activity causes dyspnoea.
Class IV	Inability to carry on any physical activity. Dyspnoea at rest.

Orthopnoea

Exertional dyspnoea may proceed to breathlessness at rest.

Paroxysmal Nocturnal Dyspnoea

Paroxysmal nocturnal dyspnoea may occur as the first manifestation of hypertensive heart disease, aortic valve disease or mitral valve disease. Nocturnal absorption of oedema fluid increases the intravascular volume. The patient may be wakened with gasping respiration associated with an irritating cough.

Acute Pulmonary Oedema

Acute left ventricular failure can be a dramatic illness which may lead to pulmonary oedema owing to rapid development of pulmonary capillary hypertension with acute and marked transudation of fluid into the pulmonary alveoli. This usually follows an acute rise in the left ventricular volume and the left ventricular end-diastolic pressure. When the pulmonary capillary pressure reaches a value greater than the plasma oncotic pressure (25–30 mmHg), transudation of fluid occurs and pulmonary oedema develops. Acute respiratory distress results, with marked ventilatory impairment secondary to reduced gas exchange and increased work associated with breathing. Hypoxia occurs secondary to an increased resistance of air flow in and out of the alveoli. In addition there is alveolar flooding with fluid, which reduces the diffusion of gases from alveolar air into capillary blood. In addition, reduced pulmonary compliance further increases the work-load of the respiratory muscles. The mucous membranes are engorged by oedema fluid, leading to bronchoconstriction (cardiac asthma). Increased mucous production may precipitate coughing, and pink frothy sputum may be produced.

In acute pulmonary oedema, the patients looks anxious and generally complains of a sense of suffocation. There is increased sympathetic discharge, with sweating and peripheral vasoconstriction. There is tachypnoea. Additional heart sounds may be present, and rhonchi, bronchospasm and rales are sometimes widespread.

Exertional Fatigue and Weakness

Exertional fatigue and weakness are manifestations of poor muscle and organ perfusion. Increased vascular stiffness, secondary to fluid retention, prevents the appropriate increase in skeletal muscle blood flow despite maximal metabolic vasodilatation during exercise (Nellis et al. 1980; Zelis et al. 1968). The anaerobic threshold is lowered and there is a shift to anaerobic metabolism, resulting in lactic acidaemia and an oxygen debt.

Signs of left heart failure are often those of the intrinsic cause of left ventricular dysfunction, such as valvular or hypertensive heart disease. There may be abnormalities of the pulse, apex beat and heart sounds. Non-specific signs include tachycardia with pulsus alternans, cardiomegaly, gallop rhythm with third or fourth heart sounds and basilar rales indicative of pulmonary congestion.

Symptoms and Signs of Right Heart Failure

Right heart failure may occur secondary to left heart failure or develop from a primary intracardiac cause, including mitral stenosis, pulmonary valve stenosis, tricuspid regurgitation or congenital heart disease. Symptoms are secondary to increased right heart pressure, with resulting systemic venous distention involving the gut and liver and causing peripheral oedema. Clinical signs include elevated jugular venous pressure and, often, functional tricuspid regurgitation. A left parasternal heave of right ventricular hypertrophy is usually evident, with a loud pulmonary second sound.

Investigations in Cardiac Failure

Electrocardiography

Routine electrocardiography is extremely useful in the assessment of patients with cardiac failure. In particular it may:

1. Confirm the cardiac rhythm. This is particularly useful in the presence of a brady- or tachyarrhythmia which may have precipitated or exacerbated the cardiac failure. If the rhythm is sinus, then P wave activity may indicate right or left atrial hypertrophy.
2. Indicate right or left ventricular hypertrophy from the configuration of the QRS complex. This may be of particular value in confirming right ventricular hypertrophy in cor pulmonale and in assessing target organ involvement in systemic hypertension.
3. Identify specific changes indicating myocardial infarction or cardiac drug effects, e.g. digoxin.

Chest X-ray

Routine chest X-ray is useful in confirming the cardiac size and may also give a qualitative indication of cardiac chamber or main vessel enlargement. Pulmonary congestion may be evident, with upper lobe blood diversion and enlarged lymphatics in the lower lobes.

Echocardiography

Echocardiography is a useful non-invasive technique which can assess:

1. Chamber dilation (left atrium, right ventricle, left ventricle).
2. Valvular disease. Echocardiography is particularly useful in mitral stenosis, aortic stenosis or regurgitation and occasionally tricuspid or pulmonary valve disease.
3. Left ventricular function; this is determined from measurement of left ventricular end-diastolic and end-systolic diameters.

Invasive Investigations

Right heart catheterisation using flow-directed (balloon-tipped) catheters is useful in measuring pulmonary artery and pulmonary wedge pressures both in patients with acute and in those with chronic cardiac failure. Serial measurements of pressure and cardiac output are extremely useful in assessing the response to therapy.

Combined right and left heart cardiac catheterisation with left ventricular angiography, aortography and coronary arteriography may be indicated for diagnostic purposes, but are of particular value in assessing those patients in whom surgical management may be required.

Management of Cardiac Failure

The treatment of cardiac failure is determined by the severity of the clinical presentation, which may vary from life-threatening pulmonary oedema to mild congestive changes with peripheral oedema. In many instances, particularly in the presence of congenital or valvular heart disease, the eventual treatment will be surgical.

The general approach to the treatment of cardiac failure should include:

1. Identification and treatment of precipitating factors
2. The introduction of general measures and specific anti-failure therapy
3. Long-term management (Taylor et al. 1982)

Precipitating Factors

Precipitating factors may affect the heart itself or increase peripheral circulatory or metabolic requirements (Table 9.3). They should be treated vigorously, as a previously stable clinical situation may be re-established.

Table 9.3. Precipitating factors for cardiac failure

Direct cardiac factors

Myocardial infarction
Arrhythmia — tachycardia
                bradycardia
Bacterial endocarditis
Drugs with negative inotropic activity, e.g. β-adrenoceptor blocking compounds, anti-
    arrhythmics
Pulmonary embolism
Non-compliance with anti-failure therapy

Extracardiac factors

Infection
Anaemia
Pregnancy
Thyrotoxicosis
Excessive fluid transfusion
Physical or emotional stress

General Treatment

The major aims of treatment are to augment the cardiac output and to reverse the pathophysiological changes which lead to cardiac decompensation. The therapeutic approaches attempt to (a) increase salt and water excretion using diuretics, (b) enhance the contractility of the heart by inotropes and (c) relieve pressure and volume overload by means of vasodilators.

General Supportive Measures

1. *Rest.*   The degree of rest required will obviously depend on the individual patient. Bed rest with the patient in the semi-recumbent position will reduce cardiac work and improve diuresis. Passive or active leg exercises should be encouraged to prevent the development of deep venous thrombosis. Commodes are preferable to bedpans. The aim should be progressive ambulation and optimal rehabilitation.

2. *Diet.*   There is controversy about dietary salt. The use of diuretics may make it adequate merely to refrain from adding salt at meal times. Drugs with a high sodium content should be avoided, as should those leading to salt and water retention such as carbenoxolone and the non-steroidal anti-inflammatory drugs.

In mild cardiac failure, particularly in the elderly, treatment at home is advisable if at all possible. In younger patients, however, when detailed investigation may be indicated, early hospital referral is required.

Specific Antifailure Therapy

Diuretic Therapy

A major advance in the treatment of cardiac failure has been the development of potent diuretics. These inhibit sodium reabsorption by the kidney and reduce intravascular volume, preload and hence left ventricular volume. The reduction in the sodium content of arteriolar walls reduces impedance and ventricular afterload. Myocardial contractility may be improved by a reduction in ventricular wall stiffness.

The choice of diuretic depends on the clinical situation. The thiazides are usually employed for mild failure, while the powerful or loop diuretics are used for moderate to severe failure. Combinations of diuretic therapy may also be used.

THIAZIDE DIURETICS

Thiazide diuretics act on the distal convoluted tubule and increase membrane permeability to sodium and chloride. The maximum increase in sodium excretion is some 5%–8% of the filtered load, and these agents become relatively ineffective in patients with glomerular filtration rates of less than 30 ml/min. The thiazides are rapidly absorbed from the gastrointestinal tract and most agents exhibit a diuretic action within 1 h of oral administration. Toxicity with thiazides is usually rare and may take the form of unsuspected hypersensitivity, purpura, dermatitis and blood dyscrasias.

Metabolic abnormalities may accompany their long-term use:

1. Hypokalaemia occurs following increased potassium secretion by the distal tubule. This is particularly important in cardiac failure, especially with concomitant administration of the cardiac glycosides. Potassium supplementation is usually required. The introduction of potassium-sparing diuretics or aldosterone antagonists may be helpful in patients prone to hypokalaemia.
2. Uric acid excretion is reduced and clinical gout may be precipitated.
3. Hyperglycaemia may occur and control of diabetes may be somewhat impaired.

Despite these metabolic side-effects, the thiazides are invaluable in the long-term management of mild to moderate cardiac failure.

LOOP DIURETICS

Loop diuretics are very potent, have a prompt onset of action and act by inhibiting sodium and chloride transport in the ascending limb of the loop of Henle. They are used when a prompt and effective diuresis is required. Loop diuretics have vasodilating properties and reduce preload before their diuretic activity is evident.

Frusemide is the agent in most widespread clinical use at present. It is a potent diuretic and fractional sodium excretion of more than 20% of the filtered load may be achieved. Additional diuretic actions may be secondary to reversal of shunting of blood from the cortical medullary nephrons, and in addition there may be a prostaglandin-mediated mechanism (Lal et al. 1969). Frusemide is active by both the intravenous and the oral route. It has a wide therapeutic range and its effects are proportional to its dosage. The oral dose is 40 mg and, when required, a similar intravenous dose may be administered. In the present of renal failure, high intravenous doses may be required. A dose of up to 500 mg may be effective when the glomerular filtration rate is less than 20 ml/min. In cardiac failure with oral therapy, the bio-availability may be reduced to some 50% and a potent diuresis may be obtained by changing the drug administration to the intravenous route (Dikshit et al. 1973; Nelson et al. 1982a).

Side-effects. In view of its high potency, frusemide is relatively contra-indicated in patients who are hypotensive and hyponatraemic. In males an acute diuresis may precipitate acute retention, especially if prostatic hypertrophy is present. Hypokalaemia may also occur, requiring potassium supplementation. Cephalosporin nephrotoxicity may be increased, and lithium levels may be enhanced if frusemide is given concomitantly. Further side-effects include nausea, malaise and gastric upset; occasionally allergic rashes occur and hyperuricaemia precipitates clinical gout. In elderly patients following control of acute cardiac failure, the continued severe diuresis with rapid onset and marked duration may be unacceptable and maintenance diuretic therapy with thiazides may be given as an alternative. In patients with resistant oedema, a combination of thiazide and loop diuretics may be given. Alternative agents to frusemide are ethacrynic acid and bumetanide. Ethacrynic acid is readily absorbed from the gastrointestinal tract but can also be given by the intravenous route. The metabolic side-effects are similar to those of frusemide and similar caution should be exercised in patients who are hypotensive. It is available in 25 and 50 mg tablets, usual dosage being 50–250 mg daily in divided doses. Bumetanide is a more potent diuretic than frusemide, but the maximal effect is the same.

In cardiac failure the major haemodynamic effect resulting from the use of the loop diuretics is a reduction in preload, but usually without a change in cardiac output. Recent studies suggest that bumetanide may increase the cardiac output following slight afterload reduction.

ALDOSTERONE ANTAGONISTS

Spironolactone is a competitive antagonist of aldosterone, the most potent endogenous mineralocorticoid. Spironolactone is useful in the management of congestive cardiac failure, particularly in the presence of hepatic congestion, when secondary hyperaldosteronism is usual. The mineralocorticoids augment renal tubular reabsorption of sodium and chloride but lead to increased potassium excretion by facilitation of sodium–potassium exchange. Spironolactone antagonises potassium excretion and may be a useful adjunctive therapy in patients who are hypokalaemic on other diuretic therapy. Spironolactone is effective in an average daily dose of 100 mg given in divided doses. The onset of action may be at least 48–72 h, and hence more potent diuretics are generally used if diuresis is urgently required. When spironolactone is administered in the presence of renal insufficiency, hyperkalaemia may be a problem and frequent monitoring of serum potassium is indicated. In patients with severe cardiac failure and resistant oedema, combination therapy with diuretics with different modes of action is indicated. Metolazone, whose site of action and potency is similar to that of chlorthiazide, is particularly useful in patients with severe renal impairment. It has a long duration of action of some 24–48 h and it may be of great value as adjunctive therapy to loop diuretics in patients with refractory cardiac failure.

Positive Inotropes

There has been a continued search for compounds which will improve contractility by stimulating myocardial function (Sonnenblick and Le Jemtel 1982; Scholz 1983; Katz and Smith et al. 1982). The ideal agent should have:

1. Efficacy. There should be adequate cardiac stimulation without detrimental peripheral vasoconstriction or oxygen-wasting tachycardia from reflex or direct stimulation.
2. Rapid onset of action with a wide therapeutic ratio, few side-effects and persistent activity with absence of tachyphylaxis.
3. Intravenous and oral formulations to allow both acute and long-term therapy to be administered.

Table 9.4. Drugs with inotropic activity

Drug	Mechanism
Cardiac glycosides	Action on $(Na^+ + K^+)$ ATPase
β_1-Adrenoceptor drugs Noradrenaline Adrenaline Isoprenaline Dopamine Dobutamine Prenalterol	Increased cAMP, stimulation of adenylate cyclase, increased Ca^{2+} uptake by sarcoplasmic reticulum
Methylxanthines Theophylline	Phosphodiesterase inhibition; increased cAMP Positive inotrope: venous and arteriolar dilatation
β_2-Adrenoceptor drugs Salbutamol Terbutaline Pirbuterol	Positive inotropic activity: peripheral vasodilatation leads to reduced preload and afterload

Although many compounds are available (Table 9.4) none so far fulfil all the criteria listed. Some are available for parenteral use only and are limited to acute treatment in hospital with haemodynamic monitoring.

CATECHOLAMINES

Catecholamines stimulate β-receptors on the cardiac cell surface. Their use, however, is limited by stimulation of other peripheral receptors (α or β_2). Dopamine and dobutamine are widely used in the treatment of cardiac failure following acute myocardial infarction, especially in the presence of hypotension. Prenalterol is available for intravenous usage and may be of particular value when cardiac failure develops in patients who have already been treated with β-adrenoceptor blocking compounds (Hutton et al. 1980; Klein et al. 1981). Several compounds used in clinical practice for bronchodilatation with predominant β_2-agonist properties have been shown to have positive inotropic and vasodilating properties when give orally (Bourdillon et al. 1980; Nelson et al. 1982b). These have not, however, been promoted for the treatment of cardiac failure. Beneficial inotropic and vasodilating actions have also been shown with phosphodiesterase-inhibiting compounds, including theophylline. Although widely used as bronchodilating drugs in patients with cor pulmonale, their use has been limited in patients with cardiac failure of other aetiology (Hillis and Been 1982).

CARDIAC GLYCOSIDES

The mainstay of inotropic treatment remains the cardiac glycosides. These cardioactive steroids have both positive inotropic and electrophysiological effects. The principal indication for their use is cardiac failure and atrial fibrillation. The slowing of the ventricular rate they produce is probably more beneficial than their inotropic activity. Controversy remains over their role in patients with cardiac failure who remain in sinus rhythm. Several studies have shown positive inotropic activity both with acute and chronic therapy, using both invasive and non-invasive methods of assessment (Arnold et al. 1980; O'Rourke et al. 1976, Kleimann et al. 1978; Firth et al. 1980). Population studies, however, have emphasised that cardiac glycosides may often be withdrawn without detrimental clinical effect, and their routine use in mild cardiac failure, particularly in elderly patients, must be questioned.

In high output states such as thyrotoxicosis and in pulmonary heart disease, the response to digoxin is usually disappointing.

The *mechanism of action* of cardiac glycosides is uncertain, although experimental evidence suggests that the cardiac glycosides inhibit sodium transport by binding to and inhibiting the monovalent cation transport enzyme complex sodium–potassium–ATPase (Skou 1957; Erdmann and Brown 1983). Reduction of sodium ion pumping produces an increment in the internal sodium which permits an augmentation of free calcium ion, resulting in enhanced actomyosin coupling with consequent positive inotropic action. This alteration in ion movement is considered to be the main mechanism of inotropic action.

although other actions, including a direct effect on the contractile proteins, cannot be excluded.

Various *preparations* are available, as listed below:

Digoxin is the most commonly used glycoside. It is of intermediate polarity and can be given by the parenteral (usually i.v.) or oral route. The onset of action is 15–30 min (its peak effect is achieved at 2–5 h), and its elimination half-life is 36 h. Only some 6% is metabolised by the liver, and its elimination is predominantly determined by glomerular filtration and renal excretion of the unchanged molecule.

Ouabain is the most water-soluble (polar) glycoside. It is administered by the intravenous route, being poorly absorbed orally. Its onset of action is 5–10 min (peak effect is at 30–120 min), and its average half-life is 21 h.

Digitoxin is the most fat-soluble glycoside and may be given by the intravenous or oral route. Gastrointestinal absorption is almost complete. The onset of action is 25–120 min and the peak effect is at 4–12 h. It is highly protein-bound and has extensive hepatic metabolism. Its elimination half-life is 4–6 days and is not altered by renal function.

Dosage schedules are determined by pharmacokinetic properties and factors which influence individual responsiveness. A loading followed by a maintenance dose is given. With digoxin the major determinant of the elimination half-life is renal function. The maintenance dose must therefore be reduced if renal function is subnormal and excretion is impaired. Normally digoxin has a narrow therapeutic range, i.e. 1–2 ng/ml; toxic side-effects may be seen with levels between 2 and 5 ng/ml. Potassium and glycosides compete for myocardial binding sites and hypokalaemia can exaggerate the toxic effects of glycosides, including arrhythmias. The concomitant administration of quinidine leads to an enhanced plasma level, and in these circumstances the maintenance digoxin dose may be halved (see p. 11). Ouabain may be of value in the present of atrial fibrillation with an uncontrolled ventricular rate, as its slightly more rapid onset of action may confer minor additional benefit. In patients with marked renal impairment, digitoxin may be appropriate in view of its hepatic excretion. Drug monitoring of plasma glycoside levels has been useful, especially in patients with renal impairment and suspected toxicity and to check patient compliance.

Digitalis Toxicity. The effects of digitalis toxicity remain common and are either extracardiac or cardiac. Extracardiac effects are:

1. Gastrointestinal upset with anorexia, nausea, vomiting and diarrhoea
2. Central nervous symptoms, including fatigue, somnolence, dizziness, headache and confusion; coloured halos may be seen, particularly by elderly subjects
3. Gynaecomastia, which may be seen, is an oestrogen-steroid effect

The commonest cardiac side-effects are secondary to enhanced automaticity. Arrhythmias include ventricular bigemini, while multifocal ventricular extrasystoles or tachycardia can occur. Paroxysmal atrial tachycardia (typically with A-V block) can develop. There may be heart block in conjunction with escape rhythms, due to excessive depression of the atrioventricular node. PR prolongation is frequently seen, and typical ST/T wave changes are noted on the electrocardiogram. Contra-indications to the use of cardiac glycosides include heart block and rare conditions such as hypertrophic obstructive cardiomyopathy and Wolff-Parkinson-White syndrome, in which cardiac glycosides, far from controlling arrhythmias, may actually precipitate them by accelerating anomalous pathway conduction.

Vasodilators

The most important recent innovation in the treatment of cardiac failure has been the use of compounds with vasodilating activity (Cohn and Franciosa 1977; Miller et al. 1976). These have been mainly used in patients with severe cardiac failure. Their place in the treatment of milder degrees of cardiac failure awaits further study. Earlier introduction has been suggested in an attempt to reduce the need for diuretic therapy, with its metabolic sequelae, and to avoid hyponatraemia, which may accompany long-term diuretic use.

RATIONALE

There are two methods by which vasodilators may benefit cardiac failure:

1. *Reduction of afterload*. As indicated above, compensatory peripheral vascular changes occur in cardiac failure, leading to arteriolar vasoconstriction and increased left ventricular afterload. The reduction of systemic vascular resistance and lowered impedance lead to an improved ejection fraction and stroke volume.

2. *Reduction of preload*. Ventricular function is improved by lowering left ventricular end-diastolic volume and diastolic pressure. Drugs which increase venous capacitance reduce venous return to the heart and ventricular volume.

In most patients with congestive cardiac failure, however, the haemodynamic changes are a combination of a low cardiac output and high filling pressure, and hence therapy with compounds having both arteriolar and venous dilating effects has been assessed. Many studies have attempted to develop a rational approach to the selection of vasodilating therapy. These have employed haemodynamic monitoring with measurement of the filling pressure of the left ventricle indirectly from the pulmonary capillary wedge pressure, and measurement of the cardiac output using the thermodilution technique. The baseline haemodynamic values have been used as a guide to the logical introduction of vasodilating therapy (Chatterjee et al. 1978). If the filling pressure is high and cardiac output satisfactory, then venodilators have been used. If the filling pressure is acceptable and cardiac output low, then arteriolar dilators have been used. The combination of high filling pressure and low cardiac output has warranted the use of compounds with mixed dilator effect.

Table 9.5 indicates the compounds shown to benefit the haemodynamic derangement in cardiac failure.

Table 9.5. Vasodilator drugs used in cardiac failure

Drug	Route of administration	Mode and site of action
Nitrates	Intravenous Oral Sublingual Transdermal	Direct effects on veins: high dosage may reduce arterial pressure. Predominant effect on venous capacitance vessels, with reduction in preload.
Hydralazine	Intravenous Oral	Direct action on vascular smooth muscle. Arteriolar dilatation leads to increased cardiac output, which may be accompanied by reflex tachycardia.
Nitroprusside	Intravenous	Mixed venous and arteriolar dilating activity. Particularly useful after acute myocardial infarction.
Prazosin	Oral	Postsynaptic α-receptor blocking agent. Mixed venous and arteriolar activity.
Captopril Enalapril	Oral	Angiotensin converting enzyme inhibitor. Reduces vasoconstrictor angiotensin II. May reduce vasoconstrictor activity of catecholamines. Vasodilator bradykinin may be increased. Exhibits mixed venous and arteriolar dilatation, leading to decreased preload and afterload.

PARENTERAL THERAPY

In acute cardiac failure intravenous nitrates, hydralazine or nitroprusside have been used. Intravenous administration is used to start treatment and to assess the haemodynamic response so that logical oral therapy can be introduced.

LONG-TERM ORAL THERAPY

Beneficial central haemodynamic changes and associated symptomatic improvement have been demonstrated following long-term therapy with compounds possessing vasodilating activity. These have usually been given in conjunction with diuretic therapy with or without cardiac glycosides.

Nitrates. Nitrates have a predominant effect on venous capacitance vessels. Their use has been limited as a result of generally poor oral absorption, and lack of analytical methods for their estimation has also made their logical application difficult. Most studies have been performed with isosorbide dinitrate, while more recently the use of isosorbide mononitrate has made dosage scheduling easier. Isosorbide dinitrate should be introduced in a dosage of 10 mg t.i.d. and increased according to the patient's tolerance. Mononitrate is used in a 20 mg b.i.d. dosage. Headache may accompany the introduction of therapy; however, many develop tolerance to this somewhat distressing side-effect. The use of a slow release formulation may aid compliance. The role of the transdermal route of administration remains to be established (for detailed clinical pharmacology, see Chap. 3) (Armstrong et al. 1980).

Hydralazine. Oral hydralazine has been shown to be beneficial. The starting dose is 25 mg t.i.d. and this is subsequently increased according to response. Reflex tachycardia may be less troublesome in patients treated for cardiac failure but this is a potential problem in patients if the failure is of ischaemic origin. Dosage may be increased to 75 mg t.i.d. and higher doses are seldom required (Chatterjee et al. 1976; Mathey 1980).

Prazosin. The α-adrenoceptor blocking compound prazosin has effects on both the venous and the arteriolar vascular beds. Hypotensive responses may occur following its first administration and the first dose of prazosin should be 0.5 mg given at night with the patient supine. Subsequent dosages are initially with 0.5 mg t.i.d. and are increased according to response. In cardiac failure, it is seldom for doses greater than 5 mg t.i.d. to be required. Tolerance to long-term administration has been reported. This can usually be overcome by manipulation of the dosage of prazosin and concomitant administration of diuretics (Awan et al. 1977; Packer et al. 1979; Silke et al. 1981).

Captopril. Through inhibition of angiotensin converting enzymes, captopril blocks the formation of the vaso-active angiotensin II. In cardiac failure captopril has mixed venous and arteriolar effects, with a similar spectrum of activity to prazosin. This mechanism of action shows changes which are promising in regard to long-term efficacy (Sharpe et al. 1980; Levine et al. 1980). Captopril is introduced in a dose of 12.5 mg t.i.d., increasing to a dose of 25 mg t.i.d. Side-effects of neutropenia and proteinuria have accompanied high dosing in patients with poor renal function.

Enalapril. This recently released angiotensin converting enzyme inhibitor has shown promising results in cardiac failure. It has a long duration of action, allowing twice daily dosing.

Long-Term Management

When the symptoms and signs of cardiac failure have been adequately treated, and the patient's general condition stabilised, it is important to determine the exact nature of the underlying cardiac disease, its severity and whether further investigations should be performed to assess the patient for cardiac surgery. This is particularly important in patients with valvular disease, congenital heart disease and ischaemic heart disease. Long-term rehabilitation obviously depends to a degree on the patient's occupation, whether he or she is employed, and the degree of support available if the patient is a housewife. Adequate symptomatic review and clinical examination should be undertaken and routine biochemical, haematological and drug level monitoring performed where indicated.

Treatment of Acute Left Ventricular Failure with Pulmonary Oedema

The clinical features of pulmonary oedema have already been described above. It represents a major cardiac emergency whose management may be life saving. If the pulmonary oedema appears in the absence of a prior history of cardiac failure, then occasionally the precipitating cause may require surgical treatment. Such causes are fairly rare, but include infective endocarditis with valvular damage, prosthetic valve dysfunction, atrial myxoma, aortic stenosis, acute mitral regurgitation and ventricular septal defect following acute myocardial infarction.

The treatment of pulmonary oedema includes general measures and specific treatment based on the principle of reversing relevant haemodynamic abnormalities causing the patient's symptoms:

1. Precipitating factors should be sought and aggressively treated as previously indicated.
2. The patient should be treated in the seated position with the legs lowered to reduce venous return.
3. Oxygen in high concentration should be administered.
4. Morphine will relieve distress and reduce the central nervous system drive, which will eventually alleviate venous and arteriolar constriction. In addition, a direct venous dilatory action helps to reduce preload further. Morphine 3–5 mg should be given by the intravenous route over a 3-min period and can be repeated if necessary.
5. A loop diuretic (frusemide 40–80 mg) is administered intravenously over 2 min. A direct effect will result within 5 min, be maximal at 30 min and persist for some 2 h. Frusemide has venous dilating property and will lead to a reduction in the pulmonary capillary pressures, although there will be no significant increase in cardiac output.
6. Cardiac glycosides should be administered in the presence of atrial fibrillation. Care should be taken that glycoside toxicity is not present. In the presence of tachyarrhythmias, with resulting acute cardiac failure, early electrical cardioversion is indicated.
7. Aminophylline should be administered by the intravenous route at a dosage

of 250–500 mg given over 10 min. This agent is useful since it not only reduces any associated bronchospasm but also has a direct stimulating effect on the myocardium, in addition to its vasodilatory actions. Side-effects include headaches, flushing, palpitations and occasional cardiac arrhythmia.

8. Reduction of preload may be required if these standard medical measures are inadequate. Rotating tourniquets may occasionally be employed.

In the hospital setting, haemodynamic monitoring will be required in patients who are resistant to the standard medical measures and vasodilating compounds will be introduced according to the haemodynamic measurements found.

Problems and Challenges

Modern methods of investigation have improved our knowledge of the underlying pathophysiological changes in cardiac failure. The haemodynamic abnormalities resulting from the primary cardiac disease, and the resulting compensatory changes, have been characterised and the pharmacodynamic actions of drugs assessed. Potentially beneficial haemodynamic changes can be demonstrated during acute studies; however, it is often more difficult to demonstrate symptomatic benefit. In acute pulmonary oedema, beneficial symptomatic changes may be obvious, but in lesser degrees of cardiac failure an improvement in exercise capacity may not be immediate. Further detailed studies are required to clarify the relationship between altered haemodynamics and functional capacity and thus determine how the most logical therapy for an individual might be decided upon. The influence of therapy on the prognosis of cardiac failure is unknown — there is an inadequate data base concerning the survival of untreated patients and those treated with diuretics alone. Retrospective studies have shown the mortality among patients with grade III or grade IV cardiac failure treated with digoxin and diuretics to be between 40% and 55% at 1 year of follow-up (Massie et al. 1981). There are no prospective studies available. Major ethical problems exist in studying patients with such a high mortality, and a comparative approach studying the effects of different treatments is difficult. In addition, modern treatment consists of polypharmacy, with a combination of diuretic, inotrope and vasodilator; accordingly, the individual influence of each type of drug on mortality is extremely difficult to determine. The available observational studies do not suggest that vasodilators and inotropes make a significant difference to survival.

It has been suggested that aggressive early therapy in patients with cardiac failure may prevent the progression which inevitably occurs. The early introduction of vasodilator therapy has attractions in reducing the cardiac workload and perhaps preventing adverse dilatation and hypertrophy. Tolerance has been noted in many studies following long-term use of inotropes and vasodilators. Further information is required concerning the mechanism.

Despite these limitations, sufficient information is now available and can be obtained in each individual to allow the introduction of logical therapy. Continued research into other management strategies is required to allow further pharmacological manipulation of the integrated cardiovascular system in order to produce long-term symptomatic and prognostic benefit.

References

Armstrong PW, Armstrong JA, Marks GS (1980) Pharmacokinetic-haemodynamic studies of nitroglycerin ointment in congestive heart failure. Am J Cardiol 46: 670–676

Arnold SB, Byrd RC, Meister W et al. (1980) Long-term digitalis therapy in left ventricular function in heart failure. N Engl J Med 303:1443–1448

Awan NA, Miller R, De Maria AN, Maxwell KS, Newmann A, Mason DT (1977) Efficacy of ambulatory systemic vasodilator therapy with oral Prazosin in chronic refractory heart failure. Circulation 56: 346–354

Bourdillon PDV, Dawson JR, Foale RA, Timmis AD, Poole-Wilson PS, Sutton GC (1980) Salbutamol in treatment of heart failure. Br Heart J 43: 206–210

Chatterjee K, Parmley WW, Massie B et al. (1976) Oral hydralazine therapy for chronic refractory heart failure. Circulation 54: 879–883

Chatterjee K, Massie B, Rubin S et al. (1978) Long-term outpatient vasodilation therapy of congestive heart failure: consideration of agents at rest and during exercise. Am J Med 65: 134–145

Cohn JN, Franciosa JA (1977) Vasodilator therapy of cardiac failure. N Engl J Med 297:27–31; 254–258

Davis JO, Freeman RH (1976) Mechanisms regulating renin release. Physiol Review 56: 1–56

Dikshit K, Vyden JK, Forrester JS, Chatterjee K, Prakash R, Swan HJC (1973) Renal and extra-renal haemodynamic effects of furosemide in congestive heart failure after myocardial infarction. N Engl J Med 288: 1087–1090

Erdmann E, Brown L (1983) The cardiac glycoside-receptor system in the human heart. Eur Heart J 4 (Supple A): 61–65

Fabiato A, Fabiato F (1979) Calcium and cardiac excitation-contraction coupling. Ann Rev Physiol 41: 473–484

Firth BG, Delmar CJ, Corbett JR, Lewis SE, Parkey RW, Willerson JT (1980) Effect of chronic oral digoxin therapy on ventricular function at rest and peak exercise in patients with ischaemic heart disease. Am J Cardiol 46: 481–490

Hillis WS, Been M (1982) Phosphodiesterase inhibitors, haemodynamic effects related to the treatment of cardiac failure. Eur Heart J 3: 97–103

Hutton I, Murray RG, Boyes RN, Rae AP, Hillis WS (1980) Haemodynamic effects of prenalterol in patients with coronary heart disease Br Heart J 43: 134–137

Katz AM, Smith VE (1982) Regulation of myocardial function in the normal and diseased heart: modification by inotropic drugs. Eur Heart J 3 (Suppl): 11–19

Klainer LM, Gibson TC, White KL (1965) The epidemiology of cardiac failure. J Chron Dis 18: 797–814

Kleimann JH, Ingels NB, Daughters G, Stinson EB, Alderman EL, Goldmann RH (1978) Left ventricular dynamics during long-term digoxin treatment in patients with stable coronary artery disease. Am J Cardiol 41: 937–943

Klein W, Brandt D, Maurer E (1981) Haemodynamic assessment of prenalterol: a cardioselective beta-agonist in patients with impaired left ventricular function. Clin Cardiol 94: 325–329

Lal S, Murtagh JG, Pollock AM, Fletcher E, Binnion PF (1969) Acute haemodynamic effects of frusemide in patients with normal and raised left atrial pressure. Br Heart J 31: 711–717

Levine TB, Franciosa JA, Cohn JN (1980) Acute and long-term response to an oral converting enzyme inhibitor captopril, in congestive heart failure. Circulation 62: 35–41

Malliani A (1982) Cardiovascular sympathetic afferent fibres. Rev Physiol Biochem Pharmacol 94: 11–74

Mason DT (1967) Control of peripheral circulation in health and disease. Mod Concepts Cardiovasc Dis 36: 25–28

Massie B, Ports T, Chatterjee K (1981) Long-term vasodilator therapy for heart failure: clinical response and its relationship to haemodynamic measurements. Circulation 63: 269–278

Mathey D (1980) Hydralazine in chronic left heart failure. Cardiology 65: 55–57

Miller RR, Williams DO, Mason DT (1976a) Pharmacological mechanisms for LV unloading in clinical congestive heart failure: differential effects of nitroprusside, phentolamine and nitroglycerin on cardiac function and peripheral circulation. Circ Res 39: 127–133

Miller RR, Vismara LA, Williams DO, Amsterdam EA, Mason DT (1976b) Pharmacological mechanisms for left ventricular unloading in clinical congestive heart failure. Circ Res 39: 127–133

Mills CJ, Cabe IJ, Mason DT (1970) Pressure flow relationships and vascular impedance in man. Cardiovasc Res 4: 405–417

Nellis SH, Flaim SF, McCauley K, Zelis R (1980) Alpha-stimulation protects exercise increment in skeletal muscle oxygen consumption. Am J Physiol 238: 331–339

Nelson GIC, Silke B, Ahuja RC, Taylor SH (1982a) Arterial dilatation or venodilatation following frusemide in acute heart failure following myocardial infarction. Clin Sci 63: 3P

Nelson GIC, Silke B, Barker MCJ, Saxton CAPD, Taylor SH (1982b) A new beta-2 adrenoceptor agonist (pirbuterol) in the treatment of ischaemic heart failure. Eur Heart J 3: 238–245

Nicholls MG, Espiner EA, Donald RA, Hughes H (1974) Aldosterone and its regulation during diuresis in patients with gross congestive heart failure. Clin Sci Mol Med 47: 301–315

O'Rourke RA, Hening H, Theroux P, Crawford MH, Ross J Jr (1976) Favourable effect of orally adminstered digoxin on left heart size and ventricular wall motion in patients with previous myocardial infarction. Am J Cardiol 37: 708–716

Packer M, Meller J, Gorlin R, Herman MV (1979) Haemodynamic and clinical tachyphylaxis to prazosin mediated afterload reduction in severe chronic congestive heart failure. Circulation 59: 531–539

Scholz H (1983) Pharmacological actions of various inotropic drugs Eur Heart J 4: 161–173

Sharpe DN, Douglas JE, Coxon RJ, Long B (1980) Low dose captopril in chronic heart failure: acute haemodynamic effects and long-term treatment. Lancet II: 1154–1157

Silke B, Hendry WG, Taylor SH (1981) Immediate and sustained haemodynamic effects of prazosin during upright exercise in man. Br Heart J 46: 663–670

Skou JC (1957) The influence of some cations on an adenosine triphosphate from peripheral nerves. Biochem Biophys Acta 23: 349–401

Sonnenblick EH, Le Jemtel TH (1982) Newer inotropic agents in congestive heart failure. In: Braunwald E, Mokk MB, Watson J (eds) Congestive heart failure, current research and clinical applications. Grune-Stratton, New York, pp 291–302

Sonnenblick EH, Spiro D, Spotnitz HM (1964) Ultrastructural basis of Starling's law of the heart; role of sarcomere in determining ventricular size and stroke volume. Am Heart J 68: 336–346

Spann JF, Buccino RA, Sonnenblick EA (1967) Contractile state of cardiac muscle obtained from cats with experimentally produced ventricular hypertrophy and heart failure. Circ Res 21: 341–354

Taylor SA, Silke B, Nelson GK (1982) Principles of treatment of left ventricular failure. Eur Heart J 3: 19–43

Watkins L Jr, Burton JA, Cant JR, Smith FW, Barger AC (1976) The renin angiotensin aldosterone system in congestive failure in conscious dogs. J Clin Invest 57: 1606–1617

Wikman-Coffelt J, Parmley WW, Mason DT (1979) The cardiac hypertrophy process: analysis of factors determining pathological v physiological development. Circ Res 45: 697–707

Zelis R, Mason DT, Braunwald E (1968) A comparison of the effects of vasodilator stimuli on peripheral resistance vessels in normal subjects and in patients with congestive heart failure. J Clin Invest 47: 960–970

Zelis R, Delea CS, Comeman et al. (1970) Arterial sodium content in experimental congestive heart failure. Circulation 41: 213–216

Zelis R, Flaim SF (1982) Alterations in vasomotor tone in congestive heart failure. Prog Cardiovasc Dis 24: 437–459

10 Hypertension

Our attitude to hypertension has changed dramatically in the past 30 years. This has been reflected in terms of investigation, in terms of medical and surgical management and in the development of hypertension as a speciality. While hypertension developed initially as a hospital-orientated problem, the trend now is towards "shared care" or general practitioner management. The search for aetiology of primary (also known as idiopathic and misleadingly as "essential") hypertension previously dominated the assessment of patients. Hypertensive patients — young or old, male or female — underwent a battery of investigations such as intravenous pyelography, radio-isotope renography and at times aortography. Complex biochemical investigations were also included. Investigation is now more selective. It is extremely complex when necessary, but overall has become simpler. The need for treatment can be based on general criteria:

Stage 1:   Raised blood pressure. No organ involvement. *Consider therapy.*

Stage 2:   Raised blood pressure. Organ involvement (e.g. LV hypertrophy). *Treatment indicated.*

Stage 3:   Raised blood pressure. Organ failure or damage (e.g. cardiomegaly, blood urea raised). *Treatment mandatory.*

Aetiology

In the large majority (more than 90%) of hypertensives no definite cause for the raised blood pressure is found and the diagnosis of primary or idiopathic hypertension is made. The underlying mechanism has been sought in terms of disordered baroreceptor function, alterations in cardiac output or plasma volume and abnormalities in catecholamine metabolism or the renin–angiotensin system. In early idiopathic hypertension the haemodynamic variables can often be explained in terms of a raised cardiac output. In the older patient, circulating volume is reduced, cardiac output is lower and peripheral resistance is higher.

In normal circumstances:

Blood pressure (BP) = cardiac output (CO) x systemic vascular resistance (SVR)

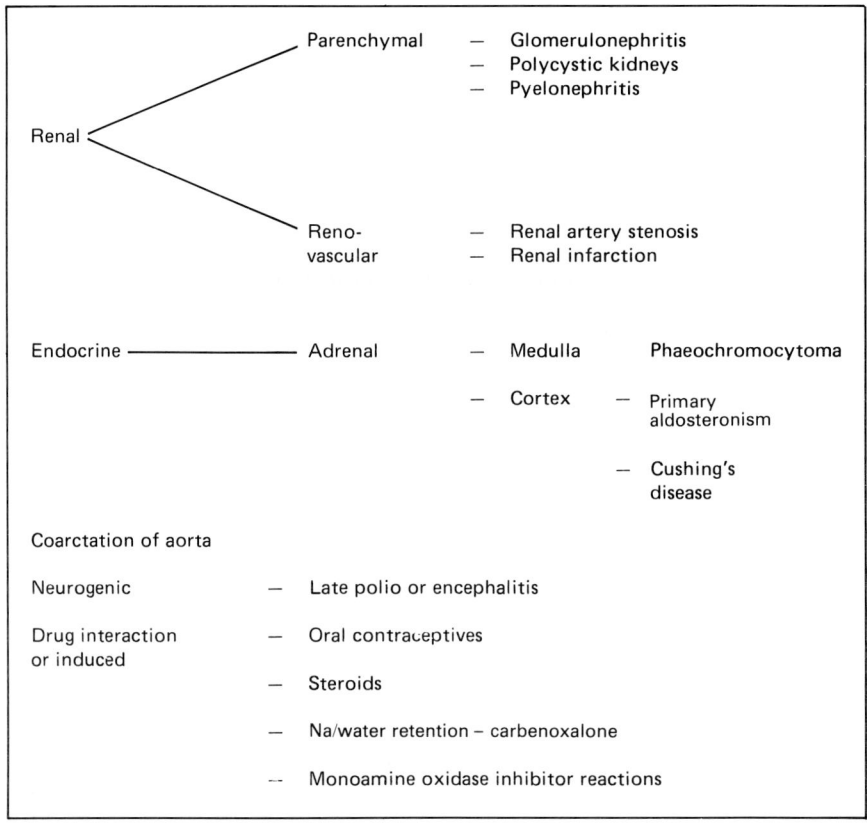

Fig. 10.1. Possible causes of secondary hypertension.

In early hypertension (often labile) the cardiac output can increase:
BP = ↑ CO x SVR
In longstanding hypertension, the cardiac output is normal and systemic vascular resistance is raised:
BP = CO x SVR ↑

There are many causes, although all are uncommon, of secondary hypertension. The search for these and their mechanisms has contributed greatly to our knowledge of blood pressure and its control (Fig. 10.1).

Risks

Data from life insurance statistics indicate that the higher the blood pressure, the poorer the prognosis. Small differences in blood pressure can make a considerable difference to mortality. Each 10 mmHg rise in systolic pressure is associated with a 30% rise in mortality and morbidity. Population studies, such as Framingham have also provided considerable information as to the significant consequences of raised blood pressure. The definition of hypertension used in this study was an initial systolic pressure of more than 159 mmHg or diastolic pressure of more than 94 mmHg. Patients who were hypertensive had an increased mortality compared to normotensives from stroke (7 times greater), cardiac failure (4 times greater) and coronary disease (3 times greater). However, the increased risk does not apply uniformly. Kannel (1977) has shown that the risk from any given level of blood pressure is unevenly distributed and closely tied to the presence and severity of concomitant risk factors such as cigarette smoking, raised cholesterol and abnormal glucose tolerance.

The risks of hypertension are now also known to be as closely linked to the height of the systolic pressure as to the diastolic level (Kannel et al. 1971). Most clinical studies, however, have concentrated on the diastolic pressure as an index of need for treatment and a measure of the effect of treatment. Blood pressure should therefore not be regarded as an isolated variable but as one factor — an important one — in the assessment of the individual patient.

Benefits of Treatment

Several large trials of the effectiveness and benefit of treatment have been undertaken. The results of the Veterans Administration studies (1967, 1970) showed benefits to male patients whose basal diastolic blood pressure was in the range 115–129 mmHg and 90–114 mmHg. In the latter study, the benefits were largely in the group with a diastolic pressure of more than 105 mmHg.

The effect of treatment on patients with blood pressure 90–104 mmHg was assessed by the Hypertension Detection and Follow Up Programme (1979) in the United States and the Australian therapeutic trial (Management Committee 1980). The HDFP and the Australian study have shown statistically significant reductions in cardiovascular system (CVS) mortality in treated mild hypertension (Table 10.1). It has been suggested that the HDFP study is a trial of more intensive medical therapy rather than treatment of hypertension since there was also a 13% decrease in non-CVS mortality. The Australian study was designed as a straightforward trial of drug therapy. There was a decrease in CVS mortality but not in non-CVS mortality, so that the benefit was attributed to antihypertensive treatment. However, the benefit in terms of coronary disease was of borderline significance and there was no clear benefit for younger men and women. A further interesting observation was that those placebo-treated patients whose diastolic blood pressure fell to below 100 mmHg had fewer CVS complications than those whose pressure was brought down to similar levels by active therapy. One possible explanation is

Table 10.1. Mortality in therapeutic trials of mild hypertension

	Mean end-diastolic pressure (mmHg)[a]	Mortality	
		CVS	Non-CVS
HDFP			
Stepped care	83.4 (−12.9)	6.4	5.7[b]
Referred care	87.8 (− 8.6)	8.7	6.6[b]
Australian trial			
Treated	88.3 (−12.2)	1.1[c]	2.5[c]
Control	93.9 (− 6.6)	2.6[c]	2.4[c]

[a] Figures in parentheses are the falls in blood pressure (mmHg)
[b] Per 100 patients at 5 years
[c] Per 1000 patients

an increased risk from drugs causing biochemical changes. In this context Rose's dictum (1981) is important, i.e. if a preventive measure exposes many people to a small risk then the harm is likely to outweigh the benefits since these are received by the relatively few. The MRC trial of treatment of mild hypertension (1985) suggested that treatment may reduce stroke incidence although coronary events and overall mortality were unaffected. This study emphasises the importance of additional risk factor modification, especially cigarette smoking. Guidelines for the treatment of mild hypertension in adults have recently been proposed (WHO, Editorial 1983), mild hypertension being defined as a diastolic pressure (phase V) persistently between 90 and 105 mmHg. It is suggested that the finding of a casual diastolic pressure above 90 mmHg implies the need to repeat the measurement on at least two further occasions over a period of 4 weeks. If the diastolic pressure then falls below 100 mmHg, further measurements should be made over a period of 3 months; if at the end of this time the level remains above 95 mmHg, antihypertensive therapy is indicated. Other factors also influence the decision to treat or not to treat. Those favouring treatment include (a) associated high systolic pressure; (b) any evidence of left ventricular hypertrophy and (c) a strong family history of a stroke or premature coronary disease. At an age of more than 70, by contrast, the need for treatment is debatable as benefits of treatment of mild hypertension have *not* as yet been established for this age group, although studies are in progress.

Investigations

Insofar as mild hypertension is concerned, the WHO group suggest a full history and physical examination to identify any possible cause for the increased blood pressure as well as to assess any effect on the heart, eyes and kidneys. Urinalysis, especially for blood, sugar and protein, is required and microscopy is also worthwhile. A history of dysuria merits further investigation. ECG, chest X-ray, serum potassium and urea or creatinine complete the investigations.

Aim of Treatment

The aim of treatment is to lower the diastolic blood pressure to below 90 mmHg. There are several ways to achieve this.

Patients need guidance and help to understand their raised blood pressure and to gain their confidence and co-operation. They need information as to *why* their blood pressure is raised (even when the exact aetiology is unknown), *how long* treatment will be needed and *why* there is any need for treatment at all. Time is needed for a thoughtful discussion on plans and goals in terms of assessment, treatment and follow-up. Possible adverse features of antihypertensive therapy should always be considered and not glossed over (Personal paper 1977). A decision usually needs to be made about *target* blood pressure. Should an attempt always be made to lower blood pressure to as near 120/80 as possible? It is best to be realistic. While a blood pressure of 120/80 may be achieved from an initial level of 165/100, it can be hard to achieve even 140/90 in someone whose initial pretreatment levels were 200+/120+. Attempts at too rigorous control can mean unacceptable side-effects and be the reason for defaulting from follow-up. By all means try for the most effective control, but be realistic enough to appreciate that the ideal is not always practical.

General Management

Non-pharmacological Methods

There is increasing interest in, and also some controversy over, non-pharmacological methods of treating raised blood pressure. These methods include weight reduction, salt restriction, reduction of alcohol intake and "relaxation".

Weight Reduction

Weight reduction is indicated on general health grounds but the effects are limited and only in mild hypertension will weight reduction obviate the need for additional treatment.

Salt Restriction

Salt restriction as a treatment for hypertension is not new. The rice diet used by Kempner in 1948 was very low in sodium. It was a drastic regime and did lower the blood pressure but not for long, since prolonged compliance on the patient's part was almost impossible. Less severe restriction of sodium intake to 70–100 mmol daily has more recently been reported to lower diastolic blood pressure by around 7 mmHg from an initial 95–109 mmHg level. (Morgan et al. 1978). Parfrey et al. (1981) compared a short-term 5-day sodium intake of 350 mmol with an intake of 10 mmol of sodium daily for a subsequent 5-day period. Blood pressure fell with the low sodium diet in those who had initially high blood pressure levels but there was little change in the others. On the other hand, Watt et al. (1983) could find little effect of sodium restriction on blood pressure. They felt it was not likely to be relevant in the management of hypertension in general practice. The role of potassium may be important. Animal studies have suggested a protective effect from added potassium and investigations are now in progress to assess this in man. However, salt intake in the general population in the Western World is now so high that considerable efforts would be needed to reduce it to a level that might affect blood pressure significantly.

Alcohol

Chronic alcoholism raises blood pressure and abstinence can be effective in restoring more normal levels. Excess alcohol intake can also impair the response to treatment.

"Relaxation"

Relaxation techniques can be enjoyable but their effect on blood pressure tends to be transitory. For some hypertensive patients transcendental meditation can certainly be worthwhile but it is time consuming and difficult to achieve consistent results.

Others

In the overall management of hypertension it would certainly seem prudent to adopt the policy of controlling as many risk factors as possible and this could include, in addition to the above, the stopping of cigarette smoking, the lowering of raised cholesterol values and the increasing or maintenance of physical activity.

Pharmacological Methods (Fig. 10.2)

As mentioned above, the aim is to restore a raised blood pressure to normal levels, but this is not always possible. A balance may have to be struck between

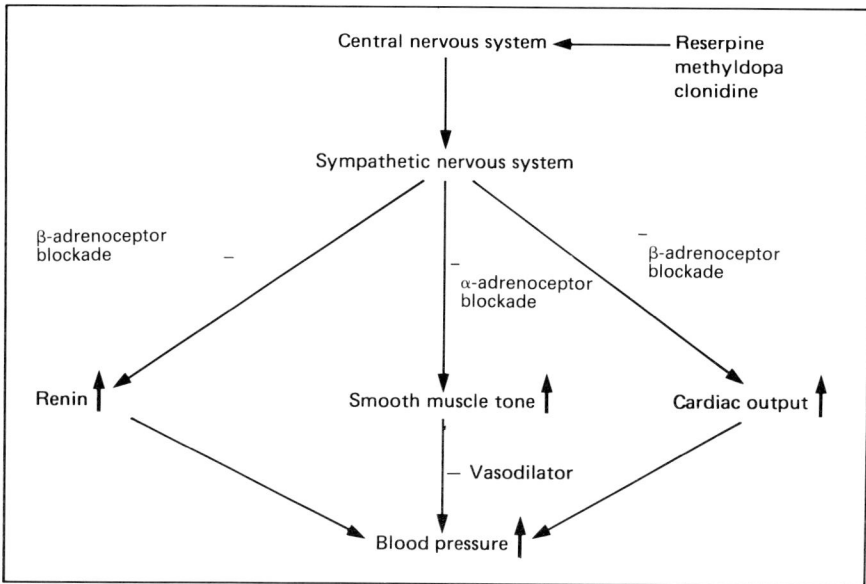

Fig. 10.2. Regulation of blood pressure and the main pathways of pharmacological intervention.

what is practical and what is ideal. Optimally also the treatment given would be aimed at correcting a previously defined specific abnormality of, for example, renin, cardiac output, peripheral resistance or catecholamines. We are possibly approaching this stage but have not yet reached it so far as the majority of hypertensive patients are concerned. Treatment remains empirical although fortunately usually effective.

Should we aim at restoring blood pressure to normal in as many patients as possible or should we set a goal — a target blood pressure that achieves an acceptable reduction although not a return to normal levels? The first approach may be theoretically preferable but does run the risk of reducing compliance because adverse effects develop. Is it better for the community to have ten patients moderately controlled rather than five who have excellent control and five others who have defaulted from any treatment whatsoever? Most clinicians would settle for moderate control.

Mild Hypertension

Mild hypertension can be arbitrarily defined as a basal blood pressure of 140–160/90–110 mmHg. Management is probably best based on the stepped care concept. The first step using β-adrenoceptor blockade or thiazide diuretic is usually adequate.

Over the next few years it seems likely that the thiazides will decrease in popularity — mainly because of their possible long-term adverse metabolic and cardiac effects. There is likely to be increasing interest in the role of calcium channel blockers as first-line therapy and also as to whether or not an acceptable angiotensin converting enzyme inhibitor can be developed for use in this situation.

Does it matter if a β-adrenoceptor blocking compound or a thiazide diuretic is chosen? Many patients will respond to either. The pattern of possible adverse effects has to be considered; thus the patient with peripheral vascular disease, heart failure or asthma is not a candidate for β-adrenoceptor blockade.

Diuretics to be considered include hydrochlorothiazide, at a dosage of as low as 12.5 mg daily, and bendrofluazide, at a dosage of 5 mg daily. The dose–response curve is flat. Increasing the dose does not enhance the blood pressure-lowering effect but does increase the metabolic side-effects in terms of lowered potassium and increased uric acid and perhaps increased dysrhythmias.

β-Adrenoceptor blocking drugs all lower blood pressure, and preparations are available to allow once or twice daily administration. The choice between a non-cardioselective compound such as propranolol, a cardioselective compound such as metoprolol or atenolol, and one with more prominent intrinsic sympathomimetic activity (ISA) such as pindolol depends not only on how well they control blood pressure but also on possible adverse effects. The cardioselective compounds impair exercise tolerance but to a lesser extent than the non-selective and they can also be used in diabetes mellitus. Those compounds with pronounced ISA also have less effect on exercise tolerance and on the peripheral vasoconstriction reported with non-selective β_1- and β_2-blockade and to a lesser extent where selective β_1-blockade is used.

Our current practice is to use either atenolol 50 mg once daily or metoprolol 50 mg twice daily as first-line therapy. These are lower doses than sometimes recommended but they have advantages. Firstly a percentage of patients can be controlled on this dose and be free from side-effects. If they do not respond in 1–2 weeks then the dose can be increased. Introducing higher doses of β-blockade from the onset may control the blood pressure but is also associated with more adverse reactions and can engender suspicion in the patient's mind as to the benefits of treatment.

Calcium channel blocking compounds are now being suggested as monotherapy in mild hypertension. Both nifedipine and verapamil appear effective but *large number, long-term* studies are needed.

Cost should never be overlooked. The thiazides are cheap. Only if you are convinced that a more expensive alternative is better for the individual should it be used.

Moderate Hypertension

The definition, in terms of blood pressure, is again arbitrary but can be regarded as 160–200/110–130 mmHg in a patient with no evidence of retinal haemorrhages or exudates to indicate accelerated hypertension requiring urgent treatment. There is no doubt as to the benefit of treating blood pressure of these levels, but control should be achieved gradually over a few weeks rather than suddenly. Hypertension may have been present for years, and abrupt reduction is unnecessary and may be dangerous. Cerebral blood flow can be critically lowered.

There are several possible *first-step treatments*. Monotherapy may still be possible, especially in previously untreated patients. β-Adrenoceptor blockade in suitable patients seems most logical at present. Any of the β-blocking compounds can be used. Our own practice is to restrict ourselves to a few compounds with which experience has been gained over the years, such as propranolol 40 mg b.i.d. (increasing quickly to 80 mg b.i.d. or more if necessary), propranolol LA 160 mg, atenolol 100 mg, metoprolol 100 mg b.i.d. or metoprolol SA 200 mg daily. Diuretics are seldom successful as single therapy since the reduction in blood pressure achieved by them alone is usually insufficient. *Step 2* is to combine β-adrenoceptor blockade with a thiazide diuretic. Using this combination around 70% of patients can be controlled satisfactorily. Other regimes have been suggested, including methyldopa (starting dose 250 mg t.i.d.) alone or with diuretic, labetalol (alone or with diuretic) and clonidine.

We no longer use clonidine since we were unable to achieve satisfactory blood pressure control without adverse effects. Methyldopa has been widely used in the past with acceptable results, and certainly many patients can be satisfactorily controlled — although adverse effects are not infrequent. We would consider methyldopa when there are contra-indications to β-blockade. It is more satisfactory in females since impotence can be a problem in males when the dose rises above 750 mg daily. An important question not yet resolved is whether or not calcium channel blockers will provide effective long-term antihypertensive management in this group of patients. Short-term studies suggest very satisfactory blood pressure control using either nifedipine or verapamil. It would be a considerable advance if their use was to become established. Nifedipine is available as the standard 10 mg preparation or as nifedipine retard 20 mg. Our initial experience suggests that the fall in blood pressure may be excessive when the long-acting preparation is used as initial treatment. Our current policy is to begin with nifedipine 10 mg t.i.d. and change to the retard preparation later if need be. Similarly, we would start with verapamil in a dosage of 80 mg b.i.d. increasing to 160 mg b.i.d. in the majority. The commencing dose may be reduced to 40 mg b.i.d. in the elderly. There is a similar situation with regard to the angiotensin converting enzyme inhibitors. They may well be useful as single therapy or combined with diuretic, but this remains to be established on a long-term basis.

If blood pressure control remains unsatisfactory on β-adrenoceptor blockade plus diuretic, then a *third-step drug* has to be considered (or alternatively a complete re-appraisal made of management and treatment). What should the third drug be? The choice is wide. Until recently the main contenders included:

Hydralazine (25 mg b.i.d. initially, increasing to 100 mg b.i.d.)
Methyldopa (250 mg t.i.d., up to 1000 mg b.i.d.)

Prazosin (first dose 0.5 mg in the evening, then 1 mg b.i.d.
  increasing to 10 mg b.i.d.).

Any of these may be useful but it can be difficult to lower the blood pressure to near normal without adverse effects. It may be necessary to accept a target blood pressure with a substantial reduction in pressure rather than complete control. In a recent study in Glasgow (McAreavey et al. 1983), hydralazine gave the best blood pressure control with fewer adverse effects, but no compound tested (methyldopa, prazosin, hydralazine, minoxidil and labetalol) could be regarded as completely satisfactory third drug treatment. Studies are now in progress to assess calcium channel blockers and converting enzyme inhibitors against hydralazine as third drug therapy, but the information as to the most suitable is not yet available.

Severe, Accelerated Phase and Malignant Hypertension

Severe hypertension can be defined as a diastolic pressure >130 mmHg but without papilloedema, retinal haemorrhages or exudates. Malignant hypertension usually has a considerably raised diastolic pressure (although not always > 130 mmHg) but is classically characterised by papilloedema; it is now recognised that retinal haemorrhages and/or exudates are also ominous and equivalent features.

Hypertension can present as severe or as malignant hypertension. In addition, a previously mild to moderate situation may suddenly deteriorate, enter an accelerated phase, and develop increased blood pressure and retinal damage. This deterioration may be due to a sudden renal complication and investigation as well as treatment is required. In severe hypertension the height of the blood pressure is important but not all-important. It is too easy to be galvanised into premature and excessive therapy when confronted by pressures of these levels. The fundi have a vital role in assessing the need for rapid emergency lowering of blood pressure. In the absence of papilloedema and retinal haemorrhages or exudates, a high diastolic pressure is not in itself an indication for emergency treatment. It may have been at this level for some considerable time and too rapid a reduction can do more harm than good. Cerebral blood flow can be reduced and cerebral infarction occur — the very complication one is seeking to prevent (Ledingham and Rajagopalan 1979). A once daily treatment schedule with a long-acting β-adrenoceptor blocking compound such as atenolol 100 mg, propanolol LA 160 mg or metoprolol SA 200 mg will usually suffice to control blood pressure over a period of days, with a satisfactory and adequate fall to 100–110 mmHg occurring within 24–72 h. Those who have hypertension associated with papilloedema, retinal haemorrhages or exudates are in a different category. They should be regarded as medical emergencies and admitted at once to hospital. Loss of vision, often unfortunately permanent, can occur at any time.

Parenteral Medication.   This is usually undertaken as a short-term measure to control the excessive pressure until simultaneously administered oral therapy — again usually a β-adrenoceptor blocking compound ± a diuretic — takes effect. Parenteral therapy is *not* required in every patient with malignant hypertension but may well be needed when it is associated with acute hypertensive left ventricular failure or hypertensive encephalopathy.

Diazoxide (50–150 mg i.v. — given rapidly as a bolus to avoid protein binding and inactivation) was previously used extensively but in general the falls in pressure were too rapid, unpredictable and uncontrollable and it is no longer recommended unless the alternatives below are not available. Labetalol, as a combined α- and β-blocker, has been used intravenously with good results. A 50 mg intravenous dose may be given over 1 min. This can be repeated at 5-min intervals to a total dose of 200 mg to achieve satisfactory control. Alternatively, an intravenous infusion with a concentration of 1 mg labetalol/ml can be given at the rate of 2 mg/min and maintained at a rate achieving satisfactory blood pressure.

Our treatment of choice is nitroprusside (Nipride). This combined venous and arterial vasodilator is quickly and reliably effective. There is considerable variation in the dosage and individual titration is required. In general the dose begins at 0.5 μg/kg body weight per minute with an average rate of administration of 3 μg/kg per minute. Nitroprusside has the advantage of a very short duration of action, and blood pressure can be stabilised within minutes at the desired level and then maintained by adjusting the rate of infusion.

Recent developments in the management of hypertensive emergencies have centred on the use of nifedipine. Beer et al. (1981) assessed sublingual nifedipine in the acute treatment of 43 patients with moderate (<110 mmHg diastolic pressure, $n = 17$) or severe (>110 mmHg diastolic pressure, $n = 26$) hypertension. The blood pressure began to fall in 1–5 min, with maximum effects at 20–30 min and a return to placebo baseline values in 4–5 h. There were no major adverse reactions. Bertel et al. (1983) used 10–20 mg of oral nifedipine in the management of 25 patients with high blood pressure requiring emergency treatment; after 30 min the systolic pressure had fallen from 221 ± 22 to 152 ± 20 mmHg, while the diastolic pressure fell from 126 ± 14 to 89 ± 12 mmHg. The fall in blood pressure correlated with initial pressures. Side-effects were minor and in four out of five patients cerebral blood flow increased. If confirmed, this could be a valuable new method of treating hypertensive emergencies.

Considerable advances in the treatment of severe and malignant hypertension have been made. There is no controversy as to the merits of treatment; the benefits are clear-cut. A disease that, untreated, has a 90% mortality, has been transformed into one in which careful and thoughtful management yields a reasonable long-term prognosis.

Hypertension in the Elderly

Hypertension is an important risk factor for cardiovascular disease in the elderly, as it is in the younger age groups. Kannel and Gordon (1978) reported data from Framingham indicating that in subjects between 65 and 74 years old, those who were hypertensive had an annual incidence of cardiovascular disease three times greater than those who were normotensive. In addition, the systolic pressure is of greater importance in the elderly. It is known to have as much or more prognostic significance than does the diastolic pressure. In the elderly the systolic pressure may be high in the presence of a normal diastolic pressure or the systolic pressure may be disproportionately higher than the raised diastolic pressure. The indications for antihypertensive treatment and its benefits remain undecided. There is general agreement that those with a sustained diastolic pressure of more than 115 mmHg require treatment. For patients with diastolic pressures persistently above 100 but less than 110 mmHg, the presence of complications, target organ involvement or a systolic pressure of more than 180 mmHg usually suggests that treatment should be considered. Isolated systolic pressure is no rarity but is a problem. It often fails to respond to even aggressive treatment or the associated fall in diastolic pressure reduces organ blood flow and increases side-effects (O'Malley and O'Brien 1980). The results from the European Working Party on High Blood Pressure in the Elderly trial (1985) are now available. These differ from those anticipated from previous studies. Mortality from coronary disease was reduced while no effect was seen on the incidence of cerebrovascular events.

Many aspects of pharmacokinetics are altered in elderly patients. Drug absorption, however, is not, being usually a passive process. The effects of β-blockers in the elderly have recently been reviewed by Hutchison and Campbell (1983). The ability of the liver to metabolise drugs declines with advancing years, which may, of course, alter the clearance of β-blockers eliminated largely by hepatic metabolism. There may also be a reduction with age in cardiovascular sensitivity to β-adrenergic receptor stimulation. The mechanism remains uncertain but may relate to reduced numbers of receptors with affinity for β-blockade or there may also be a reduced production of cyclic AMP. There is evidence that higher and more variable propranolol levels may occur in the elderly and that this may be associated with a greater increase in side-effects unless care is taken.

Compliance in the elderly must be considered. Compliance falls in all age groups with increasing complexity of dose schedule, and while simplicity of regime is always desirable, it is of even more importance in the elderly.

The main groups of compounds to be considered are:

1. β-Adrenoceptor blocking compounds
2. Calcium channel blocking compounds
3. Diuretics

β-Adrenoceptor blocking compounds are undoubtedly effective. Care has to be taken in patient selection, and cardioselective drugs in initially smaller doses than usual are used — atenolol 50 mg daily or metoprolol 50 mg twice daily.

Calcium channel blocking drugs may well become the treatment of choice. It has been suggested that calcium channel blocking agents will be the treatment in the elderly while β-blockers will be more suitable for the younger age groups. The initial impression of the effectiveness of calcium channel blockers is based on somewhat small numbers of patients overall, although so far either verapamil or nifedipine seem satisfactory. Our policy is again to start with smaller doses than are usually recommended, using verapamil 40 mg twice daily and increasing as need be. The dose may be increased but not the frequency of administration.

Diuretics are useful in lowering blood pressure but do have the disadvantage that hypokalaemia may be a definite problem in the elderly. Rather than routinely use potassium supplementation and risk hyperkalaemia, a potassium-sparing diuretic either alone or in combination can be used (such as thiazide + triamterene or thiazide + amiloride).

The goal for therapy is difficult to define in terms of absolute levels but probably should be in the area of 160/100 mmHg. Attempts to lower blood pressure beyond these limits is likely to cause side-effects out of proportion to any clinical benefit.

Hypertension in Pregnancy

Hypertension continues to cause substantial foetal and neonatal mortality. Pregnancy-associated hypertension tends to be a more frequent problem than idiopathic hypertension present before and made worse by pregnancy.

There has been controversy as to the best method of treatment. Indeed, there has been controversy with regard to treating mild to moderate pregnancy-associated hypertension by active antihypertension compounds rather than by bed rest and sedation. Those advocating active treatment generally agree that thiazides are unsuitable because of adverse foetal effects, including thrombocytopenia, and that calcium channel blocking agents have not yet been shown to be safe for use in pregnancy.

Methyldopa has its advocates, as do β-adrenoceptor blocking compounds. Methyldopa has been reported to reduce the incidence of mid-trimester abortions in women with idiopathic hypertension but apparently does not influence the onset of pre-eclampsia or the perinatal outcome (Redman et al. 1976). β-Adrenoceptor blocking drugs were initially felt to be unsuitable because of foetal bradycardia and metabolic effects such as hypoglycemia, but studies with metoprolol (Sandstrom 1978) reported an improved foetal outcome when compared with hydralazine, and oxprenolol has also been reported to reduce pregnancy-associated intra-uterine growth retardation when compared with methyldopa (Gallery et al. 1979). Valuable studies of atenolol (Rubin et al. 1983) and labetalol (Walker et al. 1983) have now been reported. Atenolol (100 mg) given once daily to 120 women with mild to moderate pregnancy-associated hypertension significantly reduced blood pressure, prevented proteinuria and reduced the number of hospital admissions. There were no adverse effects on mother and baby. Maternal side-effects were less than those reported with methyldopa (Redman et al. 1977). Labetalol also produced satisfactory blood pressure control without adverse effects, and it has been suggested that foetal heart rate and blood sugar are better maintained with the combination of α- and β-blockade rather than with pure β-adrenoceptor blocking compounds.

The options for treatment of hypertension in pregnancy have thus increased. Methyldopa, β-adrenoceptor blocking compounds and compounds with both α- and β-blocking properties can be considered and each has its advocates.

Specific Anti-hypertensive Therapy

Diuretics

Oral diuretics have been a mainstay of the treatment of hypertension for almost 30 years. They have been used either alone or as a part of a more complicated regime. They have, however, long-term metabolic effects which are potentially adverse and this gives cause for concern. An oral diuretic is no longer an automatic choice for initial therapy.

Mechanism of Action

There are two main theories as to their mechanism of action:

1. That it is related to sodium and water loss and to reduced plasma volume and body weight
2. That they act as peripheral vasodilators independent of their diuretic effect.

It is possible that these two effects may be combined. The initial fall in blood pressure may be due to a reduced plasma volume (especially in the evening), but the lowered blood pressure persists even when plasma volume returns to almost pre-treatment levels. It has been suggested that an accumulation of salt and water in the walls of the peripheral arterioles increases peripheral resistance. There may also be a long-term effect on renal prostaglandin synthesis.

Classification

Diuretics can be classified in several ways, including site of action, diuretic potency and antihypertensive effect. There are three main classes:

1. Benzothiadiazines (thiazides) and related compounds (Table 10.2)
2. Loop diuretics such as frusemide (Table 10.3)
3. Potassium-sparing diuretics such as triamterene, amiloride and spironolactone

Table 10.2. Thiazide diuretics and indapamide preparations

Drug	Daily dose	Tablet size (mg)	Proprietary names
Chlorothiazide	500–1000	500	Saluric
Hydrochlorothiazide	50–100	25, 50	Hydrosaluric, Esidrex
Hydroflumethiazide	50–100	50	Hydrenox
Bendrofluazide	5–10	2.5, 5	Aprinox, Centyl, Neo-Naclex
Cyclopenthiazide	1	1	Navidrex
Polythiazide	1	1	Nephril
Chlorthalidone	50	50, 100	Hygroton (longer acting 24 h)
Xipamide	20–40	20	Diurexan
Indapamide	2.5	2.5	Natrilix

Table 10.3. Examples of loop diuretics

Name	Daily oral dose
Frusemide	Varies. Start with 40 mg. May need more in resistant hypertension — 80–160+
Bumetanide	Varies. Start with 0.5 mg. May need 1–2 mg+
Ethacrynic acid	100 mg. Rarely used in hypertension

THIAZIDES

Class I diuretics have had by far the largest role in hypertension. The thiazides are rapidly absorbed from the gastrointestinal tract, initiate a diuresis in 2 h and are excreted unchanged. They act on the distal part of the ascending limb of the loop of Henle and at the beginning of the distal convoluted tubule. Several compounds are available and all are equally effective when given in equipotent dosage. Thiazides lower both systolic and diastolic blood pressure by about 10 mmHg in both the supine and the erect positions. Postural hypotension is rare. As a rule 2–3 days elapse before the blood pressure starts to fall and a maximum effect is at 2–3 weeks. The dose–response curve is flat, and increasing the dose has little effect on blood pressure but causes a marked rise in the incidence of adverse effects.

The antihypertensive action is maintained over 24 h. Bendrofluazide is given once a day while chlorthalidone has a longer action and is given only 3 times per week.

Adverse Effects. Thiazides present an increased sodium load to the distal tubule and increase potassium loss by an exchange with sodium. A noticeable decrease in serum potassium occurs in more than 30% of patients. Whole body counting measurements have suggested that this fall in serum potassium does not necessarily reflect a fall in total body potassium although there may be a shift in ion concentrations. Potassium supplements were initially given as a routine with thiazides to reduce hypokalaemia. They have been used less often recently because of the presumed innocence of moderate hypokalaemia. This may not be so. Significant dysrhythmias can develop. There is also evidence that acute cardiac infarction in patients with hypokalaemia is more likely to be associated with serious ventricular dysrhythmias, including ventricular fibrillation, and that adrenaline release may augment this hypokalaemia. In patients receiving both digoxin and a diuretic it would seem sensible to try and maintain the serum potassium and attempt to reduce the chance of arrhythmia developing. Other adverse features of the thiazides include hyperuricaemia due to blocking of uric acid secretion in the proximal tubule. Gout may occur. Glucose tolerance is impaired by reduced insulin release. This occurs slowly and insidiously but is persistent and tends to increase with time. Antidiabetic treatment is only seldom required but the disturbed glucose metabolism may have more subtle long-term metabolic implications. The MRC trial of thiazides and propranolol in mild hypertension revealed a surprising incidence of impotence (15%) in young males treated with thiazides (MRC Working Party on Mild to Moderate Hypertension 1981). This seems to be reversible after a few weeks withdrawal of such treatment. Lipid values also change. There is a rise in triglyceride and total cholesterol. This may be due to a triglyceride-associated VLDL cholesterol rise rather than to LDL cholesterol increase. The currently fashionable HDL falls but the importance, if any, of this remains unknown.

Indapamide and Xipamide.   These two compounds, which are structurally related to chlorthalidone, may have a role, albeit modest, in the management of hypertension. The action of indapamide is uncertain. In its usual dosage of 2.5 mg daily it does not cause a diuresis and the blood pressure-lowering effect (around 10 mmHg both systolic and diastolic) is attributed to a vasodilator action possibly effected by reducing the initial inward calcium current. Adverse metabolic effects are said to be rare but results are preliminary and in a relatively small number of patients. The definitive role of indapamide is uncertain.

Xipamide is a chlorthalidone-like structure derived from a salicylate. In its usual dose of 20 mg daily it both lowers blood pressure and causes a diuresis. Long-term use may result in significant hypokalaemia. It does not seem likely to become a major force in antihypertensive management.

Loop Diuretics

These are powerful diuretics which may be used in resistant hypertension, especially when associated with renal failure. They are not used in the management of mild hypertension and rarely in moderate hypertension. Loop diuretics commonly available are shown in Table 10.3.

These compounds are quickly absorbed and achieve peak plasma levels in about 1.5 h after ingestion. They are largely bound to plasma proteins. Frusemide is eliminated unchanged in the urine (except in the presence of severe renal failure, when faecal excretion increases). Bumetanide and its metabolites are excreted in urine, and ethacynic acid is extensively metabolised and again excretion is mainly renal.

The action of loop diuretics is to reduce sodium resorption in the ascending limb of the loop of Henle, with a lesser effect on the proximal tubule. As diuretics they differ from the thiazides in that the response increases with the dose. This has advantages and disadvantages. They are extremely effective as diuretics and antihypertensives even when renal failure is severe (glomerular filtration rate < 10 ml/min) but volume and electrolyte depletion are more likely to develop.

Adverse Effects.   The adverse effects of the loop diuretics are mainly related to the dose, in that an excess of any of them is associated with hyponatraemia and hypovolaemia. It should be noted that they are ineffective in the presence of significant hyponatraemia. It is easy to suspect that the lack of response is due to inadequate drug administration and to increase the dosage. This is the wrong thing to do. The electrolyte imbalance should be corrected as first priority. Hypokalaemia does occur but is less frequent than with the thiazides. Serum uric acid increases and glucose tolerance may be impaired. Sensitivity reactions, including purpura and bullous rashes, occur but are infrequent. Deafness, usually but not always temporary, and tinnitus are also adverse effects which may develop when these compounds are used in high dosage, especially with ethacrynic acid. This is especially so in the presence of renal failure, and care should be taken in these circumstances. Ethacrynic acid should rarely be used and always with caution.

POTASSIUM-SPARING DIURETICS

The potassium-sparing diuretics include spironolactone (dose 50–200 mg), amiloride (dose 5–20 mg) and triamterene (dose 50–200 mg). They act on the distal tubule and promote potassium retention. Spironolactone, but not the others, antagonises the action of aldosterone. While amiloride and triamterene have not found wide acceptance as antihypertensive compounds, spironolactone is effective in controlling raised blood pressure due to primary hyperaldosteronism and is useful before corrective adrenal surgery. It can also be used in long-term management of such patients when surgery is not feasible or is contra-indicated. The combination of propranolol (80 mg) and spironolactone (50 mg) has also recently been assessed in the management of idiopathic hypertension. The lowering of blood pressure by this combination is greater than when either is used singly. Although expensive, the combination may find a role in clinical practice. Serum potassium levels should be monitored, especially if there is any question of impairment of renal function. It is important to remember that when spironolactone is used as additional therapy, potassium supplements used with thiazide diuretic should always be withdrawn since significant hyperkalaemia may develop. Even with a low dosage of spironolactone the possibility of gynaecomastia in young males must be remembered. This is due to the steroid configuration of the drug. It has not been a problem in short-term studies but more long-term data are needed. Spironolactone is a relatively expensive drug and should be reserved for special situations.

Calcium Channel Blockers and Hypertension

Mechanism of Action

The recognition of the central role of calcium in muscle contraction has been followed by the development of calcium channel blocking agents for use in clinical practice. Their role as antihypertensive agents is attracting increased attention. It has been claimed that they may be tackling hypertension specifically at the site of the primary abnormality. This could make them preferable to other compounds in the management of raised blood pressure. The relationship of calcium and vascular smooth muscle as discussed below has been well presented elsewhere (Editorial 1983).

Contraction of skeletal and vascular smooth muscle involves the interaction of two contractile proteins — myosin and actin. This interaction involves the energy-dependent generation of cross bridges from the thick myosin molecule to the thin actin filament, with consequent sliding and overall shortening. The formation of cross bridges is dependent on the concentration of free calcium ions in the intracellular fluid adjacent to the contractile protein. However, vascular smooth muscle has to maintain a steady tonic contraction as well as rapidly responding to constrictor stimuli. This has led to the hypothesis that two types of cross bridge are involved. The second process is associated with a much slower turnover rate of cross bridges — these more stable links have therefore been defined as "latch bridges" since they maintain contraction at much lower energy cost. The formation of latch bridges is more sensitive to calcium. Thus when smooth muscle contraction is stimulated there is a transient increase of intracellular calcium sufficient to activate the myosin kinase and to generate phosphorylated cross-bridges. As calcium levels fall, these are converted to latch bridges to provide sustained contraction.

The regulation of free intracellular ionised calcium is therefore important to vascular tone, resistance and blood pressure. Calcium enters the cell through calcium-permeable channels in the plasma membrane and calcium is released from intracellular sites in which it is normally stored — particularly the sarcoplasmic reticulum, the mitochondria and the inner surface of the plasma membrane. Calcium enters through channels created by protein which penetrate plasma membrane lipid. These channels are linked to specific receptors so that, when an agonist molecule is encountered, additional calcium channels can be recruited as cellular entry of calcium increases. Further potential sensitive channels can also open when membrane potential is reduced. Since changes in the conductance of calcium are much slower to develop than changes in sodium permeability during depolarisation, calcium channels are described as "slow channels".

Nifedipine and verapamil have had most clinical usage and affect calcium channel entry in both cardiac and vascular smooth muscle. At the dosage employed in clinical work nifedipine usually has no electrophysiological effect whereas verapamil slows conduction through the A-V node. There may well be other differences between these compounds. Verapamil, for example, has an action upon α-adrenergic receptors in several tissues (Motulsky et al. 1983).

In theory calcium antagonists are likely to prove valuable antihypertensive agents, especially if their ability to lower blood pressure is combined with a low incidence of adverse effects. Is it justifiable to claim that calcium antagonists specifically reverse the underlying abnormality of idiopathic hypertension? This is doubtful. Most forms of hypertension are characterised by increased peripheral resistance and this could reflect changes in free calcium within the smooth muscle cell. It has been suggested that this could be a primary abnormality in idiopathic hypertension and perhaps — although this is not yet established — a factor in some secondary forms of hypertension. However, it is possible that altered calcium handling may be a late development rather than a cause of the raised blood pressure. Robinson et al. (1983) examined the vascular response to local intra-arterial infusions of vasodilators. The decrease in resistance produced by verapamil was substantially greater in patients with hypertension than in normal subjects, while the reverse response occurred with sodium nitroprusside. The authors suggested that the response of the peripheral blood vessels to verapamil reflected an abnormality of smooth muscle calcium handling in these patients. However, such results cannot be used to support the notion that calcium antagonists reverse a pathogenetic change. It seems unlikely that their effect would be limited to fine adjustment of intracellular calcium in order to maintain smooth muscle tone. The frequency of excessive vasodilation with nifedipine and the consequent flushing and tachycardia does not seem compatible with restoration of vascular tone to normal levels. Initial evidence suggests that calcium channel blockers can be effective as third-line therapy in conjunction with a β-adrenoceptor blocking compound and a diuretic, as second-line therapy or as monotherapy. In theory when considered as monotherapy, verapamil is preferable to nifedipine in view of its tendency to slow rather than speed the heart rate. Nifedipine may be added to β-adrenoceptor blocking compounds as second-line treatment. These agents may well shortly rival β-adrenoceptor blocking compounds and diuretics as first choice treatment in hypertension.

The rationale for the use of calcium channel blocking compounds in hypertension is their property of arterial vasodilatation. By their action on the peripheral circulation a reduction in systemic blood pressure can be achieved, accompanied by an increase in plasma renin and at times with nifedipine by an increase in heart rate. It seems logical to suppose that calcium channel blocking compounds might prove to be valuable in the management of hypertension associated with coronary heart disease. The haemodynamic and electrophysiological effects of the commonly used calcium channel blocking compounds nifedipine and verapamil are shown in Table 10.4.

Nifedipine

Clinical Use. As with other antihypertensive compounds, the degree of reduction in blood pressure is related to the initial level. The higher the pressure, the greater the fall. Nifedipine 10 mg will lower blood pressure within 1 h and the effect will last from 8 to 12 h. A three times daily regime has been reported to provide adequate control (Olivari et al. 1979). Nifedipine has an additive effect

Table 10.4. Haemodynamic and electrophysiological effects of nifedipine and verapamil

	Nifedipine	Verapamil
Heart rate	0	Slightly ↓
Blood pressure	↓ ↓	↓ ↓
Cardiac output	↑	↑ Slightly
Coronary dilatation	+ +	+ +
Peripheral dilatation	+ + +	+ +
Negative inotropism	+ −	+
AV block (AH interval)	0	+ +

when given with propranolol or methyldopa. Murphy et al. (1983) assessed 15 patients whose diastolic blood pressure was above 95 mmHg despite treatment with atenolol and diuretic. Nifedipine was added in increasing doses of 10, 20 and 30 mg three times a day for 2 weeks. Blood pressure fell progressively at each dose level. Although there was some dose–response relationship this was rather flat overall in that trebling the dose of nifedipine increased the effect on blood pressure by only 50%. There was no change in heart rate (perhaps because of the atenolol), with a small but significant reduction (in the statistical if not necessarily the clinical sense) of 0.3 mmol/litre in serum potassium. The level of reduction of blood pressure was similar to that reported by Bayley et al. (1982). The reason for the fall in serum potassium is not certain but it could be that the baroreflex-induced catecholamine release seen with nifedipine promotes β_2-adrenergic receptor-mediated potassium influx into the cells.

In malignant hypertension nifedipine has been claimed to be effective in lowering the systemic blood pressure within 15 min of sublingual administration, having a duration of action of 3–4 h. This could prove to be an important indication, especially when associated with left ventricular failure.

A long-acting preparation of nifedipine, nifedipine retard, is now available as a 20 mg tablet. It has been reported that satisfactory blood pressure control can be achieved by the use of 20 or 40 mg twice daily. We have found, especially in mild hypertension, that introducing nifedipine retard as monotherapy can be associated with hypotension, headache, dizziness and flushing. We therefore start with standard nifedipine 10 mg three times a day and if the compound is well tolerated, change over to the retard preparation if required.

Adverse Effects.   There are no absolute contra-indications but care may need to be taken in the presence of large doses of β-adrenoceptor blocking drugs since heart failure can occur. Care should be taken in patients with aortic and mitral valve stenosis.

Caution is required when digoxin is being administered concomitantly. Nifedipine increases digoxin levels by up to 50% and thus may precipitate digoxin toxicity. As previously mentioned, side-effects of dizziness, flushing and ankle swelling may occur. These are related to the vasodilatory properties of nifedipine.

Verapamil

Verapamil is a papaverine derivative. After oral administration absorption is rapid and 90% complete. However, due to marked first pass hepatic metabolism it has a low bio-availability of 10%–20% and a half-life of around 7–12 h.

Clinical Use.   Although known for years, only recently has the antihypertensive action of verapamil been clinically exploited. Oral doses of 120–160 mg of standard formation verapamil were given to 16 patients with moderate hypertension (Gould et al. 1982). In this study both verapamil and nifedipine were shown to produce a consistent reduction in intra-arterial blood pressure at rest and to reduce the response to dynamic and isometric exercise. Nifedipine had no effect on heart rate while verapamil (due to an uncertain mechanism) caused a small but definite reduction of around 6 beats per minute.

Verapamil should be introduced in either a twice or thrice daily dosage. Once control is established then the dose is maintained on a twice daily schedule. Slow release preparations are being developed. Effective blood pressure control has been achieved using doses of 80–160 mg twice daily (Table 10.5). In those studies in which blood pressure control was assessed with intra-arterial monitoring, 24 hour blood pressure control has been shown with conventional verapamil. No good correlation was found however between the effect on blood pressure, the patient's age and the drug level. Buhler (1982) has reported satisfactory blood pressure control with verapamil in a series of 43 patients. This group also found the decrease in mean blood pressure to be directly related to the patient's age and pre-treatment blood pressure but inversely related to the pre-treatment renin. This differs from the effects of β-adrenoceptor blockade, where there is an indirect correlation with the patient's age but a direct correlation with renin levels. *This led Buhler to suggest that a calcium channel blocker, such as nifedipine or verapamil, should be first-choice treatment for the older and low renin patients while a β-adrenoceptor blocking compound should be first choice therapy for the younger and high renin patients.*

Table 10.5. Preparations and dosage of nifedipine and verapamil

Compound	Proprietary name	Preparation	Dosage
Nifedipine	Adalat	Capsules 5, 10 mg	10 mg t.i.d. then 20 mg t.i.d. (maximum 100 mg
	Procardia	Tablets 20 mg	daily)
		Retard 20 mg	20 mg b.i.d. 40 mg b.i.d.
Verapamil	Cordilox	Tablets 40, 80, 120, 160 mg	80 mg b.i.d. up to 320 mg daily
	Securon	Tablets 80, 120 mg	80–120 mg b.i.d

Adverse Effects.   Verapamil should be used with great caution in the presence of β-adrenoceptor blockade. It should certainly not be given intravenously when adequate β-blockade has been established. Bradycardia with A-V block may develop. It has been suggested that oral β-adrenoceptor blocking compounds and oral verapamil can be given together. This is uncertain. Care still has to be taken since very low heart rate and A-V block can occur even in the presence of a normal coronary circulation. Nor should intravenous verapamil be given to patients on digoxin. Cardiac glycoside levels may be increased by 50%–75%, probably by reduction in both renal and non-renal excretion. Because of its hepatic metabolism the dosage of verapamil should be reduced in patients with liver disease. Constipation may also occur from time to time.

β-Adrenoceptor Blocking Compounds

The introduction of β-adrenoceptor blockade to the management of hypertension was initially slow but has now become popular and is regarded by many as first-line treatment.

Prichard and Gillam (1969) reported the first large-scale study of the antihypertensive effects of propranolol. Zacharias and Cowen (1970) showed that the combination of propranolol and bendrofluazide satisfactorily controlled blood pressure in 232 of 311 hypertensive patients. All currently available β-adrenoceptor blocking drugs reduce arterial pressure. Although the mechanism or mechanisms of action still remain undecided and controversial, it seems reasonable to assume that there is an association with β-blockade. The additional properties such as membrane-stabilising action, partial agonist activity (intrinsic sympathomemetic activity) and cardioselectivity do not seem to contribute to the blood pressure-lowering action.

Mechanisms of Action

The possible mechanisms of antihypertensive action include:

1. Haemodynamic changes
2. Reduction in plasma renin
3. Resetting of baroreceptors
4. Central nervous system effects
5. Action at presynaptic receptors to prevent neurotransmitter release

Haemodynamic Factors.   Several studies have measured heart rate, blood pressure and cardiac index and have derived peripheral resistance (equivalent terms are systemic vascular resistance or afterload) before and after β-adrenoceptor treatment of hypertension. When given intravenously, heart rate and cardiac output fall while blood pressure shows little change. The β-blocking compounds prevent β-mediated vasodilatation in peripheral arterioles produced by endogenous catecholamines and sympathetic activity. There is an initial rise in peripheral resistance that maintains the blood pressure. When β-blockers are given orally, in the short-term blood pressure does fall due to the reduction in heart rate and cardiac output outweighing the effect on peripheral resistance. With long-term use, circulatory adjustments take place. Heart rate and cardiac output remain low while there is a return of peripheral resistance towards — although probably not below — pretreatment levels.

Reduction in Plasma Renin Activity (PRA). Stimulation of the renal sympathetic nerves results in renin release. Buhler et al. (1972) proposed that the antihypertensive action of propranolol was due to suppression of renin release. The reduction in arterial pressure correlated with a decrease in plasma renin. Hollifield et al. (1976) made an important contribution. Propranolol, in a dosage of 160 mg daily, significantly lowered mean blood pressure in those with high or normal PRA but not in those with low PRA activity. However, blood pressure fell in both low and high renin hypertension when larger daily doses (320–960 mg) of propranolol were used, suggesting that β-adrenoceptor blockade lowers blood pressure by both renin-dependent and renin-independent factors.

Resetting of Baroreceptors. The suggestion that resetting of the baroreceptors occurs with β-adrenoceptor blocking treatment is not new (Prichard and Gillam 1969). The experimental evidence, however, is slight and has proved difficult to validate in the intact human (Hansson et al. 1974).

Central Nervous System Effects. Blood pressure falls after the direct administration of propranolol into a cerebral ventricle of conscious or anaesthetised animals (Dollery et al. 1973). It is uncertain whether this effect is relevant in man. It has been suggested that the vivid dreams reported during β-adrenoceptor blockade with propranolol may be indicative of a central effect. Lewis and Haeusler (1975) studied the effect of intravenous propranolol in conscious rabbits in which electrodes had previously been implanted in the greater splanchnic nerve. Control infusion of saline had no effect on either arterial pressure or splanchnic nerve activity. Propranolol reduced both arterial pressure and splanchnic activity, while practolol reduced only pressure. They suggested that a consequence of the reduction of cardiac response to stimuli could be diminution in automatic input to the central nervous system, decreasing its activity and eventually its mean level of output.

Action at Presynaptic Receptors to Prevent Neurotransmitter Release (Langer 1976). It is suggested that circulating adrenaline stimulates the presynaptic β-receptors to promote neurotransmitter release into the synaptic cleft. This action of adrenoceptor blockade and indeed metoprolol has been shown to prevent the pressor action of exogenous adrenaline (Tung et al. 1981).

Clinical Use

It would be desirable to treat hypertension on the basis of specific haemodynamic and biochemical profiles (Koch-Weser 1973). This is not often feasible and treatment usually has to be initiated on an empirical basis.

In borderline, mild and moderate hypertension the aim of treatment is to restore as near normal pressures as possible with as few side-effects as possible. Patients who are hypertensive but asymptomatic will not readily accept side-effects that interfere with normal life. There are good reasons why β-adrenoceptor blockade can be considered as first-line therapy for many patients. Any of the currently available compounds appears to be effective in all grades of hypertension. Treatment can be given on a once daily or at the most a twice daily basis. Satisfactory levels of control can be achieved by β-blockade in around 70% of patients when given alone, and in perhaps 80% when given with a diuretic. Surges in blood pressure produced by physical and emotional stress can be reduced by β-blockade (Lorimer et al. 1980). Equally important is the prolonged control of blood pressure with no postural hypotension and no post-exercise hypotension.

β-Adrenoceptor blocking compounds can be added to existing regimes to improve blood pressure control and to permit a reduction in dosage and lessening of side-effects. Triple therapy, involving β-blockade, diuretic and vasodilator, seems to be an effective and logical treatment of difficult to control hypertension.

The role of β-blockade in hypertension associated with coronary disease may be especially relevant. Whether or not β-blockade reduces the chance of a cardiac event is uncertain but seems possible. The range of currently available β-adrenoceptor blocking compounds and their properties is shown in Fig. 10.3 and Table 10.6.

Adverse Effects

β-Adrenoceptor blocking compounds should be used with care and understanding. Because of their pharmacological properties they can precipitate heart failure and undue bronchospasm in those with obstructive airways disease. It should be emphasised that heart failure with β-blockade in hypertension is rare and is usually the result of faulty patient selection or administration of an excessive dose. The most dramatic change in the sympathetic environment of the heart takes place when treatment is begun. Subsequent increases represent only small pharmacological increments and there is no abrupt change in the cardiac sympathetic environment. Hypertensive patients who have a history of heart failure or who have considerable cardiomegaly should not be given β-blockers initially, although these may be cautiously introduced later as adjuvants to blood pressure control. Bronchospasm can occur in 2%–5% of patients given non-cardioselective drugs. It should be remembered that cardioselective drugs are not cardiospecific. Cardioselective compounds do increase airways resistance although to a lesser extent, and this can also be improved by bronchodilators.

Other side-effects include lethargy, cold extremities, reduced effort capacity, gastrointestinal disturbances and impotence. Propranolol has also been associated with vivid dreams. Symptoms of peripheral vascular disease may worsen. The mechanism may be unopposed α-vasoconstriction secondary to

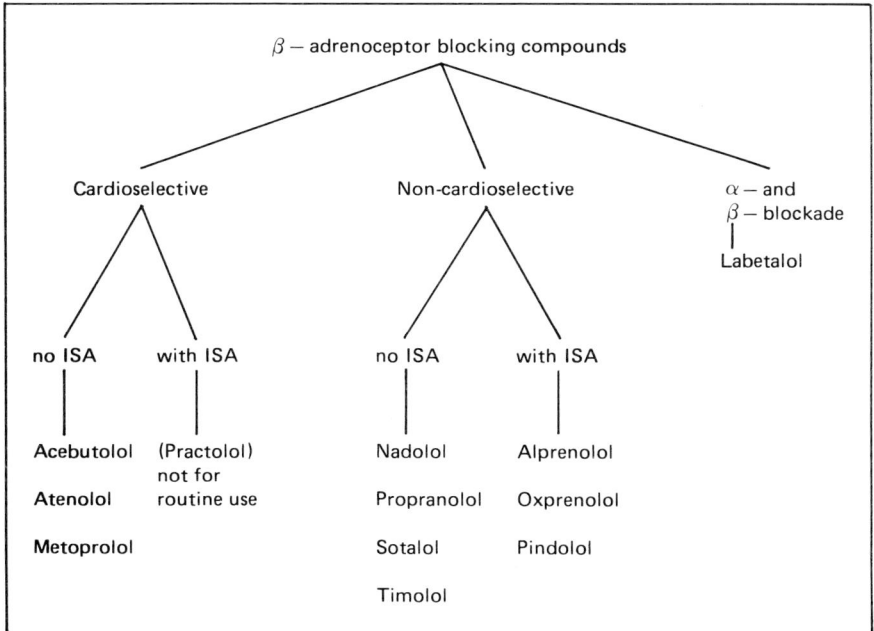

Fig. 10.3. Classification of β-adrenoceptor blocking compounds.

β-blockade. There is evidence to suggest that compounds with intrinsic sympathomimetic activity may have an advantage in certain of these areas. Peripheral blood flow is maintained and physical effort capacity is not impaired. It is also interesting to note that racial differences in response to therapy have been reported (Veterans Administration Cooperative Study Group on Antihypertensive Agents 1982): In a study of 683 men, propranolol and hydrochlorothiazide were equally effective in whites while hydrochlorothiazide was more effective in blacks.

Ganglion Blocking and Adrenergic Neurone Blocking Compounds

The first compounds used in the management of severe hypertension were the ganglion blocking compounds such as hexamethonium and pentolinium. They act by occupying receptor sites on autonomic ganglia (Fig. 10.4) and by stabilising postsynaptic membranes against the action of acetylcholine liberated from presynaptic nerve endings. These compounds lowered blood pressure and reduced mortality from renal failure and heart failure but at the cost of major and often unacceptable side-effects. It would not have been possible to use such compounds in less severely ill patients.

Adrenergic neurone blocking agents such as guanethidine and bethanidine

Table 10.6. Properties of some currently available β-adrenoceptor blocking compounds

Drug	Daily dose	Tablet size	Proprietary names	% protein bound	Approx. plasma half-life (h)	Urine recovery, % of oral dose	% of drug unchanged	Slow release prep.
Non-selective β-Blockers								
Alprenolol (not in U.K.)	400–900	–	Aptine	85	2–3	90	41	Yes
Nadolol	80–240	40–80	Corgard	30	15–37	25	95	–
Oxprenolol	160–320	20, 40, 80, 160	Trasicor	80	2	75–95	5	Yes
Pindolol	10–45	5–15	Visken	57	3–4	95	40	–
Propranolol	160–320	10, 40, 80, 160	Inderal	95	3–4	96	4	Yes
Sotalol	160–600	40, 80, 160, 200	Sotalol β-Cardone	54	15	75	95	–
Timolol	10–60	10	Betim Blocadren	10	5–6	66	25	–
Cardio-selective β-blockers								
Acebutolol	400–800	100, 200, 400	Sectral	30–40	$2-11^x$ (11^x — metabolite)	38	56	–
Atenolol	50–200	50–200	Tenormin	25–30	6–15	80–90	80–90	–
Metoprolol	100–200	100–200	Betaloc Lopresor	12	3–4	95	5	Yes
Combined α- and β-blockers								
Labetalol	300–600	100, 200, 400	Trandate	50	4	60	5	–

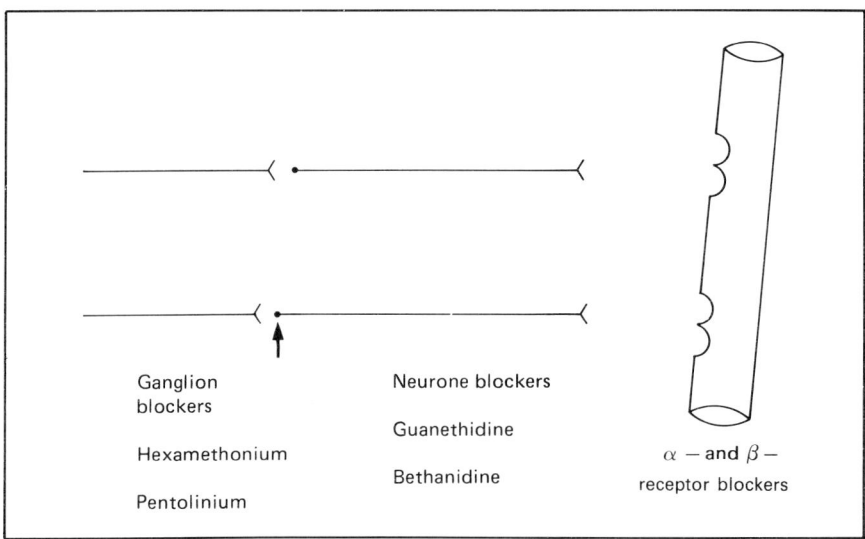

Fig. 10.4. Peripherally acting autonomic ganglia; adrenergic neurone and adrenoceptor blocking compounds.

were then introduced. They too have now been superseded. The major effect of guanethidine is inhibition of the response to sympathetic adrenergic nerve stimulation. Guanethidine is taken up, accumulates in adrenergic nerve endings and displaces noradrenaline from intraneuronal storage granules so that the amount of available noradrenaline is drastically reduced. Guanethidine suppresses equally responses mediated by α- and β-adrenergic receptors.

The absorption of guanethidine varies considerably from 3%–30% but tends to be constant in individuals. Excretion is by the kidney and the drug has a long action so that once daily administration is sufficient but effects may persist for more than a week after stopping treatment. The starting dose is 10 mg daily and up to 50 mg has been given. Side-effects are cumulative and severe. They include postural hypotension, (made worse by alcohol, heat or exercise) and failure of ejaculation. Diarrhoea can also occur.

Bethanidine has similar effects but a much shorter duration of action, necessitating a three times daily regime. This group of drugs has now also been replaced.

Centrally Acting Drugs

Reserpine, methyldopa and clonidine are the best known centrally acting drugs. All have been popular in the past and methyldopa continues to be widely used. Reserpine should not now be used, and even methyldopa is likely to find its use at best static and more likely to decline. More recently introduced compounds have advantages.

Reserpine

Reserpine is the principal alkaloid of *Rauwolfia*, a climbing shrub used extensively and effectively for many years by Indian physicians.

Clinical Use.   Cheap and initially popular, reserpine is now seldom prescribed. It interferes with the intracellular storage of catecholamines, probably by competitively antagonising the uptake of noradrenaline by isolated chromaffin granules. There may also be a lesser peripheral vasodilatory effect. It is readily absorbed with a slow onset of effect but a prolonged action. Blood pressure falls slowly over 2–3 weeks, with a probable reduction in both peripheral resistance and cardiac output. The initial dosage is small — 0.1 mg daily. This can be increased cautiously to up to 0.25 mg t.i.d.

Adverse Effects.   Side-effects have prevented the continued widespread use and acceptance of reserpine in the Western world. Weight gain is common and oedema can occur, as can abdominal cramps and diarrhoea. More important is drowsiness and sedation with a definite risk (around 6%) of significant depression. An increased risk of carcinoma of the breast has also been suggested but this remains uncertain. Overall, reserpine cannot be recommended for use in the management of hypertension.

Methyldopa

Methyldopa (L-α-methyl-3,4dihydroxyphenylalanine) has been popular in the management of hypertension since 1960. It is still widely used, though not now often regarded as a drug of first choice. There have been several theories as to its mechanism of action. Since methyldopa inhibits the decarboxylation of both dopa (L-aromatic amino acid decarboxylase) and 5-hydroxytryptophan, it was first suggested that this effect results in decreased noradrenaline stores and consequently reduces vasomotor activity. This was shown to be incorrect and attention then turned to the "false transmitter" theory. Because methyldopa is metabolised to α-methylnoradrenaline it was proposed that this compound is stored in sympathetic nerve endings and displaces noradrenaline. However, α-methylnoradrenaline is itself a vasoconstrictor and can be readily released from nerve endings. The present concept of the action of methyldopa is that there is a direct effect on the brain stem near the vasomotor centre, where α-adrenoceptors are found. Stimulation of these centres leads to a reduction in blood pressure. α-Methyldopa readily penetrates the blood–brain barrier, and α-methylnoradrenaline stimulates α_2-adrenoceptors to reduce blood pressure.

Pharmacokinetics.   After oral administration about 50% is absorbed. A proportion of this is metabolised in the liver and excreted in the urine as conjugates. Only about 10% of the dose is metabolised to α-methylnoradrenaline. A considerable proportion of the drug is excreted unchanged in the urine with a plasma half-life of about 1.5 h. There is also a second phase of elimination at a much slower rate and this is important in renal failure since accumulation may develop.

The haemodynamic effects show considerable variation in individual patients. In the acute situation blood pressure falls because of lower cardiac output and heart rate with little effect on peripheral resistance. In a long-term study reported by Lund-Johansen (1972) the main effects were again on heart rate and cardiac output other than peripheral resistance. Upon exercise, heart rate and blood pressure both rose, probably indicating that the centrally mediated effects can be overridden by other regulatory mechanisms.

Clinical Use.   Methyldopa was a most welcome introduction in 1960. In comparison with previous therapy it was effective, it had only mild postural effect, and its side-effects, although not negligible, were less severe. For many years methyldopa was regarded as first choice therapy. Although still widely used, it has been superseded by β-adrenoceptor blocking compounds and is threatened by the newly introduced vasodilators. Nonetheless, it continues to have a role.

The initial dose is usually 250 mg 3 times a day, although 125 mg 3 times a day can also be effective. The average daily dose is 1.0 g, but more can be given if required, up to 2 g. Side-effects increase markedly above a daily dose of 1.0 g. Blood pressure is controlled both lying and standing with a slight further fall of around 10 mmHg on becoming upright. Methyldopa can be used in conjunction with diuretics or β-adrenoceptor blocking drugs. A parenteral preparation (50 mg/ml) is available. It was initially introduced as a means of urgently controlling blood pressure, although more suitable agents are now available.

Adverse Effects.   The major adverse effects of methyldopa are a feeling of sleepiness and a separate and distinct feeling of lassitude or weariness. These can occur at any dose level but are more frequent above 1.0 g daily. Nasal stuffiness can occur. The main adverse effect in males is impotence. This is especially prevalent in young males, well over 50% of whom may be affected. This side-effect was once a major reason for clinic default. Most young men preferred to be hypertensive than impotent.

In a study comparing metroprolol and methyldopa in the management of hypertension, Lorimer et al. (1980) found that a β-blocker and methyldopa were equally effective in controlling blood pressure but that metoprolol was more effective in controlling blood pressure response to stress and exercise. There was no postexercise hypotension with either drug. The main difference was with side-effects. These were much higher in the methyldopa group both in terms of withdrawal from the study and in less severe symptomatic adverse reactions.

Methyldopa also causes certain adverse effects which may have "an immune basis". Over 20% of patients can develop a positive direct antiglobulin (Coomb's test). However, this is usually innocuous and of little clinical significance since subsequent haemolytic anaemia is uncommon. Positive antinuclear factor (ANF) and rheumatoid factor have been reported. Reversible abnormalities of liver function (raised AST, ALT) can develop, and although persistent liver damage is rare it can occur (Goldstein et al. 1973).

These adverse effects and caveats as to use might suggest that methyldopa is difficult to use in clinical practice. This is not so. Many patients are satisfactorily controlled for long periods. Methyldopa, however, can no longer be regarded as the ultimate in therapy. It can be improved on.

Clonidine

Clonidine is a potent antihypertensive drug related clinically to tolazoline. It had a period of considerable popularity but is at present used less frequently and is not now a drug of first choice.

Mechanism of Action. The intravenous injection of a few µg/kg of clonidine produces an initial brief rise and then a fall in blood pressure. The rise in pressure is probably due to direct stimulation of α-adrenergic receptors. However, peripheral actions are inadequate to explain the total effect of clonidine, and it has a considerable central action in addition. It has been suggested that clonidine stimulates central α-adrenergic receptors that are inhibitory to sympathetic nerve activity and that vasomotor activity in the medulla oblongata is reduced. Certainly clonidine can cause marked sedation and reduces centrally, although not peripherally, induced salivation.

In man the acute effects of both parenteral and oral administration are associated with a fall in cardiac output rather than in peripheral resistance. Haemodynamic effects of chronic administration are less clear, with a relative bradycardia but no major changes in peripheral resistance or cardiac output. Glomerular filtration rate and cerebral blood flow also fall slightly, as does the plasma renin.

Clinical Use. Because of the small dose (µg), little is known of the pharmacokinetics of clonidine, but it is rapidly absorbed and its antihypertensive effects are seen within 30–60 min, reaching a peak at 2–4 h. Maintenance therapy is given 3–4 times a day.

Clonidine is available in 100 µg tablets with a daily requirement that varies between 400 and 2000 µg. New methods of administration are being evaluated. They involve skin application with a constant absorption rate to maintain blood levels. An intravenous preparation of 150 µg/ml is also available. Although more usually used for maintenance treatment, clonidine has also been used to lower the blood pressure quickly in hypertension "urgencies" (Anderson et al. 1981). These authors studied 36 severely hypertensive patients who were given a loading dose of 300 µg followed by 100 µg hourly to a total dose (if needed) of 700 µg. The average dose of clonidine required was 450 µg and control was maximal at 5 h, with blood pressure falling from the initial 212/139 to 151/103 mmHg. Although apparently effective, such a regime has not found widespread acceptance. When urgent treatment is necessary, compounds such as labetalol, nitroprusside and perhaps nifedipine seem preferable.

Adverse Effects.   Clonidine frequently has adverse effects, the commonest being severe sleepiness, a dry mouth and constipation. Long-term administration may reduce but does not abolish these side-effects. Rashes and pruritus may also occur. Clonidine should always be withdrawn slowly and never abruptly since this may cause a severe rebound hypertension requiring urgent management by α- and β-adrenoceptor blocking drugs. There are also interactions with tricyclic antidepressants which abolish the blood pressure-lowering effect of clonidine. Overall, therefore, the use of clonidine has declined, although there is no doubt that it has been a very satisfactory agent in a relatively few selected patients.

α-Blockers

Mechanism of Action

α-Blockers cause dilatation of both arterial and venous sides of the circulation and thus reduce afterload (decreased peripheral resistance) and preload (venous return). They do this by catecholamine antagonism at α-receptor sites.

There are at least two types of α-receptor. α_1-Receptors are those found on postsynaptic membranes such as arteriolar and venous smooth muscle. Vasoconstriction occurs when these receptors are stimulated by catecholamines. Peripheral α_2-receptors have also been identified on presynaptic nerve terminals (Motulsky and Insel 1982). Their stimulation by catecholamines (such as noradrenaline released into the synaptic cleft) results in a diminished release of noradrenaline from the nerve terminal. It is probable that α_2-receptors may also be found postsynaptically and that in this site they respond particularly to circulating catecholamines. There are also α_2-receptors in the central nervous system. In this situation the receptors are found primarily on postsynaptic nerve cell membranes and their stimulation results in diminished sympathetic outflow (Fig. 10.5).

Phentolamine and phenoxybenzamine affect both α_1- and α_2-receptors. Attempts have been made to utilise these compounds in hypertension but their action is short and tolerance develops. They may be occasionally used to control blood pressure in a patient with excess catecholamine production such as is caused by a phaeochromocytoma, but usually in the short-term and in association with anaesthesia and surgery. They have been used in combination with a β-blocker (Beilin and Juel-Jensen 1972) but resulted in significant orthostatic hypotension and intestinal upset. The use of α-blockers has been superseded. In the management of hypertension the most frequently used compounds with α-blocking properties are prazosin, labetalol and indoramin. The latter two have effects other than α-receptor blockade.

Prazosin

Prazosin was initially regarded as a direct vasodilator. It is now known that this is wrong. It dilates peripheral arterioles by selectively blocking the α_1- or

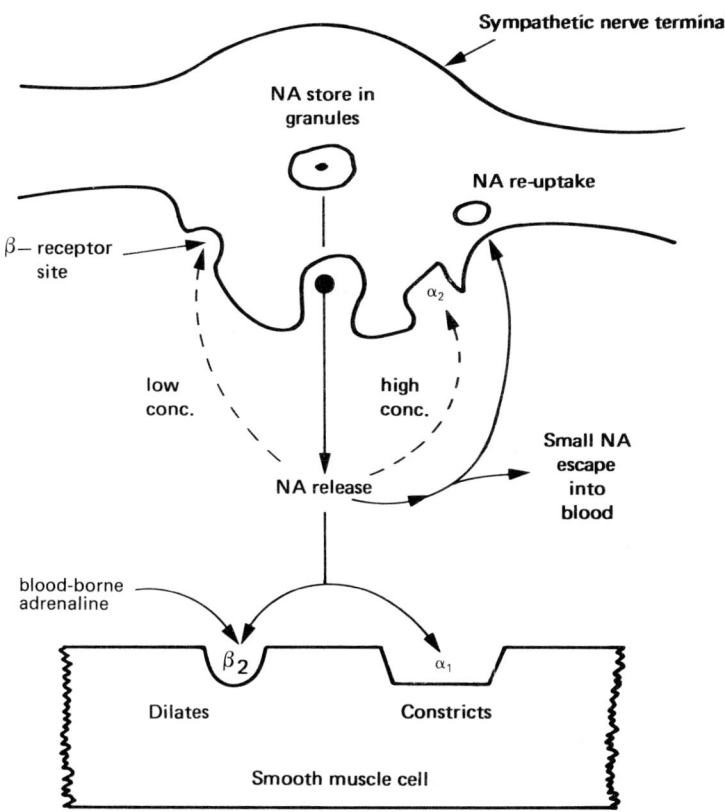

Fig. 10.5. Simplified diagram of noradrenaline release from a sympathetic nerve terminal, to show the feedback loops (*dotted line*) which control the rate of release. Initial low concentrations increase the rate of release, but at concentrations about 100 times greater the rate of release is inhibited by the presynaptic α-receptor. (Modified from Langer 1976).

postsynaptic α-adrenoceptors in the periphery. There is also an action on the venous circulation.

Pharmacokinetics.   Prazosin is readily absorbed and considerable first pass liver metabolism occurs, with about 50%–70% reaching the systemic circulation unchanged. It is more than 95% bound to albumin and eliminated almost entirely by subsequent hepatic metabolism. Dosage may need to be varied in those with lowered albumin concentration since this increases the unbound and pharmacologically active levels; similar caution in respect of dosage is needed when cirrhosis is present. The haemodynamic effects are a reduction in systemic vascular resistance, a slight increase in cardiac output and a less than expected although not negligible increase in heart rate.

Clinical Use.   It is important that the first dose be small (0.5 mg is recommended). It should be taken in the evening, preferably after going to bed. This is because dizziness and syncope occur in an appreciable number of patients if the starting dose is too high. A dramatic fall in blood pressure may occur, although the underlying mechanism remains unclear. This effect is particularly noticeable when diuretics and β-blockers have already been given but it can occur in the absence of these compounds. The "first dose" effect is not a problem if it is remembered and avoided. Subsequently prazosin is given twice daily, starting with 0.5 mg and increasing as required every 3–4 days by 2–4 mg increments to a total of around 20 mg or more daily. Although dosages above 20 mg daily can be given, those levels are the exception rather than the rule and are required only in severe or refractory hypertension. Prazosin is used mainly as a third-line drug following prior administration of a β-blocker and diuretic. Attempts have been made to use it as monotherapy. Alternative α-blockers such as terazosin, which may be given once daily, are being developed. Encouraging success rates have been achieved in initial clinical trials.

Adverse Effects.   These relate predominantly to first dose effect. Nausea, malaise and a sense of fatigue can also occur. In our hands this has been much more of a problem when prazosin has been used alone rather than in combination.

Indoramin

This is a relatively new compound in terms of management of hypertension. Its final role has not yet been established. Blood pressure reduction is probably due to selective antagonism of α_1-adrenoceptors. Additional actions are antagonism of serotonin and histamine, with a possible but uncertain role in blood pressure reduction.

Pharmacokinetics.   There is considerable hepatic first pass metabolism, with 90% being protein bound, and subsequently also elimination by the liver.

Clinical Use.   Widespread experience has not yet been gained in its use but indoramin seems to be of comparable efficiency to methyldopa and prazosin. The initial dose is 25 mg twice daily and this can be increased every 2 weeks to 50 mg twice daily initially and finally 100 mg twice daily. Unlike with prazosin, there is no first dose hypotension.

Adverse Effects.   These may be important. They include sedation, failure of ejaculation and fluid retention, which can be relieved by diuretic administration. It is unlikely that indoramin will become a first line drug, but it may have a role in patients who are difficult to control or in whom there are contraindications to β-adrenoceptor blocking compounds.

Labetalol

Theoretically, a drug which combines the effects of α-adrenoceptor blockade by reducing peripheral resistance and of β-adrenoceptor blockade by decreasing heart rate and cardiac output, might be expected to be of value in the management of hypertension. Labetalol is such a drug (Robertson 1982). It is a mixture of four stereo-isomers which combine α- and β-adrenoceptor antagonist activity. Labetalol is a more powerful β- than α-blocker (3:1 after oral and 7:1 after intravenous administration). It has β-blocking activity similar to propranolol and α-blocking properties similar to prazosin, although it is less potent than either. Haemodynamically, labetalol reduces peripheral systemic resistance, heart rate and blood pressure with little effect on cardiac output.

Pharmacokinetics.   Labetalol is rapidly and completely absorbed and undergoes extensive first pass hepatic metabolism. Clearance is by liver metabolism to produce a series of metabolites, some active and some inactive. It has a half-life of some 4-7 h. Reduced elimination is seen in patients with cirrhosis.

Clinical Use.   Labetalol has to be given 2–3 times daily. The starting dose is 100 mg three times a day, although in severe hypertension it can be given as 200 mg twice daily plus bendrofluazide 5 mg daily. Depending on the response, dosage can be increased rapidly to about 1000 mg daily. Higher doses of up to 2 g have been given but are associated with side-effects of nausea and of postural hypotension. Labetalol is effective in both the supine and the erect position, but probably as a consequence of its vasodilating properties, does produce a postural fall in blood pressure.

Intravenous labetalol is also available and is effective in the emergency reduction of blood pressure when 50 mg is given intravenously over 1 min. Blood pressure reduction is rapid and, depending on effect, further injections of labetalol can be given.

Adverse Effects. In higher doses nausea and giddiness occur but are infrequent. The side-effects are those of β-blockade modified by α-blockade and conversely of α-blockade modified by β-blocking effects. Since the predominant action involves β-blockade, adverse reactions are similar to those of non-selective β-adrenoceptor blocking compounds, and labetalol should be avoided or used with caution in the presence of obstructive airways disease, heart failure and peripheral vascular disease.

An unusual and unexplained side-effect after intravenous administration is scalp tingling. This is not important but can be alarming for the patient unless explained and anticipated.

Labetalol has been a useful adjunct to the management of hypertension but it has been less successful than hoped. The apparent advantage of a degree of α-adrenoceptor antagonist activity has not been sufficient to displace the conventional β-blocking drugs from their role in management.

Vasodilators

Vasodilators relax vascular smooth muscle, either directly or indirectly through adrenergic neurones. Vasodilators may act on veins, arteries or both. In hypertension blood pressure is lowered by reducing peripheral vascular resistance. The newer vasodilators (Table 10.7) include:

Hydralazine and minoxidil with a direct action on arteriolar smooth muscle

Angiotensin converting enzyme (ACE) inhibitors

Prazosin — an α_1-blocker — see previously

Nifedipine or verapamil as calcium channel blockers — see previously

Table 10.7. Dosage of antihypertensive therapy

	Daily dose	Tablet size	Proprietary names
Vasodilators			
Hydralazine	75–200	25, 50	Apresoline
Prazosin	6–20	0.5, 1, 2, 5	Hypovase
Minoxidil	10–50	2.5, 5, 10	Loniten
CNS-active drugs			
Methyldopa	500–2000	125, 250, 500	Aldomet, Dopamet
Clonidine	0.1–1.2	0.1, 0.3	Catapres
Angiotensin converting enzyme inhibitors			
Captopril	37.5–150 (start with low dose)	25, 50, 100	Capoten

Hydralazine

Hydralazine was introduced more than 30 years ago. Its popularity has fluctuated. An initially wide use declined as immunological problems became apparent. As these have become better understood, so the effectiveness of hydralazine has again become apparent and appreciated.

Mechanism of Action. The major action of hydralazine is direct relaxation of vascular smooth muscle with preferential dilatation of arterioles as compared to veins. Labelled hydralazine has a high affinity for the walls of muscular arterioles. Given acutely in volunteers, hydralazine causes an abrupt fall in systemic vascular resistance with a slight increase in cardiac output and only minor heart rate changes. In patients with hypertension systemic vascular resistance again falls, cardiac output again increases and there is a considerable heart rate change. There is a reflex tachycardia, while salt and water retention occur due to renin stimulation. When hydralazine is given chronically, blood pressure and vascular resistance remain low while heart rate increases by 10% or more. Exercise cardiac output increases normally, with an increase in renal blood flow and maintenance of glomerular filtration rate. Overall the underlying haemodynamic changes of hypertension are corrected.

Pharmacokinetics. Hydralazine is well absorbed, with maximum blood levels some 3–4 h after oral administration. Pharmacological effects correlate well with plasma concentration. Extensive metabolism takes place in gut and liver. The major metabolic pathways include conjugation with glucuronic acid and N–acetylation. The latter is an important process. The enzyme acetyltransferase catalyses N-acetylation and levels of this enzyme are genetically determined as an autosomal recessive trait. Those who are slow acetylators of hydralazine will have higher plasma levels of unchanged drug, especially when it is given in doses above 200 mg per day. Adverse effects become more common with higher levels since, for example, after a given dose "slow acetylators" will achieve plasma concentrations almost twice those of the more usual "fast acetylators" (Zacest and Koch-Weser 1972). Hydralazine is eliminated rapidly but active metabolites tend to prolong its action.

Clinical Use. Hydralazine is available for intravenous and oral use. The intravenous preparation (20 mg/ml) may be used to lower blood pressure rapidly. It is given slowly, with a maximum dose of around 40 mg. Its effect is variable, there may be tachycardia and angina can occur in those with underlying coronary disease. Other agents are now available to cause smoother and more predictable rapid control of blood pressure.

Orally the initial dose is 25 mg twice or three times a day and this can be increased to 100 mg twice daily over a period of weeks. Larger doses should be given only if there is no alternative and if the acetylator status of the individual has been determined.

Hydralazine is not suitable for monotherapy since it causes unpleasant reflex tachycardia and flushing. It is usually used as a constituent of triple therapy where a β-blocker is given to control heart rate and a diuretic is given to reduce fluid retention. With these constraints and in this role hydralazine remains an acceptable antihypertensive agent.

Adverse Effects. Many of the adverse effects reflect the action of the drug and are related to tachycardia (palpitation) and vasodilatation (headache, flushing, nasal congestion). Skin rash, polyneuritis and pancytopenia have been reported. The principal adverse feature is that of a hypersensitivity syndrome associated with a positive antinuclear factor. This may present as an acute rheumatoid state, or less frequently as a syndrome indistinguishable from systemic lupus erythematosus (SLE). This is predominantly found in slow acetylators taking more than 200 mg daily but has been reported with a lower dosage. The symptoms and signs regress after withdrawal of hydralazine, but treatment with corticosteriods may be necessary. This possibility emphasises the need for vigilance in the use of hydralazine. Although it remains a useful drug it is likely eventually to be replaced by other vasodilators lacking this hazard.

Minoxidil

Pharmacokinetics and Administration.   Minoxidil is an arterial vasodilator acting directly on smooth muscle in the arterial wall (Lowe 1983). Oral administration results in virtually complete absorption, with a peak plasma concentration at about 60 min and a maximal effect on blood pressure within a few hours. The plasma half-life is 4 h, but the effect on blood pressure is longer than this and can be prolonged to up to 3 days due to tissue binding. Metabolism of minoxidil is mostly hepatic, which allows it to be used in renal failure although care must be taken with time of administration since it can be readily dialysed out.

Clinical Use.   Minoxidil can be given once or twice daily. The starting dose is 2.5 mg b.i.d., increasing by 5–10 mg every few days to a usual maximum of 50 mg (occasionally more). If rapid reduction of blood pressure is needed, it can be given more frequently.

There is no doubt that minoxidil is effective. In severe refractory hypertension it may be of great value in lowering and controlling blood pressure. Renal function can improve (Taverner et al. 1983). Drowsiness, impotence and postural hypotension are absent but there are other problems which militate against its widespread use.

Adverse Effects.   Various adverse effects occur with minoxidil:

1. The lowering of blood pressure brings about a reflex tachycardia which can cause palpitation. β-Adrenoceptor blocking compounds are therefore given in conjunction (propranolol 80 mg or atenolol 100 mg).
2. Pronounced fluid retention and weight gain occur unless concomitant diuretics are given. Thiazides are not sufficiently effective and frusemide is often needed.
3. Hypertrichosis (excessive hair) on the face, arms and legs often develops and is usually (though surprisingly not always) an unacceptable side-effect for women. It is not permanent but gradually disappears a few weeks after stopping treatment.
4. Breast tenderness, gastrointestinal distention and more importantly pericardial effusion may develop. This may be asymptomatic and can be a problem in renal failure, when removal of pericardial fluid may be necessary. The development of breathlessness or an increase in heart size on chest X-ray are indications for echocardiography to detect the presence and amount of pericardial fluid.

An apparently disquieting observation is the rapid development of T wave inversions in the ECG in more than 60% of patients within a few days of starting minoxidil. It was feared this could be a reflection of acute myocardial ischaemia associated with blood pressure reduction but this does not seem to be so. It is usually asymptomatic and an incidental finding. Changes in ion concentration have been suggested but not proven.

Angiotensin Converting Enzyme (ACE) Inhibitors

The renin–angiotensin–aldosterone system is intimately involved in the regulation of vascular tone and the inhibition of angiotensin converting enzyme is a relatively new approach to the management of hypertension (Fig. 10.6). The octapeptide angiotensin II is formed by the action of converting enzyme on the inactive precursor decapeptide angiotensin I. Angiotensin II raises blood pressure directly by vasoconstriction. Converting enzyme inhibitors prevent the conversion (by competitive inhibition) of angiotensin I to angiotensin II.

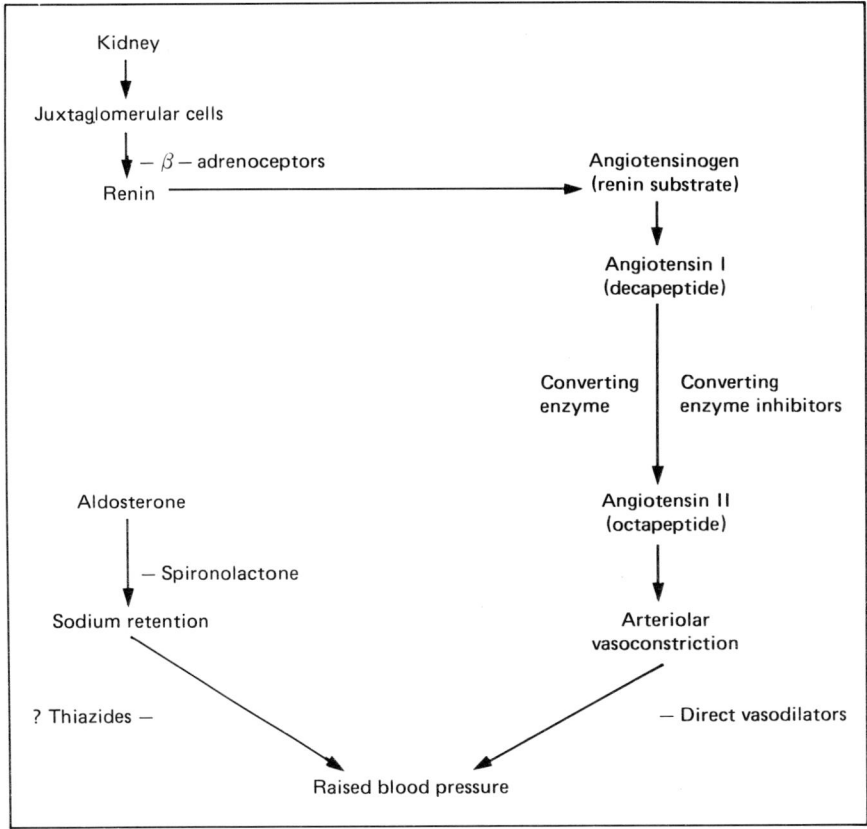

Fig. 10.6. Renin–angiotensin system in hypertension.

Captopril is at present the converting enzyme inhibitor in clinical use although others (such as enalapril) are rapidly being developed.

Use in Hypertension

It is now clear that ACE inhibitors are effective in a large proportion of patients with idiopathic hypertension. They have properties additional to those opposing the vasoconstrictor action of angiotensin, including actions at the synapse and in the vessel wall. Captopril reduces noradrenaline released at any given rates of nerve stimulation. Inhibition of bradykinin metabolism may also raise the concentration of vasodilator kinins, although the clinical significance of this is not yet apparent (Vidt et al. 1982).

Captopril

Captopril is a proline derivative containing a sulphydryl group. It is well absorbed after oral administration. The pharmacokinetics remain uncertain since accurate measurement of captopril and its metabolites is difficult. It is likely that both hepatic and renal mechanisms are involved. Captopril and the newer compound enalapril (which has a longer action) both reduce plasma angiotensin II and aldosterone levels, with reciprocal increases in plasma renin and angiotensin I. The early fall in blood pressure is mainly due to a reduction in peripheral vascular resistance largely mediated via angiotensin II. Although the predominant effect is arteriolar, there may also be an action on venous capacitance vessels. It should be noted, however, that other mechanisms may be involved, since infusion of exogenous angiotensin II does not completely restore the blood pressure to previous levels (Morton et al. 1982). Whether this additional effect is due to bradykinin, prostaglandins, sympathetic nervous system or resetting of baroreceptors remains unresolved. The degree of blood pressure response depends on sodium balance and the activity of the renin–angiotensin system. Converting enzyme inhibitors should be most effective when the angiotensin II is raised. This is indeed the case. Large and sudden falls in blood pressure may occur in the presence of sodium depletion or intensive diuretic treatment and when renovascular disease is present. Converting enzyme inhibitors also lower the blood pressure in those with idiopathic hypertension by reducing peripheral resistance and filling pressure without development of tachycardia (Rubin and Reid 1983).

Clinical Use. Captopril was initially advocated for management of renovascular hypertension and hyperaldosteronism. It then became a third choice drug as a vasodilator in the stepped care of idiopathic hypertension and is now being assessed as monotherapy in mild to moderate hypertension. A principal effect of this class of compounds could be enhancement of the antihypertensive effect of diuretics (which cause an increase in renin and angiotensin II). In certain patients with refractory hypertension the combination of a diuretic and converting enzyme inhibitor has been found to be effective (Atkinson et al. 1980).

Captopril is usually given in three divided daily doses. In those already receiving a diuretic the starting dose should be low (6.5 mg) since the initial response may be a dramatic fall in blood pressure. The subsequent dose is around 25 mg t.i.d., with an increase to 150 mg t.i.d. over 2–6 weeks depending on blood pressure response. Those with renal impairment require less. Recent reports have also indicated that milder degrees of hypertension may be successfully treated using considerably lower daily doses. Enalapril, which is being introduced to clinical practice, has a longer half-life and may be needed only once per day (dosage 10–20 mg).

Adverse Effects.   Orthostatic hypotension is rare, as is reflex tachycardia. Plasma potassium increases (probably as a consequence of lowered aldosterone) and potassium supplements are not needed and should be stopped. Rashes, loss of taste and gastrointestinal disturbances are relatively frequent (5%). These usually resolve when treatment is stopped. Early reports also raised the possibility of major adverse effects (in around 1% of patients), including proteinuria, membranous glomerulonephritis and bone marrow depression. These effects have usually been seen in those on high dosage (> 450 mg per day) and with underlying pre-existent renal or immunological disease. Lower doses are likely to reduce major side-effects considerably to a level at which captopril could be considered for more widespread use, rather than being confined to those with severe hypertension resistant to conventional treatment.

The major side-effects are almost certainly related to chemical structure rather than mode of action. They are similar to those reported with penicillamine, a drug which also has a sulphydryl group. The results of studies using converting enzyme inhibitors without a thiol group will be of considerable interest and importance.

Parenteral Therapy — Rapid Lowering of Blood Pressure

Diazoxide

Diazoxide was previously widely used in the management of hypertensive emergencies when rapid lowering of blood pressure was needed. However, it has largely been superseded.

Diazoxide is closely related to the thiazide diuretics and has a profound effect on the peripheral blood vessels. An intravenous injection of diazoxide in a hypertensive subject produces a prompt fall in systolic and diastolic blood pressure along with an increase in cardiac output and a reflex tachycardia. The major action is by dilatation of arterioles and a reduction in peripheral resistance.

Clinical Use.   Intravenous injections have to be given rapidly as a bolus or the effect is lost. This is due to diazoxide being 90% bound to plasma protein and an inadequate concentration reaching vascular smooth muscle if equilibration with proteins occurs. The effect on blood pressure lasts 4–12 h and repeat injections can be given. Overall the blood pressure reduction is unpredictable and can be difficult to control. The side-effects of diazoxide do not interfere with its short-term use but do prevent it being an acceptable long-term anti-hypertensive treatment. It is available as 20-ml ampoules containing 300 mg diazoxide. Care should be taken to avoid extravasation since the solution is alkaline and tissue damage may occur.

Oral diazoxide is available as 50 mg tablets. It has in the past been used as an oral treatment of refractory or severe hypertension and it certainly can be extremely effective in lowering blood pressure. However, the side-effects include fluid retention, nausea, diabetes mellitus and hyperuricaemia, and diazoxide is now seldom required as long-term oral management of even refractory hypertension.

Nitroprusside

Sodium nitroprusside is a powerful vasodilator. It is not new but it is being used more and more often as improvement in techniques of measuring circulatory haemodynamics (venous pressure, pulmonary wedge pressure, arterial pressure and cardiac output) have made it possible to monitor and control a rapidly changing clinical situation.

Mechanism of Action.   The effects of nitroprusside are similar to those of nitrate in that the action is directly on vascular smooth muscle and probably due to the nitroso linkage. Both resistance (afterload) and capacitance (pre-load) vessels are affected, and a rapid fall in both venous and arterial pressures develops with intravenous administration. There is a compensatory increase in cardiac output and a reflex tachycardia.

Clinical Use.   The fall in blood pressure with nitroprusside is dramatic but it can be controlled. The reduction is dose related and transient owing to the rapid conversion within the body of nitroprusside to thiacyanate. Stopping the infusion means a return to pre-treatment blood pressure levels in 5–10 min. Adverse effects are usually associated with vasodilation and low blood pressure and include nausea, sweating and headache. Nitroprusside is a very effective means of quickly lowering the blood pressure to a desired level. It should not be used casually. It is a compound for hospital use and preferably for use in a specialised unit familiar with its administration and control. At the very least, frequent measurements of heart rate and blood pressure are needed. Standard sphygmomanometer methods are usually adequate and intra-arterial measurements are not required.

Sodium nitroprusside is available as a 50 mg per vial water-soluble powder which can be made up to 500 ml with distilled water. The solution decomposes in light and should be protected by opaque shielding such as that provided by silver foil. No other drugs should be added to the nitroprusside solution, which is given slowly by controlled continuous intravenous infusion with the rate of administration determined by the blood pressure. The adult dose is usually around 200 μg/min and should not exceed 800 μg/min. Nitroprusside is essentially a short-term solution to high blood pressure but is extremely effective and possibly the drug of first choice in this situation.

References

Anderson RJ, Hart GR, Crumpler CP, Reed WG, Mathews CA, (1981) Oral clonidine loading in hypertensive urgencies. JAMA 246: 848–850

Aoki K, Kondo S, Mochizuke A, Yoshida T, Kato S, Takikawa K (1978) Antihypertensive effect of cardiovascular Ca^{++} antagonists in hypertensive patients in the absence and presence of beta adrenergic blockade. Am Heart J 96: 218–226

Atkinson AB, Brown JJ, Lever AF, Robertson JIS (1980) Combined treatment of severe intractable hypertension with captopril and diuretic. Lancet II: 105–107

Bayley S, Dobbs PJ, Robinsin BF (1982) Nifedipine in the treatment of hypertension: report of a double blind controlled trial. Br J Clin Pharmacol 14: 509–512

Beer N, Gallegos I, Cohen A, Klein N, Sonnenblick E, Frishman W (1981) Efficacy of sublingual nifedipine in the acute treatment of systemic hypertension. Chest 79: 571–574

Beilin LH, Juel-Jensen BE (1972) Alpha and beta adrenergic blockade in hypertension. Lancet I: 979–982

Bertel O, Conen D, Radv EW, Muller J, Lang C, Dubach UC (1983) Nifedipine in hypertension emergencies. Br Med J 286: 19–21

Buhler FR, Laragh JH, Baer L, Vaughan ED, Brunner HR (1972) Propranolol inhibition of renin secretion. N Engl J Med 287: 1209–1214

Buhler FR, Hulthen UL, Kiowski W, Muller FB, Bolli P (1982) The place of the calcium antagonist verapamil in antihypertensive therapy. J Cardiovasc Pharmacol 4 [Suppl]: 350–357

Dollery CT, Lewis PJ, Myers MG (1973) Central hypotensive effect of propranolol in the rabbit. Br J Pharmacol 48: 343

Editorial (1983) Lancet II: 22–24

European Working Party on high blood pressure in the elderly (1985) Mortality and morbidity results from the Working Party on high blood pressure in the elderly trial. Lancet II: 1349–1354

Gallery EDM, Saunders DM, Munyor SM, Gyopy AZ (1979) Randomised comparison of methyldopa and oxprenolol for treatment of hypertension in pregnancy. Br Med J I: 1591–1594

Goldstein GB, Lam KC, Mistilis SP (1973) Drug induced active chronic hepatitis. Am J Digest Dis 18: 177–184

Gould BA, Horning RS, Mann S, Balasubramanian V, Raftery EB (1982) Slow channel inhibitors verapamil and nifedipine in the management of hypertension. J Cardiovasc Pharmacol 4 [Suppl]: 369–373

Guidelines for the treatment of mild hypertension: memorandum from a W.H.O./I.S.H. meeting (1983) Lancet I: 457–458

Hansson L, Zweifler AJ, Julius S (1974) Propranolol therapy in essential hypertension. Observations on predictability of therapeutic response. Int J Clin Pharmacol 10: 79–86

Hoffman BB, Lefkowitz RJ (1980) Alpha-adrenergic receptor subtypes. N Engl J Med 302: 1390–1397

Hollifield JW, Sherman K, Vander Zwagg R, Shand DG (1976) Proposed mechanisms of propranolol's antihypertensive effect in essential hypertension. N Engl Med 295: 68–73

Hutchison S, Campbell LM (1983) Beta-blockers and the elderly. J Clin Hosp Pharm 8: 191–194

Hypertension Detection and Follow-up. Program Co-operative Group (1979) Five year findings of the hypertension detection and follow-up program. Reduction in mortality of persons with high blood pressure, including mild hypertension. JAMA 242: 2562–2571

Kannel WB (1977) An overview of the risk factors for cardiovascular disease In: Genest S, Koiw E, Kuchel OED (eds) Hypertension, physiopathology and treatment. McGraw Hill, New York

Kannel WB, Gordon T (1978) Evaluation of the cardiovascular risk in the elderly: The Framingham Study. Bull N Y Acad Med 54: 573–591

Kannel WB, Gordon T, Schwartz MG (1971) Systolic versus diastolic blood pressure and risk of coronary heart disease. The Framingham Study. Am J Cardiol 27: 335–346

Koch-Weser J (1973) Correlation of pathophysiology and pharmacotherapy in primary hypertension. Am J Cardiol 32: 499–510

Langer SZ (1976) The role of alpha and beta presynaptic receptors in the regulation of noradrenaline release elicited by nerve stimulation. Clin Sci Sl (Suppl 3): 421–426

Ledingham JGG, Rajagopalan B (1979) Cerebral complications in the treatment of accelerated hypertension. Q J Med 48: 25–41

Lewis PG, Haeusler G (1975) Reduction in sympathetic nervous activity as a mechanism for hypotensive effect of propranolol. Nature 256: 440

Lorimer AR, Barbour M, Hillis WS, Lawrie TDV, Stoker JB, Sreeharan N, Leanage RV, Linden RJ (1980) Long term comparison of metoprolol and methyldopa in the treatment of hypertension. Clin Cardio 3: 36–39

Lowe GDO (1983) Vasodilators: minoxidil and drugs used in peripheral vascular and cerebral disorders. Br Med J 286: 1262–1264

Lund-Johansen P (1970) Haemodynamic changes in long term diuretic therapy of essential hypertension. Acta Med Scand 187: 509–518

Lund-Johansen P (1972) Haemodynamic changes in long term alpha methyldopa therapy of essential hypertension. Acta Med Scand 192: 221–226

Lund-Johansen P (1979) Haemodynamic consequences of long term beta-blocker therapy: a 5 year follow-up study of atenolol. J Cardiovasc Pharmacol 1: 487–495

McAreavey D, Ramsey LE, Latham L, Lorimer AR, McLaren D, Reid JL, Robertson JIS, Robertson MP, Weire RJ (1983) The "third drug" trial. J Hypertension 1 (Suppl 2): 116–120

MacKay A, Isles C, Henderson I, Fife R, Kennedy AC (1981) Minoxidil in the management of refractory hypertension. Q J Med 198: 175–190

Management Committee (1980) The Australian therapeutic trial in mild hypertension. Lancet I: 1261–1267

Medical Research Council Working Party (1985) MRC trial of treatment of Mild Hypertension: principal results. Br Med J 291: 97–104

Morgan T, Adam W, Gillies A, Wilson M, Morgan G, Carney S(1978) Hypertension treated by salt restriction. Lancet I: 227–230

Morton JJ, Tree M, Casals-Stenzel J (1982) Effect of infused captopril on blood pressure and the renin angiotensin aldosterone system in normal dogs subjected to varying sodium balance. Am J Cardiol 49: 1395–1400

Motulsky HJ, Insel PA, (1982) Adrenergic receptors in man. N Engl J Med 307: 18–29

Motulsky HJ, Snavely MD, Hughes RJ, Insel PA (1983) Interaction of verapamil and other calcium channel blockers with $_{1\,2}$ adrenergic receptors. Circ Res 52: 226–231

MRC Working Party on Mild to Moderate Hypertension (1981) Adverse reactions to bendrofluazide and propranolol for the treatment of mild hypertension. Lancet II: 539–543

Murphy MB, Scriven AJI, Dollery CT (1983) Role of nifedipine in treatment of hypertension. Br Med J 287: 257–259

Olivari MT, Bartorelli C, Polese A, Fiorentini C, Moruzzi P, Guazzi MD (1979) Treatment of hypertension with nifedipine, a calcium antagonistic agent. Circulation 59: 1056–1062

O'Malley K, O'Brien E (1980) Management of hypertension in the elderly. N Engl J Med 302: 1297–1401

Parfrey PS, Markandu ND, Roulston JE, Jones BE, Jones JC, McGregor GA (1981) Relation between arterial pressure, dietary sodium intake and renin system in essential hypertension. Br Med J 283: 94–97

Personal Paper (1977) Trials and tribulations of a symptom-free hypertensive physician receiving the best of care. Lancet II: 291–292

Prichard BNC, Gillam PMS (1969) Treatment of hypertension with propranolol. Br Med J I: 7–16

Redman CWG, Beilin LJ, Bonnar J, Dunsted MK (1976) Foetal outcome in trial of antihypertensive treatment in pregnancy. Lancet II: 753–756

Redman CWG, Beilin LJ, Bonnar J (1977) Treatment of hypertension in pregnancy with methyldopa — blood pressure control and side effects Br J Obstet Gynaecol 84: 419–426

Robertson JIS (1982) Labetalol: The nineteen eighties. Br J Clin Pharmacol 13 [Suppl 1]: 137–141

Robinson BF, Dobbs RJ, Bayley S (1983) Response of forearm resistance vessels to verapamil and sodium nitroprusside in normotensive and hypertensive men: evidence for a functional abnormality of vascular smooth muscle in primary hypertension. Clin Sci 63: 33–42

Rose G (1981) Strategy of prevention: lessons from cardiovascular disease. Br Med J 282: 1847–1851

Rubin PC, Reid JL (1983) Alpha-blockers and converting enzyme inhibitors. Br Med J 286: 1192–1195

Rubin PC, Clark DM, Sumner DJ, Low RA, Butters L, Reynolds B, Steedman D, Reid JL (1983) Placebo-controlled trial of atenolol in treatment of pregnancy-associated hypertension. Lancet I: 431–436

Sandstrom B (1978) Antihypertensive treatment with the adrenergic beta receptor blocker metoprolol during pregnancy. Gynecol Invest 9: 195–204

Taverner D, Bing RF, Heagerty A, Russell GI, Pohl JEF, Swales JD, Thurston H (1983) Improvement of renal function during long term treatment of severe hypertension with minoxidil. Q J Med 206: 280–287

Tung LH, Rand MJ, Majewski H (1981) Adrenaline-induced hypertension in rats. Clin Sci 61 (Suppl 7): 191–193

Veterans' Administration Co-operative Study Group (1967) Effects of treatment of morbidity in hypertension. JAMA 202: 1028–1034

Veterans' Administration Co-operative Study Group (1970) Effects of treatment of morbidity in hypertension. Results in patients with diastolic blood pressure averaging 90 through 114 mmHg. JAMA 213: 1143–1152

Veterans' Administration Co-operative Study Group on Antihypertensive Agents (1982) Comparison of propranolol and hydrochlorothiazide for the initial treatment of hypertension. JAMA 248: 1996–2003

Vidt DG, Bravo EL, Fouad FM (1982) Captopril. N Engl J Med 306: 214–219

Vilsvik JA, Schannin J (1976) Effect of atenolol on ventilatory function in asthma. Br Med J II: 453–455

Walker J, Greer I, Calder AA (1983) Treatment of acute pregnancy-related hypertension: labetalol and hydrallazine compared. Postgrad Med J 59 (Suppl 3): 168–170

Watt GCM, Edwards C, Hart JT, Hart M, Walton P, Foy CW (1983) Dietary sodium restriction for mild hypertension in general practice. Br Med J 282: 432–436

11 **Rheumatic Fever**

Rheumatic fever is an acute or subacute pyrexial illness with systemic effects and widespread inflammatory lesions in the connective tissues involving the joints, heart, blood vessels and hypodermis. It was previously the commonest cause of heart disease in patients under 50 years of age (Stollerman 1975). There has been a dramatic decline in the incidence and prevalence of the disease in the developed countries (Rammelkamp et al. 1952). This is more likely to have been caused by socio-economic improvements in nutrition and housing with a resulting benefit in general health rather than by advances in medical treatment (Gordis 1973).

Rheumatic fever occurs predominantly in young people; it is commonest in the age range of 5–15 years, and is rare before 4 years and after 50 years. It is initiated by infections with Lancefield's group A haemolytic streptococcus. A clear-cut clinical illness of tonsilitis, nasopharyngitis or otitis media is evident in 70% of patients. After a latent period of 7–35 days (mean 19 days) the manifestations of rheumatic fever appear. In those with no previous clinical illness, serological examination usually confirms an immune reaction with an elevated titre of streptococcal antibodies. However, in epidemics of strep-tococococcal infection only some 3% develop rheumatic fever, suggesting that constitutional or hereditary factors determine an individual's immune response (Stollerman et al. 1965).

Pathology

The affected tissues show widespread connective tissue involvement, with the development of Aschoff nodules. These are granulomas of epithelioid cells with central necrosis and lymphocytic perimeters. These may heal completely or go on to fibrosis with resulting local damage. They may affect the heart, causing a pancarditis, and be scattered through the endocardium, myocardium and pericardium (Virmani and Roberts 1977). The valve leaflets have oedematous nodules, being mostly present in the mitral (75%–80%) and aortic valves (30%). The synovial joint linings may be similarly affected, as may the lungs, pleura and subcutaneous tissues.

Clinical Presentation

The mode of onset is variable. In adults the attack is frequently abrupt, occurring 10–21 days after streptococcal infection. In children the onset is commonly insidious, with subacute features. Epistaxis and abdominal pain are relatively common features in children. The diagnosis is made following the simultaneous appearance of characteristic clinical manifestations. The major signs have the greater importance in establishing the diagnosis (Jones 1944).

Major Features

Carditis

Carditis is the most important clinical presentation as it may lead to chronic rheumatic heart disease or to death. It usually occurs in children and adolescents but may be mild and overlooked if the other symptoms are not present. The major cardiac manifestations are:

1. *Cardiomegaly* reflecting dilatation (predominantly of the left atrium and left ventricle) and the degree of inflammatory involvement.

2. *Organic cardiac murmurs*
a) An apical systolic murmur reflects mitral valve involvement with oedema leading to mitral regurgitation. This may be accompanied by an apical mid-diastolic murmur (Carey-Coombs) which is low pitched and often transient.
b) A soft aortic diastolic murmur may be present, indicating aortic involvement.

3. Congestive cardiac failure may occur with right and left heart failure. Right heart failure is commoner in children. Cardiac failure is rare (5%–10%) in first attacks and usually occurs during a recurrence. Additional heart sounds are common.

4. Occasionally arrhythmias occur with extrasystoles or atrial fibrillation. Conduction defects with delayed A-V conduction are common, especially first degree heart block. Second and third degree heart block occasionally occur.

Arthritis

Arthritis is the usual presenting symptom in adults. Gradual or sudden joint pains are associated with evidence of inflammation, and there is swelling, redness, heat tenderness and limitation of movement. Migratory or fugitive polyarthritis effects the large joints, including the knees, elbows, ankles and wrists; hip and spinal involvement is rare. The arthritis subsides, without permanent deformity, in 1–5 weeks.

Chorea

Chorea presents as continuous, non-repetitive, semi-purposive jerky movements of the limbs, trunk and facial muscles. It occurs particularly in the young, is rare after puberty and affects females more than males. Chorea may occur without other manifestations of rheumatic fever (50% of cases); however, even in the absence of other features 20% of patients develop chronic rheumatic heart disease.

Subcutaneous Nodules

Subcutaneous nodules are common in children (occurring in 20%), in whom they present as firm, painless subcutaneous lesions varying in size (0.5–2 mm). They are localised over fascia and tendon sheaths, particularly over the bony prominences of the elbows, the dorsum of the hands, the malleoli and the occiput. Although similar to the nodules found in rheumatoid arthritis, they are less persistent and are often associated with the presence of carditis.

Erythema Marginatum

Although other skin manifestations may occur, including marked sweating and erythema nodosum, erythema marginatum is a major criterion. It presents as annular or irregular areas with a clear centre, and affects the proximal area of the limbs and the trunk. The rash may be transient, or may persist after the features of active inflammation have subsided.

Minor Features

Minor features are non-specific and help to establish the diagnosis when associated with the major criteria.

1. *Fever* is a reflection of the inflammatory process. There is no specific pattern and the temperature is usually in the range of 38.5°–40°C.
2. *Arthralgia* is commonly present as a migratory joint discomfort, but without specific signs of inflammation.
3. Malaise, asthenia, anorexia and weight loss are present, while abdominal pain may occur in young children.

Diagnosis

Clinical Findings

In classical rheumatic fever the diagnosis, when suspected, is easy to make. There is a decreasing incidence, however, and atypical presentations are now common.

Laboratory Investigations

There is non-specific evidence of inflammation, with an elevated ESR and increased C reactive proteins. Leucocytosis (10–15 000) is common, with an associated normochromic and normocytic anaemia. The anti-streptolysin 'O' (ASO) is high and usually rises during the course of the disease. Throat cultures are positive for haemolytic streptococcus in some 50% of cases.

Treatment

General Management

The general management of rheumatic fever depends on the severity of the illness and the resulting clinical manifestations. Physical rest has an essential role in treatment but may be difficult to enforce, particularly in the young patient group. The general nursing management is that of an acute febrile illness. Patients should be nursed in the upright position and receive a light diet. Bed rest must be absolute and be continued for the duration of the acute illness, i.e. until fever and other clinical signs of activity subside. This may be gauged by pulse monitoring, including the sleeping pulse. Simple laboratory investigations are also useful. Serial estimation of the sedimentation rate gives an index of activity. The ECG should be repeated until it is normal or until fixed changes are established. Echocardiography allows serial assessment of the heart size and may be helpful in excluding pericardial effusion or valvular dysfunction. Bed rest may be required for 1–2 weeks or for up to several months if evidence of carditis is present. Mobilisation is gradual, leading to a positive and purposive rehabilitation.

Antirheumatic Therapy

The choice is not critical and lies between salicylates and corticosteroids, although combination therapy may be used. In general salicylates are the first choice. Both drugs blunt the tissue response but do not affect the underlying cause. Symptomatic relief is usually quickly achieved.

Salicylates

The early use of soluble aspirin leads to relief of fever and controls other toxic manifestations, with relief of pain and joint effusions. Aspirin is usually introduced in the absence of carditis, and steroids may be used in more serious cases or as additional therapy if early symptomatic relief is not obtained. Soluble aspirin 6–9 g daily should be given in divided doses to adults (70 kg or more). Within 24–48 h after adequate doses of salicylate, there is usually considerable or complete relief of pain, swelling, immobility, local heat and redness of the involved joints. Children should be given 100–125 mg/kg/day in divided doses every 4–6 h. The dose should be tailored to obtain therapeutic blood levels of 30–35 mg/100 ml (250–350 μg/ml). Salicylates may be taken with milk if gastrointestinal symptoms are present. Concomitant ingestion of sodium bicarbonate reduces absorption. The duration of therapy depends on the clinical response. Seventy-five to eighty per cent show symptomatic control in 6 weeks, while over 90% respond within 12 weeks. In a small proportion of cases (5%) therapy may be continued for up to 6 months. Salicylates should be discontinued when the patient has been free of symptoms for at least 1 week. The initial high dose can be reduced in stepwise fashion at weekly intervals. The dose should gradually be reduced if the course has been prolonged or if any evidence of relapse is evident (United Kingdom and United States Joint Report on Rheumatic Heart Disease 1960, 1965).

General Pharmacology. Salicylates have an antipyretic analgesic and anti-inflammatory activity. They inhibit the biosynthesis and release of prostaglandins by blocking their formation at the first step by action on cyclo-oxygenase. They work as mild analgesics and are effective against pain of low to moderate intensity. In general there is no change in sensory perception; however, there may be a central (hypothalamic) site of action. Their antipyretic action again appears to be related to inhibition of prostaglandin synthesis.

Aspirin is rapidly absorbed from the gastrointestinal tract. Therapeutic levels may be obtained within 30 min, with a peak at 2 h and then gradual reduction. The absorption from the stomach depends on the pH and on the dissolution rates of the tablet formulation. It is transformed in the hepatic endoplasmic reticulum and mitochondria to its predominant metabolic product, salicyluric acid. The metabolites are excreted mainly by the kidney and this is influenced by the pH of the urine. Salicylates have many side-effects related to action on other systems:

1. Gastrointestinal bleeding in conjunction with gastric erosions is common; it may be a reflection of reduction of a prostaglandin protective activity. Nausea and vomiting may be common, and may in part be a central effect.

2. Tinnitus and hearing loss are closely related to the plasma level. They are

common in the early high dose stage of therapy, but are reversible within 2–3 days upon cessation of treatment.

3. Respiratory effects: The administration of salicylates leads to increased total body oxygen consumption which may be a reflection of uncoupling in the periphery of oxidative phosphorylation. In addition there is direct stimulation of the respiratory centre which leads to hyperventilation. The respiratory alkalosis which results is compensated by excretion of bicarbonate. In overdose further metabolic problems may be manifest.

4. The use of salicylates may be accompanied by a prolongation of the bleeding time. This does not appear to be a direct influence on clotting factors but rather the result of an action on platelet cyclo-oxygenase.

Hypersensitivity reactions occur. Aspirin is highly protein bound and drug interactions may occur with other drugs with similar properties.

Corticosteroids

The use of corticosteroids remains controversial; however, they are often used in the presence of persistent carditis. When required, prednisolone should be given at a dose of 20–40 mg daily. When carditis is evident, sodium and water retention may be a problem and dietary restriction of sodium may be required. Diuretic therapy may also be introduced. Steroids should be continued until symptoms are resolved; the dose can be de-escalated initially to two-thirds. If signs of relapse occur, then the previous dose should be re-introduced.

Rebound activation of the disease may occur when antirheumatic therapy is discontinued. Most episodes develop within a few days and usually within 2 weeks. The episode may be severe, with associated pericarditis or even cardiac failure. Rebound activation may be avoided by gradually tapering the steroid dosage or by introducing salicylates as the steroids are discontinued (Combined Rheumatic Fever Study Group 1965).

Antibiotic Therapy

Penicillin should be introduced in the acute attack as soon as throat swabs have been obtained for culture. Adequate early treatment should be given using benzyl penicillin by the parenteral route. Long-term antibiotic therapy must be maintained for prophylaxis.

Long-Term Prophylaxis

Streptococcal infection should be avoided by reducing personal contact at times of risk. If possible, home conditions should be improved. If streptococcal infections occur in closed communities, e.g. army camps or student hostels, mass penicillin prophylaxis should be undertaken. Long-term penicillin prophylaxis leads to a reduction in positive throat cultures and reduces overt infection. Therapy should be continued for at least 5 years or until age 21, whichever is the longer. The route of administration depends on the likelihood of compliance as protection is obviously best achieved by continuous chemoprophylaxis. Intramuscular injections of long-lasting penicillins (1.2 mega units benzathine penicillin DG) may be given monthly. The recurrence rate of rheumatic fever with this regime is some 1 in 250 cases. Oral prophylaxis using penicillin V appears to be somewhat less reliable and should be used in those patients who have had a single clinical episode or involvement. Erythromycin may be used in patients who have penicillin sensitivity. The risk or recurrence decreases with age and with an increasing time interval from the previous attack.

References

Combined Rheumatic Fever Study Group (1965) A comparison of the short-term intensive prednisolone and acetylsalicylic acid therapy in the treatment of acute rheumatic fever. N Engl J Med 272: 63–70

Gordis L (1973) Effectiveness of comprehensive care programs in preventing rheumatic fever. N Engl J Med 289: 331–335

Jones TD (1944) The diagnosis of rheumatic fever. JAMA 126: 481–484

Jones Criteria (revised) for guidance in the diagnosis of rheumatic fever (1965) Circulation 32: 664–668

Rammelkamp CH, Denny FW, Wannamaker LW (1952) Studies on the epidemiology of rheumatic fever in the armed services. In: Thomas L (ed) Rheumatic fever. Minneapolis, University of Minnesota Press, pp 72–89

Stollerman GH (1975) Rheumatic fever and streptococcal infection. Grune and Stratton, New York

Stollerman GH, Siegel AC, Johnson EE (1965) Variable epidemiology of streptococcal disease and the changing pattern of rheumatic fever. Mod Concepts Cardiovasc Dis 34: 45–48

United Kingdom and United States Joint Report on Rheumatic Heart Disease (1960) The evolution of rheumatic heart disease in children. Five year report of a co-operative clinical trial of ACTH, cortisone and aspirin. Circulation 22: 503–515

United Kingdom and United States Joint Report on Rheumatic Heart Disease (1965) The natural history of rheumatic fever and rheumatic heart disease. Ten-year report of a co-operative clinical trial of ACTH, cortisone and aspirin. Circulation 32: 457–475

Virmani R, Roberts WC (1977) Aschoff bodies in operatively excised atrial appendages and in papillary muscles. Frequency and clinical significance. Circulation 55: 559–563

12 Chronic Valvular Disease of the Heart

Chronic valvular disease is most commonly the result of rheumatic damage following single or repeated attacks of rheumatic fever. There is resulting rigidity or deformity of the valve cusps, with fusion of the commissures and shortening or fusion of the chordae tendineae of the mitral and tricuspid valves. This leads to valvular stenosis or incompetence, although both may coexist. Following rheumatic damage the mitral valve is affected alone in 50%–60% of cases; combined aortic and mitral involvement occurs in 20%, and aortic involvement in some 10%. The tricuspid valve is usually only affected in patients who also have aortic and mitral valve involvement (Reichek et al. 1973). Sixty per cent of patients who present with rheumatic valvular disease give a prior history of rheumatic fever. They may, however, present with cardiac murmurs found on routine examination. Follow-up is required by physical examination and serial X-rays, electrocardiograms and echocardiography. Cardiac catheterisation is indicated during assessment for surgery.

Mitral Valve Disease

Mitral Stenosis

Mitral stenosis is the result of rheumatic damage in the vast majority of patients. There is a three-to-one female to male predominance, and three-quarters of the females are less that 45 years old.

Pathophysiology

Rheumatic damage leads to significant disruption of the mitral valve apparatus, with fusion of the valve cusps forming a funnel-shaped orifice. The valve cusps are thickened and deformed, and the chordae tendineae are short and thick. These pathological changes occur within some 2 years after acute rheumatic fever and most patients present with clinical symptoms within a further 10 years. The normal valve orifice is some 4–6 cm^2; when it is less that 2 cm^2 mild stenosis is present, and stenosis is severe when the orifice is less that 1 cm^2. This is usually associated with a mitral valve diastolic gradient of some 20 mmHg, leading to inadequate left ventricular filling, a reduced cardiac output and increase in the left atrial, pulmonary venous and pulmonary capillary pressures (Cohen and Gorlin 1972).

Clinical Presentation

These haemodynamic changes lead to pulmonary congestion with possible development of:

1. *Dyspnoea.* When severe, this may present as orthopnoea with paroxysmal nocturnal episodes. Dyspnoea may be worsened following acute physical effort, emotional stress, respiratory infection, fever, pregnancy or the onset of atrial fibrillation.

2. *Atrial fibrillation.* This develops in 50%–80% of patients and may present with sudden onset of severe dyspnoea with pulmonary oedema.

3. *Systemic embolisation.* Twenty to thirty per cent of patients develop systemic emboli affecting the cerebral, visceral or peripheral arteries.

4. *Haemoptysis.* This may be minor, with blood-stained sputum, and associated with nocturnal dyspnoea and acute pulmonary oedema. Minor haemoptysis may suggest pulmonary infarction or be associated with bronchitis. Alternatively it may be severe if there is rupture of a bronchial vein secondary to pulmonary hypertension.

5. *Pulmonary hypertension.* This develops with the backward transmission of an increased left atrial pressure, and in addition reactive arteriolar constriction occurs, with eventual organic obliterative changes in the pulmonary vascular bed. Right ventricular hypertrophy arises and in these circumstances almost half the patients develop right heart failure.

The signs and typical investigative findings in mitral stenosis are shown in Table 12.1.

Natural History

There is a latent period after rheumatic damage of some 10–20 years; thereafter there is usually deterioration in general clinical well-being over the following 5–10 years. Data are scanty for the presurgical era; however, in patients with grade III effort dyspnoea there was 62% survival at 5 years and 38% survival at 10 years. With grade IV symptoms there was only a 15% survival at 5 years (Rapaport 1975). In general, when symptoms occur there is a period of rapid progression of the disease. In those patients with moderate or severe symptoms related to mitral stenosis, cardiac surgery should be considered.

Table 12.1. Signs and typical investigative findings in mitral stenosis

Inspection	Malar flush; JVP elevated if there is right heart failure.
Pulse	Small volume, often atrial fibrillation.
Palpation	"Tapping" apex beat; possible diastolic thrill; left parasternal heave if pulmonary hypertension present.
Auscultation	Loud abrupt M_1; opening snap after second heart sound. Low-pitched rumbling diastolic murmur with pre-systolic accentuation. Auscultatory findings are attenuated in the presence of calcified valve, with quiet first heart sound and absence of opening snap.
	With atrial fibrillation pre-systolic accentuation is lost.
	A Graham-Steell murmur may be heard, representing pulmonary regurgitation in severe pulmonary hypertension.
	Auscultation performed after exercise with patient lying on left side using ball of stethoscope.
Chest X-ray and fluoroscopy	Straight left heart border. Large left atrium indenting barium-filled oesophagus in right anterior oblique position.
	Large right ventricle and pulmonary artery seen if in the presence of pulmonary hypertension.
ECG	If sinus rhythm, P mitrale in standard leads. If pulmonary hypertension, right axis deviation or right ventricular hypertrophy.
Echocardiography	Reduced movement seen of the anterior mitral valve cusp, with a reduction in the E to F slope. Parallel movement of posterior leaflet with anterior leaflet.
	Left atrial size increased.
Cardiac catheterisation	Right heart catheterisation confirms the degree of pulmonary hypertension before and after exercise. Simultaneous indirect left atrial and left ventricular pressures give the diastolic valve gradient.

Medical Management

1. *General measures*: Patients with a history of rheumatic fever should have penicillin prophylaxis as previously noted. General advice should include the avoidance of infections and strenuous exertion.
2. *Oral diuretic therapy* is required if patients are significantly symptomatic, particularly with regard to dyspnoea.
3. *Cardiac glycosides* are indicated if atrial fibrillation supervenes.
4. *Anticoagulants* are indicated in those patients who have a large left atrium, when atrial fibrillation is present and in those with a prior history of pulmonary or systemic arteriol embolism.

Surgical Management

Indications. Mitral valve surgery is indicated in patients with:

1. Major symptoms of effort dyspnoea, together with evidence of mitral stenosis and pulmonary congestion

2. Severe pulmonary hypertension and right ventricular hypertrophy
3. Episodes of systemic or pulmonary emoboli
4. Right heart failure secondary to mitral valve disease.

Procedures.   Three procedures may be indicated:

1. *Closed mitral valvotomy* is still occasionally performed using the trans-ventricular dilator. This is particularly suitable in emergency situations in which cardiac bypass may be unavailable. Transventriculator dilation is suitable in those cases in which there is no concomitant mitral regurgitation, no atrial thrombus and no valvular calcification (Mullin et al. 1972).
2. *Open valvotomy* may be performed using cardiopulmonary bypass and hypothermia. Thrombus is removed from the atrium and atrial appendage, and plastic procedures on the valve and associated apparatus may be possible. The presence of mitral regurgitation or valvular calcification usually precludes such plastic procedures. Following closed or open valvotomy, the incidence of valvular restenosis is variable, but may be as high as 60% over a 20-year follow-up period.
3. *Mitral valve replacement* is required when there is a major deformity of the valve and associated calcification or when there is any valvular regurgitation.

Mitral Regurgitation

Mitral regurgitation may result from abnormalities of the mitral valve apparatus, including the valve leaflets, chordae tendineae and papillary muscles. The leaflets are affected following rheumatic fever and form short, rigid, deformed retracted cusps with fused chordae tendineae and papillary muscles. Calcification of the mitral valve apparatus may be seen in elderly patients, in whom it may accompany aortic calcification and be accelerated by hypertension or diabetes. Functional mitral regurgitation sometimes occurs secondary to gross dilatation of the left ventricle with associated dilatation of the valve ring. Chordal rupture may lead to acute mitral regurgitation. This can occur in the absence of a non-specific cause but may also complicate bacterial endocarditis, trauma, rheumatic fever, acute myocardial infarction, hypertrophic obstructive cardiomyopathy or myxomatous proliferation. The papillary muscles are vulnerable to myocardial ischaemia (Burch et al. 1968). If this is transient, then mitral regurgitation may occur during anginal episodes. Ischaemia of the posterior papillary muscle is more frequent than that of the anterior, and necrosis may occur during acute inferior infarct following obstruction of the posterior descending branch of the right coronary artery. Frank rupture is rare. If total rupture occurs then the outcome is usually fatal, with overwhelming acute mitral regurgitation.

Pathophysiology

The regurgitant volume depends on the size of the regurgitant stream and the pressure gradient between the ventricle and the atrium. The volume of regurgitation may be lowered by reducing the left ventricular size. The left atrial volume is increased, left atrial pressure rises and this is transmitted to the pulmonary veins and pulmonary artery capillaries.

Clinical Presentation

Patients present with exertional dyspnoea and fatigue and these symptoms progress slowly over many years. Eventually, following major left ventricular dilatation, cardiac decompensation occurs, with evidence of left heart failure with orthopnoea and paroxysmal nocturnal attacks. If this failure is sustained, then right heart failure also supervenes. Atrial fibrillation may occur but its onset has a less deleterious effect in mitral insufficiency than in mitral stenosis. Systemic emboli complicate the presence of mitral incompetence in less than 5% of cases. Bacterial endocarditis may complicate the long-term course. The signs and typical investigative findings in mitral regurgitation are shown in Table 12.2.

Table 12.2. Signs and typical investigative findings in mitral regurgitation

Inspection	Apical impulse may be seen to the left of the mid-clavicular line.
Pulse	May be jerky in character and of fairly full volume.
Palpation	The cardiac apex is brisk and may be displaced to the left.
	A systolic thrill may be present at the cardiac apex.
	Left parasternal heave may be present, with pulmonary hypertension.
Auscultation	A blowing high-pitched pansystolic murmur is heard at the cardiac apex radiating to the axilla; it is heard best with the diaphragm of stethoscope.
	Third heart sound frequent.
Chest X-ray and fluoroscopy	Enlarged left ventricle and left atrium seen in the left lateral projection or in the right anterior oblique with barium.
ECG	Left axis deviation or left ventricular hypertrophy. P mitrale may be present.
Echocardiography	Cross-sectional echo may show prolapsing mitral valve leaflet.
	Other findings on M mode non-specific, with rapid anterior motion of the mitral valve and increased left ventricular and left atrial size.
Cardiac catheterisation	Right heart catheter confirms associated pulmonary hypertension.
	Left ventricular angiography confirms the degree of mitral regurgitation from systolic jet passing into left atrium.

Natural History

Patients with isolated mitral regurgitation may remain stable for many years. Some 80% survive 5 years after the diagnosis is made and 65% survive 10 years.

If combined mitral stenosis and regurgitation is present, the survival is significantly reduced, with 67% surviving 5 years and 30% surviving 10 years.

Medical Management

1. Cardiac glycosides may be helpful in reducing left ventricular volume.
2. Diuretics should be used in the presence of significant dyspnoea.
3. Afterload reduction may be introduced at an early stage in both acute and chronic mitral regurgitation to reduce aortic impedence so that left atrial regurgitant volume is reduced, with an associated reduction in the 'V' wave. The use of nitroprusside by the intravenous route may allow haemodynamic stabilisation of the patient prior to acute surgery. Long-term oral therapy with oral hydralazine or prazosin has also been shown to be beneficial (Greenberg et al. 1978).

Surgical Management

Indications. In general terms, indications for surgery must be balanced against the good natural prognosis of most patients with mitral regurgitation. The local surgical mortality should be considered, as should medical contra-indications which may lead to significant morbidity, including renal, hepatic and pulmonary disease. The main indications for operation are persistent symptoms despite full medical management, particularly if cardiomegaly is prominent and serial echocardiography confirms an increasing left ventricular end-systolic volume.

Procedures. Repair of mitral valve by reducing the size of the valve ring using a Carpentier prosthesis may be considered in children and young adults, particularly when there is functional dilatation. The principal surgical operation is mitral valve replacement. This has a mortality of some 2%–5% in patients with chronic rheumatic mitral regurgitation. A higher mortality results if valve replacement follows systemic embolisation, active infective endocarditis or a major dysfunction.

Mitral Valve Prolapse

Mitral valve prolapse has attracted increasing interest. It has been recognised to occur in varying degrees in 5%–10% of the population and can be both symptomatic and asymptomatic. It has been given various descriptive terms, including mid-systolic click syndrome, Barlow's syndrome, billowing mitral valve syndrome, floppy mitral valve and ballooning mitral cusp. The clinical findings and diagnostic features have been found in association with many cardiac and extracardiac conditions. the latter affecting connective tissues and other systems. In particular, it is found in 90% of patients with Marfan's syndrome (Table 12.3) (Barlow and Pocock 1984).

Table 12.3. Conditions associated with or causing mitral valve prolapse

Cardiac conditions	Connective tissue disorders	Probable associations
Primary mitral valve prolapse	Marfan's syndrome	Atrial septal defect
Congestive cardiomyopathy	Polyarteritis nodosum	Patent ductus arteriosus
Hypertrophic cardiomyopathy	Ehlers–Danlos syndrome	Ebstein's anomaly
Mitral valve surgery	Lupus erythematosus	Ventricular septal defect
Cardiac trauma	Muscular dystrophy	Sub-aortic stenosis
Myocarditis	Turner's syndrome	Corrected transposition
Rheumatic endocarditis	Straight-back syndrome	Prolonged QT syndrome
Left atrial myxoma		
Coronary artery disease		
Left ventricular aneurysm		
Wolff–Parkinson–White Syndrome		
Athlete's heart		

Pathophysiology

Myxomatous proliferation of the mitral valve occurs with a haphazard disruption and fragmentation of collagen fibrils. The increase in the myxoid stroma leads to prolapse of the mitral valve leaflets. The chordae and annulus may be affected, and chordal rupture may occur, which intensifies any mitral regurgitation. In Marfan's syndrome, tricuspid, aortic and pulmonary valve regurgitation may result from widespread degeneration of connective tissue. There also may be abnormalities of the thoracic spine and ribs in association with the straight-back syndrome and with a narrow anteroposterior diameter of the chest. Developmentally this may be an abnormality of structural formation of both the thorax and mitral valve during weeks 35–42 of foetal development.

Clinical Presentation

1. Patients may be symptomatic, the auscultatory findings being elicited on routine examination.
2. Episodes of palpitation may be suggestive of intermittent arrhythmias. Occasionally a history of familial sudden death may be obtained.
3. Atypical chest pain may be troublesome, perhaps with some characteristics and precipitation of cardiac pain.
4. Symptoms of dyspnoea and tiredness may reflect the presence of mitral regurgitation with haemodynamic significance.

The clinical *signs* reflect the degree of mitral regurgitation.

Complications

In patients with palpitation and mitral valve prolapse a wide spectrum of cardiac arrhythmias may be detected by 24-h tape monitoring. Supraventricular or ventricular tachyarrhythmias may also be found. These arrhythmias are usually insignificant. Episodes of ventricular tachycardia and ventricular fibrillation are, however, not unknown. These serious arrhythmias are usually associated with ST/T wave changes seen on the resting ECG. Bradyarrhythmias may also occur, with sinus node dysfunction or degrees of atrioventricular block.

Paroxysmal atrial tachycardia is the commonest arrhythmia and is associated with left-sided bypass tracks in some 60% of patients with mitral valve prolapse. If paroxysmal tachycardia has been documented, then detailed electrophysiological studies should be performed. Cardiac glycosides are contraindicated if anterograde conduction occurs through an atrioventricular bypass tract during the tachyarrhythmia. Sudden cardiac death has been reported secondary to both tachy- and bradyarrhythmias.

Investigations (Table 12.4)

The widespread availability of echocardiography has revealed several patterns of abnormal valve movement:

1. Abrupt posterior movement of either the posterior leaflet or both leaflets may be evident in mid-systole
2. Pansystolic bowing with a U or hammock shape
3. Sudden posterior collapse of the anterior mitral valve leaflet may be evident as it approaches the posterior leaflet

There is considerable variability in the relationship between the intensity of the auscultatory signs and the echocardiographic appearance. In addition there is a high incidence of the echocardiographic features in first degree relatives of

Table 12.4. Signs and typical investigative findings in mitral valve prolapse

Pulse	Normal or hyperdynamic
Apex	May be left ventricular in character; hyperdynamic.
Auscultation	Systolic click 0.14 s after first heart sound; mid to late systolic murmur, duration depends on severity of mitral regurgitation. Measures to reduce left ventricular volume lead to earlier onset of click murmur. If volume increased, onset of click murmur delayed.
ECG	Usually normal: non-specific ST/T wave changes in inferior or lateral leads. Inverted or biphasic T waves. Changes may reflect ischaemia of papillary muscles. Cardiac arrhythmias (see text).
Echocardiography	Several patterns of abnormal valve movement (see text).
Angiography	Left ventricular angiography reveals the typical appearance of prolapsing posterior leaflet into the left atrium during systole. Minor contraction abnormalities may also be evident.

patients with mitral valve prolapse. This may occur even in the absence of any clinical symptoms or signs (Brown and Anderson 1981).

Management

Mitral valve prolapse presents as a clinical spectrum in which therapy is mandatory in some cases and unnecessary in others. Asymptomatic patients with no evidence of cardiac arrhythmias, a normal ECG and absence of haemodynamically significant mitral regurgitation should be reassured but followed up over some 2–3 years.

Antibiotic prophylaxis for bacterial endocarditis should be given in the presence of a cardiac murmur and echocardiographic abnormalities (Corrigall et al. 1977).

Anti-arrhythmic therapy should be given if there is evidence of cardiac arrhythmias. Arrhythmias may be suggested by palpitations or non-specific symptoms such as light-headedness, dizziness, syncope or attacks of dyspnoea. The patient should be fully investigated by a resting electrocardiogram and 24-h tape monitoring. A stress test should be performed to attempt to precipitate arrhythmias when there is a high degree of suspicion of their intermittent presence. β-Blocking drugs have had reported success in controlling both arrhythmias and chest pain. In the unusual case associated with prolonged QT syndrome, phenytoin may be the drug of choice.

In the presence of chest pain, associated coronary artery disease should be excluded. An exercise electrocardiogram with a thallium scan should be performed where possible in order to differentiate those with and those without obstructive coronary artery disease. The administration of *nitrates* may accentuate mitral valve prolapse and these agents should be prescribed with great caution.

If haemodynamically significant mitral regurgitation is present, then haemodynamic investigations should be undertaken with the usual considerations concerning the degree of severity.

Occasionally embolic episodes may be suggested by intermittent minor cerebral events, and in these cases *anticoagulants* should be considered, possibly supplemented with antiplatelet therapy such as aspirin and dipyridamole.

Overall, however, the importance of mitral valve prolapse has been overemphasised. An incidental echocardiographic abnormality and a minor systolic murmur are not reasons for detailed investigation and intensive therapy. Only if definite symptoms are present should treatment be considered. The vast majority of patients can be reassured and left alone.

Aortic Valve Disease

Aortic Stenosis

Left ventricular outflow tract obstruction may be localised above the valve (supravalvular), below the valve (subvalvular) or may involve the valve cusps.

Rheumatic damage involves the cusps, causing retraction of the valve with sclerosis and thickening, often with extensive calcification and poststenotic aortic dilatation. Other causes of valvular stenosis include congenital bicuspid valves which, over time, develop fibrosis with increasing rigidity and calcification (Mills et al. 1978). In elderly patients stenotic valves are usually tricuspid with calcification and may be associated with atheroma of the aorta and other major arteries. Rarely rheumatoid arthritis involves the aortic valve, with nodular thickening of the valve leaflets.

Pathophysiology

The major pathophysiological change is compensatory left ventricular hypertrophy secondary to outflow obstruction. Critical obstruction occurs when there is a systolic gradient of greater than 50 mmHg, at which time the valve is often less than 0.5 sq.cm/m^2 body surface area.

Clinical Presentation

Symptoms: There may be a long presymptomatic phase; patients eventually present with:

1. Progressive left ventricular failure
2. Syncope due to cerebral ischaemia as the cardiac output may be reduced during exercise
3. Chest pain of anginal character occurring secondary to inadequate myocardial oxygenation

In left ventricular hypertrophy, abnormal compression of the coronary arteries reduces coronary perfusion pressure. The *signs* and typical *investigative findings* are shown in Table 12.5.

Natural History

There is a long latent period following rheumatic damage, during which time patients are asymptomatic. When symptoms appear, the long-term prognosis tends to be poor, and when cardiac failure presents, the prognosis is usually less than 2 years. Following syncope, it is some 3 years and after the onset of angina, the likely outcome is some 5 years' survival (Frank et al. 1973). Syncope is usually orthostatic and often occurs in the presence of systemic dilatation associated with a fixed cardiac output. In some cases premonitory symptoms may suggest that syncope is associated with arrhythmias. Transient self-terminating ventricular arrhythmias, atrial fibrillation or atrio-ventricular block may occur. Fatigue appears as a late manifestation and atrial fibrillation usually accompanies longstanding disease with secondary pulmonary hypertension.

Table 12.5. Signs and typical investigative findings in aortic stenosis

Inspection	Cardiac apex may be displaced.
Pulse	Plateau pulse. Small volume and slow rising.
Palpation	Powerful left ventricular sustained apex to the left of the mid-clavicular line.
	Systolic thrill felt over the aortic area.
Auscultation	A harsh, rough ejection systolic murmur heard at the aortic area radiating to the carotids.
	An ejection click is occasionally present preceding the murmur.
	The second aortic sound may be quiet.
Chest X-ray and	Left ventricular hypertrophy.
fluoroscopy	Prominent ascending aorta with possible post-stenotic dilatation.
	Aortic calcification seen on fluoroscopy.
ECG	Left ventricular hypertrophy.
Echocardiography	Shows possible narrowed aortic valve orifice. Calcification seen as multiple echoes. Left ventricular hypertrophy confirmed.
Cardiac catheterisation	Systolic gradient confirmed by withdrawal tracing over the aortic valve or by simultaneous aortic and left ventricular tracings using the transeptal approach.

Medical Management

1. Endocarditis prophylaxis should be used as in any other valvular disease. Asymptomatic patients should have careful follow-up, sequential ECGs, chest X-ray and echocardiogram. Patients with mild aortic obstruction will generally develop moderate obstruction and those with moderate obstruction will proceed to severe obstruction with the passage of time. Final decompensation should be anticipated. If there is evidence of major obstruction then strenuous activity should be avoided.

2. Diuretics should be introduced cautiously in breathless patients so that frank hypokalaemia may be avoided.

3. Cardiac arrhythmias should be treated vigorously as they may lead to left ventricular decompensation. If atrial fibrillation is evident, then associated mitral valve disease should be excluded. Cardiac glycosides are used for control of the ventricular response (Johnson et al. 1977).

Surgical Management

Indications.   In view of the possible long-term prognosis, the advisability and timing of surgical intervention are important. The age of the patient and the overall degree of valve deformity should be assessed. Operation should be considered in those patients who (a) have severe obstruction even if they are asymptomatic, (b) have severe obstruction with symptoms, (c) have evidence of severe left ventricular dysfunction as evidenced by hypertrophy and dilatation or (d) have progressive cardiomegaly and echocardiographic evidence of left ventricular hypertrophy.

Operative Procedures. In children and adolescents open valvotomy with commissural incision under direct vision should be considered. This may lead to initial haemodynamic improvement, but often re-operation and valve replacement will be required at a later stage. Aortic valve replacement is required in adult patients, using either a mechanical prosthesis or a tissue valve (Copeland et al. 1977).

Aortic Regurgitation

Aortic regurgitation may result from rheumatic damage to the valve cusps or, alternatively, from aortic ring dilatation.

Pathophysiology

There is a major regurgitant volume which leads to left ventricular dilatation (Table 12.6) with enhanced myocardial stretching and vigorous contraction as a compensatory mechanism. Valvular abnormalities may be the result of rheumatic heart disease but may also complicate infective endocarditis and trauma or be secondary to connective tissue disorders such as Marfan's syndrome and Ehlers–Danlos syndrome. Aortic root dilatation may be the result of aortic ectasia, cystic medionecrosis, syphilis, ankylosing spondylitis or other forms of non-specific arteritis.

Table 12.6. Signs and typical investigative findings in aortic regurgitation

Inspection	Diffuse cardiac apex may be seen displaced beyond the mid-clavicular line.
	Marked capillary pulsations or carotid arterial pulsations in neck.
Pulse	Water-hammer or collapsing pulse.
Palpation	Cardiac apex displaced to the left, with hyperdynamic heaving character.
Auscultation	Blowing early diastolic murmur heard best at the left sternal border in the third and fourth interspace.
	Heard best with patient leaning forward and breath held in expiration using the diaphragm.
Chest X-ray and fluoroscopy	Evidence of left ventricular dilatation and hypertrophy.
	Often prominent aortic lurch, with strong pulsation on fluoroscopy.
ECG	Left ventricular hypertrophy.
Echocardiography	May show prolapsing aortic leaflet.
	Regurgitant stream leads to quivering of the anterior mitral valve leaflet.
	Left ventricle dilated and possible left ventricular hypertrophy.
Cardiac catheterisation	Supra-aortic injection of contrast medium confirms the size of the aortic root and shows the degree of filling of the left ventricle.

In the early stages of development of aortic regurgitation there is an increase in left ventricular end-diastolic volume and haemodynamic compensation is maintained. The end-systolic volume, however, gradually increases and is a sensitive index of myocardial function and correlates with long-term mortality.

Medical Management

Medical measures include the introduction of cardiac glycosides and diuretics to control cardiac decompensation. Arrhythmias, if of recent onset, may cause clinical deterioration and should be treated vigorously. Vasodilating therapy should be considered. Afterload reduction may help to stabilise the patient and reduce the regurgitant volume, especially in the presence of acute valvular regurgitation. Even if the patients are asymptomatic they should be followed up on a regular basis at 6-monthly intervals with serial electrocardiograms, echocardiograms and radionuclide ventriculograms to assess whether the ventricular volume is increasing.

Surgical Management

When aortic regurgitation occurs as an acute event then prompt surgical repair is indicated as soon as the patient is stabilised (Morganroth et al. 1977). Aortic valve replacement is indicated in those patients who are significantly symptomatic, with evidence of left ventricular decompensation. The choice of valve is discussed below (Samuels et al. 1979).

Prognosis

In the presence of chronic regurgitation, moderately severe or even severe regurgitation may have a good prognosis with 75% surviving 5 years and 50% 10 years. If the patients develop symptoms then mortality is usually high within 4 years following the onset of angina and within 2 years after the onset of cardiac failure.

Tricuspid Valve Disease

Tricuspid Stenosis

Tricuspid stenosis is almost always rheumatic in origin and usually accompanies mitral and aortic valve disease. The haemodynamic changes are similar to those of mitral stenosis; however, they predominantly affect the right side of the circulation. The right atrium is dilated and hypertrophied and severe passive congestion occurs.

Clinical Presentation

If the valve gradient is greater than 5 mmHg then it is usually accompanied by marked venous congestion with elevated jugular venous pressure, peripheral oedema and ascites. The clinical signs and typical investigative findings are shown in Table 12.7. Patients present predominantly with fatigue, abdominal discomfort secondary to hepatomegaly and abdominal swelling. Marked peripheral oedema may also be evident.

Table 12.7. Signs and typical investigative findings in tricuspid stenosis

Inspection	A waves on jugular pulse.
	Skin pallor.
Pulse	Of low volume, exhibiting atrial fibrillation.
Palpation	Mid-diastolic thrill may be felt at the lower left sternal border.
	Presystolic pulsation of liver when patient in sinus rhythm.
Auscultation	Similar to mitral stenosis. Murmurs are usually loudest during inspiration.
Chest X-ray and fluoroscopy	Right atrial enlargement seen.
ECG	Wide, tall, peaked P waves.
Echocardiography	Similar features to those found in mitral stenosis may be seen if the tricuspid valve is visualised.
Cardiac catheterisation	Right atrial pressure is increased, with a dominant A wave.
	Diastolic gradient confirmed across the tricuspid valve either on withdrawal tracing or with simultaneous pressure measurement.

Management

Although salt restriction and the use of diuretics may help to relieve some of the initial symptoms and signs, tricuspid valve replacement is usually indicated in the presence of right ventricular decompensation.

Tricuspid Regurgitation

Tricuspid regurgitation is commonly associated with dilatation of the tricuspid valve ring and may accompany mitral valve disease with severe pulmonary hypertension, right ventricular infarction, congenital heart disease with severe pulmonary hypertension, primary pulmonary hypertension or cor pulmonale. Regurgitation involving the valve cusps themselves may be the result of a congenital abnormality, such as Ebstein's anomaly or common AV canal, but may also be caused by rheumatic heart disease, trauma and infective endocarditis, particularly in drug abusers; in addition it may accompany the carcinoid syndrome.

Clinical Presentation

If tricuspid regurgitation is not a reflection of pulmonary hypertension then it may be well tolerated. However, in the presence of pulmonary hypertension it is associated with reduced cardiac output, leading to right heart failure. Again, backward manifestations are manifest, with hepatomegaly, ascites and oedema. The signs and investigative findings are shown in Table 12.8.

Table 12.8. Signs and typical investigative findings in tricuspid regurgitation

Inspection	Large V waves seen on jugular pulse.
Pulse	Atrial fibrillation often present.
Palpation	Right ventricle easily palpable at the left sternal border. Occasional systolic thrill at the lower left sternal edge. Hepatic pulsation of the liver is usually found.
Auscultation	A blowing pansystolic murmur heard at the left sternal border is increased on inspiration.
Chest X-ray and fluoroscopy	Enlarged right atrium and right ventricle.
ECG	Shows right axis deviation.
Echocardiography	May not be helpful but similar features to mitral regurgitation may be seen.
Cardiac catheterisation	The right atrial pressure is elevated, with a very dominant V wave. This can be best demonstrated with simultaneous pressure tracings of right ventricle and right atrium.

Management

If no pulmonary hypertension is present then tricuspid regurgitation is well tolerated and no specific measures are indicated. Any underlying cause should be treated, and digoxin and diuretics introduced in the usual fashion. In the presence of pulmonary hypertension, a prosthetic ring to reduce the valve ring size may be introduced or annuloplasty attempted. When major decompensation occurs, tricuspid valve replacement is indicated. As the risk of right atrial thrombus and pulmonary embolism is common, biological valves should be used when at all possible (Carpentier et al. 1974).

Artificial Valves

The development and clinical application of artificial valves has greatly increased the scope of cardiac surgery in patients with valvular disease. Valves have been designed which are suitable for insertion both at the mitral or tricuspid and aortic positions. In general terms there are two groups: (a) mechanical prostheses and (b) tissue valves.

Mechanical Prostheses

1. Ball and cage valves were first introduced in 1960, and the Starr-Edwards cloth-covered valve is still widely used. In most centres, however, it has been superseded by valves with a lower profile and a larger valve orifice.
2. The Smeloff-Cutter valve has a double cage design with a larger valve orifice, but also has a ball prosthesis. Recent developments include tilting disc valves.
3. The Bjork-Shiley valve has a tilting pyrolite disc which opens to some 60° (Bjork 1969). This gives a good valve orifice to the diameter of the frame annulus.
4. The Lillehei-Kaster pivoting valve opens to some 80° and has a resulting large central flow orifice (Lillehei et al. 1971).

Prosthetic valves have good durability and have been used for up to 15 years in clinical practice. In view of their plastic and metal structure, there is a continued risk of thromboembolism. The rate of thromboembolic complication is some 3%–6% per patient year. Long-term anticoagulant therapy with warfarin is therefore required; it is introduced some 2 days after operation and requires long-term control.

Tissue Valves

Tissue valves were developed in an attempt to reduce the incidence of thromboembolism, the basic frame material being non-thrombogenic (Cohn 1978). Sterilised homografts were first introduced, but resulted in early valve failure. Fresh homografts were then developed but had a significant incidence of late failure following valvular distortion and calcification. Porcine heterografts were introduced in 1965. Early studies confirmed an early graft failure; however, when sterilised and stabilised with glutaraldehyde, a stable valve is produced. The Carpentier-Edwards modification of the basic Hancock valve is now in wide use. It consists of a stellate ring with polypropylene struts.

The use of biological valves has reduced the incidence of thromboembolism. As this is commonest during the first 2 months following valve replacement, anticoagulants are used during this time. Thereafter they may be discontinued. Anticoagulants must be continued (a) if the patient has longstanding atrial fibrillation, (b) if thrombus is removed from the left atrial appendage at the time of operation or (c) if there is a large dilated left atrium. The incidence of thromboembolic complications is less than 0.5% per patient year. Experiments with other forms of tissue valves were initially unsuccessful, but further new valves are being assessed.

Haemodynamic Properties

All valves have an in vitro orifice size smaller than the natural valve ring. This is due to the sewing ring and associated struts. The valve orifice is further reduced by endothelialisation. All valves in use at the present time therefore exhibit the effects of a mildly stenotic valve. When in the mitral position an end-diastolic gradient of some 5–10 mmHg may occur at rest. The gradient may be less with the prosthetic than with the biological valves. In the aortic position, the valve ring is smaller and persistent systolic gradients of up to 40 mmHg may be present over the aortic valve on exercise.

Choice of Valve

The choice of valve for an individual patient is difficult and clinical factors must be taken into consideration. If there is a small mitral or aortic valve ring or ventricular cavity, then the tilting disc is preferred to porcine valves.

The choice of tissue valve obviates the need for anticoagulants and this should obviously be considered in young patients, in those with a bleeding diathesis and in those in whom compliance with long-term anticoagulants may be difficult. In the case of young females with child-bearing potential, a tissue valve is obviously preferable. Unfortunately there are reports of failure of biological valves after some 9–10 years of use. Thus in young patients a further operation may be required later in life.

Thromboembolic events are less frequent when prosthetic valves are placed in the aortic rather than the mitral position, which may be a reflection of the lower incidence of associated atrial fibrillation. There is, however, a smaller root size, and the haemodynamic gradient will be greater over a relatively small valve. In addition, hydraulic stress is also increased and a degree of haemolysis may result. With prosthetic valves in the aortic position there is a 2%–7% risk of thromboembolism annually. The embolic rate is reduced to 1%–2% annually with porcine valve and this may be further reduced with anticoagulant therapy (Stinson et al. 1977).

Complications During Pregnancy

Young female patients who become pregnant while on anticoagulants with prosthetic valves in situ are particularly difficult management problems (Oakley and Docherty 1976). Our policy is to continue warfarin throughout pregnancy until just before delivery, when low-dose subcutaneous heparin may be introduced. If the patients are hospitalised this can be performed during the last 2 weeks of pregnancy. There is a risk of a teratogenic effect using warfarin; however, in general it is accepted that the risk to the child is less than the risk to the mother of having a significant thromboembolic event. Full anticoagulation should be reintroduced when possible, some 24–48 h after delivery. In patients having non-cardiac surgery, warfarin may be discontinued some 3 days before and introduced 48–72 h after surgery.

References

Barlow JB, Pocock WA (1984) The mitral valve prolapse enigma two decades later. Mod Concepts Cardiovasc Dis 53: 13–17

Bjork VG (1969) A new tilting disc valve prosthesis. Scand J Thorac Cardiovasc Surg 3: 1–10

Brown AK, Anderson V (1981) M-mode and cross-sectional (2D) echocardiograms in the diagnosis of mitral valve prolapse. Eur Heart J 2: 147–154

Burch GE, De Pasquale NP, Phillips JH (1968) The syndrome of papillary muscle dysfunction. Am Heart J 75: 399–415

Carpentier A, Deloche A, Hanania G, Furman J, Sellier P, Piwnisa A, Dubost C (1974) Surgical management of acquired tricuspid valve disease. J Thorac Cardiovasc Surg 67: 53–65

Cohen MV, Gorlin R (1972) Modified orifice equation for the calculation of mitral valve area. Am Heart J 84: 839–840

Cohn LH (1978) Surgical treatment of valvular heart disease. Am J. Surg 135: 444–451

Copeland JG, Griepp RB, Stinson EB, Shumway NE (1977) Long term follow-up after isolated aortic valve replacement. J Thorac Cardiovasc Surg 74: 875–889

Corrigall D, Bolen J, Hancock EW, Popp RL (1977) Mitral valve prolapse and infective endocarditis. Am Med J 63: 215–222

Frank S, Johnson A, Ross J (1973) Natural history of valvular aortic stenosis. Br Heart J 35: 41–45

Greenberg BH, Hassie BM, Brundage BH, Botvinick EH, Parmely WW, Chatterjee K (1978) Beneficial effects of hydralazine in severe mitral regurgitation. Circulation 58: 273–279

Johnson AD, Engler RL, Le Winter M, Karliner J, Peterson K, Tauji IJ, Daily PO (1977) The medical and surgical management of patients with aortic valve disease. A symposium. West J Med 126: 460–470

Lillehei CW, Kaster RL, Block JH (1971) Clinical experience with the new central flow pivoting disc aortic and mitral prosthesis. Chest 60: 298

Mills P, Leech G, Davies M, Leatham A (1978) The natural history of a non-stenotic bicuspid aortic valve. Br Heart J 40: 951–957

Morganroth J, Perlof JK, Zeldis SM, Dunkman WB (1977) Acute severe aortic regurgitation. Pathophysiology, clinical recognition and management. Ann Intern Med 87: 223–232

Mullin EM, Glancy DL, Higgs LM, Epstein SE, Morrow AG (1972) Current results of operation for mitral stenosis: Clinical haemodynamic assessments in 124 consecutive patients treated by closed commissurotomy, open commissurotomy or valve replacement. Circulation 46: 298–308

Oakley C, Docherty P (1976) Pregnancy in patients after valve replacement. Br Heart J 38: 1140–1148

Rapaport E (1975) Natural history of aortic and mitral valve disease. Am J Cardiol 35: 221–227

Reichek N, Shelburne JC, Perloff JR (1973) Clinical aspects of rheumatic heart disease. Progr Cardiovasc Dis 15: 491–533

Samuels DA, Curfman GD, Friedlich AL, Buckley MJ, Austen WG (1979) Valve replacement for aortic regurgitation; long-term follow up with factors influencing the results. Circulation 60: 647–654

Stinson EB, Griepp RB, Oyer PE, Shumway NE (1977) Long-term experience with porcine aortic valve xenograft. J Thorac Cardiovasc Surg 73: 54–63

13 Infective Endocarditis

Pathophysiology

The lesions of infective endocarditis are infected vegetations which usually develop on a pre-existing congenital or acquired cardiac lesion where blood is abnormally turbulent. Platelets and fibrin are deposited and can be invaded by circulating micro-organisms. Turbulence and pressure are related so that mitral and aortic valves are more often infected than are pulmonary or tricuspid valves (although lesions of the tricuspid are increasing owing to illicit drug administration), and ventricular rather than atrial septal defects. Predisposing valve lesions are usually a consequence of rheumatic heart disease but in addition valves which were previously normal or only slightly abnormal (bicuspid aortic valve, mitral valve prolapse) can become infected. Undiagnosed patent ductus arteriosus or aortic coarctation can also be involved. As the population grows older, infections on degenerate aortic valves are more often found and endocarditis on prosthetic valves is also more frequent. This is not due to an increase in the percentage of valves becoming infected but to an increasing number of surgically treated patients at risk.

Clinical Presentation

Infective endocarditis is a disease that may be acute, subacute or chronic. It is caused by a wide variety of organisms although a few are much more often found than are others.

Subacute Endocarditis

Subacute endocarditis usually presents as a low-grade fever with anorexia, weight loss and an associated cardiac murmur. The diagnosis should be considered in all patients with a fever that cannot be explained by another specific diagnosis. Inquiries should be made with regard to dental work, urological investigation or other minor surgical procedures.

Acute Endocarditis

Acute endocarditis typically presents with high fever (perhaps rigors) and a newly developed heart murmur (if one was not previously present), and often with a complication. Rapidly developing heart failure may be especially critical with infections due to a virulent organism such as *Staphylococcus aureus* or *Streptococcus pyogenes*. The organisms may spread by contiguity from the valve into the neighbouring myocardium and be associated with abscess formation and/or conduction abnormalities, with the development of heart block or arrhythmias.

Complications

Complications may develop during the course of infective endocarditis or may be the presenting feature that draws attention to the underlying condition. Complications may be regarded as cardiac or extracardiac (Table 13.1).

Table 13.1. Complications of infective endocarditis

Cardiac
Heart failure due to valve damage — aortic and/or mitral incompetence
Myocardial abscess, conduction abnormality
Myocardial infarction — coronary artery embolus

Extracardiac
Systemic or pulmonary emboli (R- sided endocarditis)
Mycotic aneurysm
Renal
CNS
Cutaneous and musculoskeletal
Anemia — non-specific or haemolytic

   The clinical presentation may be the result of cardiac involvement with heart failure, the effects of longstanding fever or the development of emboli.
   Renal abnormalities may be due to focal or diffuse glomerulonephritis or more rarely to renal embolisation. Proteinuria, cellular casts and microscopic haematuria are often present. A widespread vasculitis with skin petechiae and

renal involvement can also develop. Peripheral vascular lesions include splinter haemorrhages (which are an eagerly sought clinical feature although more often due to trauma), Osler nodes and Janeway lesions, which occur in the toes and fingers and are probably due to a vasculitis rather than to emboli. "Target"-shaped haemorrhages can occur in the fundi.

Systemic emboli may develop in any organ; they represent an additional hazard because of the presence of infected material with a possibility of development of a mycotic aneurysm and consequently an added danger of rupture.

Diagnosis

Several clinical features are helpful in establishing a diagnosis of infective endocarditis. These include a history of fever, anorexia and weight loss; additional findings include petechiae, splenomegaly and a cardiac murmur which may be of changing character as valve damage occurs. Non-specific but helpful laboratory tests include haematology since anaemia and a moderate polymorph leucocytosis occur in most patients, as does a raised ESR and urine abnormalities such as microscopic haematuria. Blood cultures are vital if the diagnosis is considered possible.

Before antibiotics were available all patients with infective endocarditis died. This was because of sepsis, heart failure or some other complication. Host defences play little part in infective endocarditis since the organisms lie deep within the vegetations, protected from phagocytosis and other defence mechanisms. The prognosis has improved but mortality and morbidity are still considerable. This emphasises the need for prevention if possible, early diagnosis and prompt effective treatment.

Although any organism can cause infective endocarditis, the majority (around 75%) are still due to *Streptococcus* and *Staphylococcus*. However, other organisms are now more frequently implicated. This is due partly to improvement in microbiological techniques and partly to nosocomially acquired infections associated with the use of intravascular prostheses, especially prosthetic cardiac valves. Another factor is an increase in tricuspid valve involvement in drug addicts following intravenous administration of illicit drugs. Such infections can be caused by various organisms, including *Staphylococcus epidermidis*, gram-negative bacilli and opportunistic organisms.

Management

The microbiologist has a crucial role. Blood cultures should always be obtained before starting treatment. Opinions differ as to when treatment should then commence. There are those who begin antibiotics when the diagnosis is suspected and blood has been sent for culture. Others prefer to obtain a precise microbiological diagnosis with identification of the organism and assessment of sensitivities so that an appropriate antibiotic can be selected. In a longstanding illness this would seem to be the correct approach, although it is mandatory that urgent treatment be started on an empirical basis when warranted by the clinical situation. If antibiotics have not been given beforehand (and unfortunately they often have) it is usually not necessary to take more than three separate samples for blood culture at 5-min intervals on 2 consecutive days. In such situations blood cultures are positive in 90% of patients and should be confirmed in two separate samples so that "false-positives" due to contamination can be avoided. Bacteraemia is constant rather than sporadic and samples do not need to be timed to peak pyrexial periods. It goes without saying that a meticulous technique is required at the time of venepucture.

The role of the microbiologist does not end with a positive blood culture and the antibiotic sensitivity of the organism. Whenever possible the minimal inhibitory concentration, the minimal bactericidal concentration and serum bactericidal titres should be measured.

The general principles of management can be summarised as follows (Wilson et al. 1982b):

1. Establish the microbiological diagnosis before starting treatment. This is especially important in chronic infective endocarditis since otherwise cardiac complications may arise as a consequence of prolonged inappropriate treatment. Once the diagnosis is made, treatment should be prompt.

2. Empirical treatment is justified in urgent situations of acute infection or rapid haemodynamic deterioration. Immediately after samples for culture have been obtained, treatment should be given to provide adequate antibiotic levels against penicillin-sensitive streptococci, penicillinase-producing staphylococci and enterococci. Penicillin G, flucloxacillin and streptomycin or gentamycin may thus be appropriate. Antibiotic levels may need to be measured so that satisfactory peak and trough levels are obtained.

In general, antibiotic therapy should be given parenterally since absorption is unpredictable after oral administration, although Gray (1975) has reported satisfactory use of oral amoxycillin in the management of pencillin-sensitive streptococcal endocarditis. Our own policy is to give antibiotics intravenously to avoid repetitive painful intramuscular injections. Treatment is by "pulse" injection 8 or 12 hourly as indicated, rather than by continuous infusion. Veins are delicate and antibiotics in high concentration may cause chemical endothelial damage; they should therefore be given through a rapid flush of saline and should not be combined with other agents in the syringe or infusion.

3. The clinician must search meticulously for signs of embolisation, vasculitis or cardiac deterioration with development of either mitral or aortic incompetence and consequent heart failure. Management of patients with infective endocarditis links physician, microbiologist and cardiac surgeon. The surgeon should not be summoned to a patient with uncontrolled infection and gross

valve disease. He should have been involved from the outset in planning the clinical management.

4. Look for a focus of infection. Dental abscesses and a history of dental work are well recognised sites of infection but even edentulous patients may have retained roots which are infected, and dental X-rays are necessary. Urine culture is worthwhile before starting antibiotic treatment. It has also been suggested that endocarditis due to *Streptococcus bovis* may be associated with colonic neoplasm, and gall-bladder and renal disease may also be occult sources of infection.

It is not possible to recommend a single treatment for all patients with infective endocarditis. It is a highly individual procedure requiring considerable clinical judgement.

Range of Infection

Infective endocarditis may be caused by a wide range of bacteria as well as by larger organisms, fungi and *Coxiella*. Viruses do not appear to be involved. The diagnosis is made on clinical grounds and confirmed by positive blood cultures or occasionally serology (*Chlamydia* and *Coxiella*). In a series reported from the Mayo Clinic for the years 1970–1979, the following organisms were implicated (Wilson et al. 1982a):

Strep. viridans 38%
Group D streptococci 20%
Staph. aureus 18%
Staph. epidermidis 4%
Gram-negative bacilli 9%
Others 7%
Culture negative 4%

Table 13.2. Incidence and causative organism in naturally occurring and extraneous endocarditis

	Naturally occurring	Extraneous

Incidence	Any time
	May follow dental or surgical
	  procedure
		Cardiac surgery (valve
		  replacement)
		Intravenous drug abuse
		Prolonged i.v. cannulation

Organism	*Strep. viridans* *Strep. faecalis* Other streptococci Diphtheroids *Chlamydia*	*Staph. aureus* *Staph. epidermidis* Gram-negative bacilli Fungi

Treatment of Penicillin-Sensitive Endocarditis

The antibiotic chosen should be bactericidal for the infecting organism. Bacteriostasis is not enough. The questions to be asked are:

1. What drug to give
2. How to give it
3. How long to give it

Penicillin G remains a highly successful drug when given in an adequate dose for an adequate time.

Recent retrospective studies have shown that high dose penicillin must be given for at least 4 weeks to be effective. Penicillin and streptomycin act synergistically in vitro against *Strep. viridans*, and the combination has been shown to be effective clinically. Thus Wolfe and Johnson (1974) reported no relapses in 35 patients treated in this way.

Amoxycillin has also been used successfully in the management of penicillin-sensitive *Strep. viridans* endocarditis (Gray 1975), and in this situation probenicid is also usually given to enhance blood levels.

Route of Administration

Penicillin can be given intramuscularly or intravenously. However, the dosages used are too large, too painful and too frequent to be given intramuscularly, and therefore intravenous therapy is preferred. High peak concentrations of antibiotics can best be achieved by giving penicillin as a repeated intravenous bolus. Because infusion fluid may inactivate the antibiotic, this should never be added to infusion bottles. A central subclavian or internal jugular venous line maintains patient mobility and avoids problems of low flow which can in turn lead to venous thrombosis or secondary infection.

Oral administration has been used successfully but most clinicians prefer to start with intravenous therapy for at least 2 weeks and our own practice is to continue with the intravenous route unless major problems arise with venous access.

Length of Treatment

Treatment needs to be continued for a considerable time. Many prefer 4 weeks although a satisfactory cure rate can be achieved using the combination of i.v. penicillin and i.m. streptomycin for 2 weeks. This obviously has benefits in terms of overall costs but does mean frequent intramuscular injections of streptomycin with the possibility of vestibular nerve damage in a small number of patients (2%). Penicillin alone should be used in those over 45 years old or with any degree of renal impairment.

Our personal choice in penicillin-sensitive *Strep. viridans* endocarditis is penicillin G 10–20 million units daily in divided doses given intravenously for 4 weeks.

If streptomycin is thought worthwhile it can be given as 7.5 mg/kg body weight (up to 500 mg) every 12 h for 2 weeks in addition to the above regime of penicillin, which would be continued for a total of 4 weeks.

Penicillin Sensitivity

Penicillin sensitivity may be known to be previously present or may develop during treatment. If there is a history of anaphylaxis or angioneurotic oedema then penicillin should not be given but another drug chosen — usually erythromycin or vancomycin. Vancomycin is not an easy drug to use. It requires to be given intravenously and can cause renal impairment. Although cross-sensitivities with penicillin are low, the cephalosporins are probably best avoided. If the history of penicillin sensitivity is vague or inconclusive, it is reasonable to treat with penicillin and await events since many patients will receive their penicillin without ill-effect and delay in treatment may have serious consequences.

Staphylococcal Infective Endocarditis

Staphylococci affect normal as well as abnormal valves. Staphylococcal infective endocarditis is a serious illness with a considerable mortality and morbidity despite prompt antibiotic treatment. Early surgery to replace the infected valve because of haemodynamic deterioration or failure to control infection has been a major advance and can be life saving. Staphylococcal bacteraemia does not necessarily mean endocarditis, and the most important clinical finding is a newly diagnosed or changing heart murmur.

In addition to involvement of native valves, prosthetic valve endocarditis is often caused by *Staph. aureus* in terms of both early (within 2 months of operation) and late infection.

Infective endocarditis in drug addicts may also be due to this organism; the tricuspid valve is most often infected and the presentation may be with cough, fever, pleuritic pain and pulmonary infiltrates on X-ray.

Treatment Outline

If the diagnosis is established by positive blood culture then an appropriate single antibiotic can be given, with an additional drug, such as gentamycin, being reserved for those with a poor response. Treatment should be for at least 4 weeks in all and perhaps 6 weeks in prosthetic valve endocarditis. In penicillin-sensitive patients penicillin G 3–4 million units i.v. is given every 4 h, while in penicillin-resistant patients flucloxacillin 1.5–2 g i.v. every 4 h or cephalothin 1.5–2 g every 4 h is given. Other regimes include vancomycin or clindamycin and should be considered following discussion with a microbiologist.

The cardiac surgeon should be involved from the outset in management since surgery may be urgently required.

Enterococcal Endocarditis

Enterococci cause 10%–20% of infective endocarditis. Enterococcal endocarditis may develop in younger women following obstetric or gynaecological procedures or in older men as a consequence of prostatic disease. Cholecystitis can also be implicated. The enterococci are group D streptococci. They are relatively resistant to most antibiotics. Penicillin given alone is bacteriostatic and not bactericidal. Fortunately almost all strains of enterococci, regardless of species, are killed synergistically by the combination of penicillin and gentamycin.

Treatment Outline

1. Penicillin G 20–40 million units i.v. daily in divided doses, *or*
2. Ampicillin 12 g i.v. daily in divided doses plus gentamycin 1 mg/kg i.v. every 8 h (check peak and trough levels)

Therapy should be given for 4–6 weeks.

If allergy to penicillin is present or develops, then vancomycin plus gentamycin may need to be considered. Nephrotoxicity can be a problem, and measurement of blood levels and continued checks of renal function are important.

Endocarditis Due to Gram-Negative Bacilli

Endocarditis due to gram-negative bacilli has been rare in the past but is now increasing in frequency both in native and in prosthetic valves. It can be caused by a wide variety of organisms, both aerobic and anaerobic. When prosthetic valves are involved, a combined approach of preliminary antibiotic treatment followed by early cardiac surgery in terms of further valve replacement can improve the prognosis considerably, although it remains a formidable medical and surgical problem.

Treatment Outline

Haemophilus infections — ampicillin 12 g i.v. daily in divided doses plus gentamycin for 3–4 weeks.

Infections due to more esoteric organisms require skilled microbiological help in the selection and control of an antibiotic regime.

Culture-Negative Endocarditis

Culture-negative endocarditis — perhaps better termed *apparently* culture-negative endocarditis — is also becoming more frequent. The failure to obtain positive blood cultures may be the result of several possibilities:

1. Previous antibiotic treatment. Cultures may remain negative for 1–2 weeks or longer after initial random treatment. Inadequate treatment is worse than no treatment at all.
2. Fastidious slow growing organisms. Cultures may take more than 48–72 h to become positive, so culture plates should not be discarded prematurely as negative. Special culture media may be necessary for identification.
3. Non-bacterial organisms, including *Coxiella* and fungi — especially on prosthetic valves and infection by *Chlamydia*.

The diagnosis can be difficult and time consuming. Additional investigations may need to include serology (*Coxiella, Chlamydia*), bone marrow culture and repeated blood cultures. Van Scoy (1982) has pointed out that a good response, with a 90% survival, can be obtained if the fever is controlled within 1 week. The prognosis is poor if the pyrexia is unresponsive for longer than this.

Treatment Outline

Treatment in the early stages must be empirical. Unfortunately this state of affairs all too often persists. When no antibiotic has been given beforehand and when cultures are negative consider penicillin G 3–4 million units i.v. 4 hourly plus flucloxacillin 1.5–2 g i.v. 4 hourly plus gentamycin 1 mg/kg i.v. 8 hourly.

A special problem is that of the infected but culture-negative prosthetic valve. No fixed regime can be laid down but vancomycin, gentamycin and even rifampicin may need to be considered. As with the other infections, surgical management may be life saving. It should certainly be considered early rather than late if the infection is uncontrolled. Even apparently minor prosthetic leaks may pose considerable haemodynamic problems.

Prophylaxis of Infective Endocarditis

Antimicrobial prophylaxis is an accepted procedure for cardiac patients with congenital or valvular heart disease and those with prosthetic valves. This includes treatment before dental work, tonsillectomy, bronchoscopy and genito-urinary and gynaecological procedures.

The possibility of infective endocarditis occurring after dental procedures is something every medical (and dental) student is taught, although the evidence is circumstantial and the risk slight (Wilson 1970). Nonetheless, the need for prophylaxis is accepted. The intention of treatment is not to sterilise the mouth but is to kill any bacteria released into the bloodstream following dental treatment (which includes scaling, filling and extraction).

Rabbit models of prophylaxis against infective endocarditis have suggested that penicillin alone is insufficient and that a combination of penicillin and streptomycin or vancomycin alone may be necessary. Such studies led to the recommendations of the American Heart Association (Kaplan et al. 1977). These recommendations are impractical and have not been widely followed since it is difficult to time injections to dental work and in addition the fear of injection has meant an avoidance of dental treatment. Regular dental treatment and good oral hygiene remain, of course, cornerstones in the prevention of endocarditis. Timing is still important with oral penicillin. Administration too early means that the mouth can be recolonised by penicillin-resistant organisms. Similarly, dental work should be completed in a single session or in sessions several weeks apart to allow penicillin-sensitive organisms to recolonise the mouth. A further set of possible recommendations has recently been published (Working Party of the British Society for Antimicrobial Chemotherapy 1982).

Treatment Outline

1. Penicillin V 2 g orally 1 h before procedure and 500 mg every 6 h for three doses, *or*
2. Amoxycillin 3 g orally 1 h before procedure, *or*
3. If allergic to penicillin, erythromycin 1 g 2 h before procedure and 500 mg 6 hourly for three doses

Procedures in hospital that are likely to be followed by bacteraemia are usually done under general anaesthesia, and antibiotics can be given parenterally:

1. Penicillin G 1 g i.m. or i.v. plus gentamycin 80 g i.v.
2. For urological or gynaecological procedures, ampicillin 1 g i.v. or i.m. plus gentamycin 80 mg i.v. or i.m., both given 1 h before procedure

It should be recognised that even the best antibiotic prophylaxis will prevent only a few patients developing infective endocarditis. Unfortunately the portal of entry of the infection in most situations is unknown; nonetheless, this does not make attempted prophylaxis any the less worthwhile.

References

Gray IR (1975) The choice of antibiotic in treating infective endocarditis. Q J Med 44: 449–458

Kaplan EL, Anthony BF, Bisno A, Durack D, Houser H, Millard MD, Sanford J, Shulman ST, Stillerman M, Taranta A, Wenger N (1977) Prevention of bacterial endocarditis. Circulation 56: 139A

Van Scoy RE (1982) Culture negative endocarditis. Mayo Clin Proc 57: 149–154

Wilson GRE (1970) Is chemoprophylaxis necessary? Proc R Soc Med 63: 267–271

Wilson WR, Guiliani ER, Geraci JE (1982a) Treatment of penicillin sensitive streptococcal infective endocarditis. Mayo Clin Proc 57: 95–100

Wilson WR, Guiliani ER, Danielson GK, Geraci JF (1982) General considerations in the diagnosis and treatment of infective endocarditis. Mayo Clin Proc 57: 81–85

Wolfe JC, Johnson WD Jr (1974) Penicillin sensitive streptococcal endocarditis in vitro and clinical observations of penicillin: streptomycin therapy. Ann Intern Med 81: 178–181

Working Party of the British Society for Antimicrobial Chemotherapy (1982) Antibiotic prophylaxis of infective endocarditis. Lancet II: 1323–1326

14 **Cardiomyopathies**

Cardiomyopathies can be defined as disorders of cardiac muscle of unknown cause. This group of cardiac disorders has been the subject of intensive investigation in the last decade and much has been learned with regard to their pathophysiology. Unfortunately the aetiology remains essentially unknown and treatment is often empirical and relatively ineffective. These conditions must be distinguished from disorders which affect the heart muscle and other organs as part of a systemic disease, for which specific forms of therapy are in some instances indicated (Table 14.1).

Classification

Goodwin (1982) has classified the cardiomyopathies into four groups:

1. Hypertrophic
2. Congestive
3. Obliterative
4. Restrictive

The last two subdivisions are rare and may not be separate entities but rather different stages of the same process; in this chapter they are discussed together, in the section "Restrictive Cardiomyopathy" (pp. 267–268).

Hypertrophic Cardiomyopathy

Pathophysiology

The major structural changes which occur in ventricular geometry and function in this condition have led it to be known variously as hypertrophic obstructive

Table 14.1. Specific heart muscle disease (modified from Goodwin 1980)

1. Infective	Viral, including Coxsackie
2. Metabolic	Endocrine
	— hyper- or hypothyroidism
	— adrenal cortical insufficiency
	— phaeochromocytoma
	— acromegaly
	Familial storage disease
	— haemochromatosis
	— glycogen storage disease
	Vitamin deficiency
	— beri beri
	Amyloid
	— primary or secondary
3. Systemic disease	Connective tissue disorders
	— SLE
	— PAN
	— rheumatoid arthritis
	— scleroderma
	— dermatomyositis
	Infiltration
	— sarcoid
	Granulomas
	— leukaemia
4. Heredo-familial neuromuscular disorders	Muscular dystrophy
	Cerebral dystrophy
5. Sensitivity or toxic reactions	Sulphonamides
	Cobalt
	Emetine
	C_2H_5OH
	Isoprenaline
	Daunorubicin, irradiation

cardiomyopathy, idiopathic subaortic stenosis and muscular subaortic stenosis. The gross pathological changes are those of muscle hypertrophy associated with fibrosis. The left ventricle is more commonly affected than the right and the hypertrophy involves the septum as well as the free ventricular wall. The endocardium may be thickened by fibrous tissue where it comes into contact with the anterior mitral leaflet. The mitral valve may be calcified and the papillary muscles are often hypertrophied. The major coronary arteries tend to be of large calibre. On light microscopy the muscle fibres are greatly hypertrophied and form circular but disorganised whorls. Electron microscopy shows changes of cellular hypertrophy and degeneration, with increased numbers of mitochondria and containing increased numbers of glycogen particles. The myofibrils show bizarre changes.

Haemodynamic Changes

Invasive and non-invasive techniques have been used to study the haemodynamic alterations in this condition. These may be considered in regard to abnormalities both of ventricular contraction and of relaxation. The hypertrophied muscle contracts vigorously in the early stage of systole, with rapid left ventricular emptying and a high ejection fraction so that the left ventricular cavity is almost completely obliterated. Ninety per cent of left ventricular stroke volume is ejected in the first half of systole, resulting in hyperdynamic flow into the aorta. A left ventricular pressure gradient often occurs at this time. The gradient appears to be secondary to apposition of the anterior mitral valve apparatus to the hypertrophied septum after the onset of systole (Simon et al. 1967). Mitral regurgitation may occur in the presence of a systolic gradient, and occasionally severe regurgitation may result in the presence of a thickened or even calcified mitral valve leaflet.

The degree of systolic gradient varies according to the ventricular volume and this may be influenced by physiological or pharmacological interventions. Any manoeuvre which reduces left ventricular volume, such as excess catecholamines, squatting, exercise or amylnitrate inhalation, increases the systolic gradient (Braunwald and Ebert 1962). Conversely, the systolic gradient may be reduced by increasing the left ventricular volume by the administration of β-adrenoceptor blocking compounds or calcium channel blockers. In ventricular diastole filling is impaired and prolonged due to poor compliance (Goodwin 1980). Ventricular relaxation is slower with great variation in diastolic function, which is poorly co-ordinated. The isovolumic contraction time and the rapid filling phase are prolonged, leading to impaired ventricular diastolic performance. This may constitute the major abnormality in hypertrophic cardiomyopathy (Lorell et al. 1982).

Clinical Presentation

Hypertrophic cardiomyopathy presents with a wide spectrum of clinical symptoms, ranging from the asymptomatic individual to those severely limited. There may be a familial tendency, with transmission by the autosomal dominant pattern and equal sex incidence.

Symptoms

1. *Dyspnoea* is common secondary to raised left ventricular end-diastolic pressure with resultant pulmonary congestion.

2. *Angina.* The pattern of cardiac pain may be typically induced by emotion or exercise or alternatively prolonged periods of pain may occur, with evidence of myocardial necrosis. The coronary arteries, however, are usually widely patent. The ischaemic pain may be the result of impaired subendocardial perfusion due to abnormal systolic and diastolic compression on the arterial arcades.

3. *Palpitation.* Continuous electrocardiographic monitoring has confirmed a high frequency of supraventricular and ventricular arrhythmias (Savage et al. 1979; McKenna et al. 1981). Frequent ventricular arrhythmias

occur in up to two-thirds of patients and may indicate a poor prognosis. Supraventricular arrhythmias are of less importance, except when atrial fibrillation develops. This may lead to marked cardiac decompensation and be difficult to control.

4. *Dizziness or syncope*.   The mechanism is unclear but it may be secondary either to mechanical derangement in obstructive cardiomyopathy or to associated cardiac arrhythmias.

Signs

The clinical signs depend on the presence or absence of an outflow tract gradient. In the presence of a gradient, three clinical signs are usually evident:

1. The pulse is jerky in character and similar to the pulse in mitral regurgitation. This reflects initial powerful ventricular contraction and the high output in the early stage of contraction.
2. The left ventricular impulse tends not to be displaced and is often double due to an additional atrial impulse prior to the powerful ventricular contraction.
3. A cardiac murmur is usually easily heard at the left sternal edge and at the cardiac apex. It has a crescendo–decrescendo character. There is an occasional systolic click but the onset of the ejection murmur is usually delayed, a short interval occurring after the first heart sound.

In the absence of a systolic gradient, the diagnosis is difficult to make. The history of angina from a relatively early age may be suggestive, but often no physical signs are present. Occasionally a double apex beat or a jerky arterial pulse may be found. A rumbling apical mid-diastolic murmur may suggest mitral stenosis. The differential diagnosis includes conditions with a similar cardiac murmur, such as aortic stenosis, mitral regurgitation or even a ventricular septal defect. In the presence of atrial fibrillation, rheumatic mitral regurgitation is often considered, since mitral stenosis may be suggested by the presence of a mid-diastolic murmur and evidence of pulmonary hypertension. Obstructive cardiomyopathy should be excluded in patients who have a history of angina pectoris in the absence of obstructive coronary heart disease.

Investigations

1. *Chest X-ray* may reveal a prominence of the left heart border, with the left ventricular configuration representing the hypertrophied free wall of the left ventricle. Left atrial enlargement may be present, seen as a double shadow at the right heart border. Interstitial oedema may be evident in the lung fields secondary to increased pulmonary venous pressure.

2. The *electrocardiogram* may be normal but may show extreme left ventricular hypertrophy with Q waves in the chest leads suggestive of a previous myocardial infarction. P wave abnormalities suggesting left atrial hypertrophy

may also be evident. The PR interval may be shorter than normal and left axis deviation of left anterior hemiblock may be evident. High voltage R waves with deep T wave inversion are not infrequent and in the presence of symptomatic angina may suggest coronary artery disease.

3. Several typical features are present in the *echocardiogram*. Left ventricular hypertrophy is usually present with an unusual distribution. The septum is thicker than normal, with a septal to left ventricular ratio of 1:3 or greater. Movement of the intraventricular septum is diminished. The posterior free wall of the ventricle shows vigorous contraction, while the left ventricular cavity is small. The mitral valve apparatus is displaced towards the septum. In the presence of a systolic pressure gradient, systolic anterior movement of the mitral valve occurs and this may come into contact with the intraventricular septum. The aortic valve leaflets show mid-systolic closure (Henry et al. 1973) and the diastolic closure rate of the mitral valve is reduced secondary to an elevation in the left ventricular end-diastolic pressure. This latter feature is a non-specific change. To establish the diagnosis, all these echocardiographic features should be present, as they may occur in isolation in association with other pathological conditions (Doi et al. 1980).

4. *Left heart catheterisation* confirms the presence of elevated systolic and end-diastolic pressures in the left ventricle. A resting outflow tract gradient is commonly present but may only appear on provocation. The outflow tract gradient may be up to 100 mmHg. In a suspected case the gradient may be provoked following the inhalation of amylnitrate or the intravenous administration of isoprenaline. In the presence of ventricular extrasystoles, post-extrasystolic potentiation of the pressure gradient is seen (Murgo et al. 1980).

Left ventricular angiography confirms the presence of massive septal thickening with narrowing of the left ventricular cavity which may obliterate the apical area. The left ventricular cavity has a crescentic contour. In the presence of an outflow tract gradient, mitral regurgitation may be present. The coronary arteriogram usually shows large patent coronary arteries.

Prognosis and Complications

Prognosis is variable and unfortunately it is difficult to predict the outcome in the individual case (Shabetai 1983). The complications include cardiac failure, cardiac arrhythmias and sudden death.

Cardiac Failure

Cardiac failure occurs in 10% of patients and often follows the onset of atrial fibrillation. This arrhythmia is a serious complication as it removes the atrial component of filling of the non-compliant ventricle. The cardiac output is reduced and the left ventricular end-diastolic pressure is increased. Systemic embolisation is common in this phase of the disease.

Cardiac Arrhythmias

Re-entry arrhythmias may occur secondary to conducting tissue abnormalities. Enhanced automaticity may also occur locally due to high concentrations of catecholamines and be responsible for atrial and ventricular arrhythmias (Goodwin and Krikler 1976).

Sudden Death

Sudden death is obviously the most serious complication. It may occur at any time and may be the first symptom. Some features, however, may be of predictive value. Sudden death is more likely in the presence of the following:

1. Symptoms occurring in childhood, particularly if there is a strong family history (McKenna et al. 1981; Maron et al. 1978)
2. Arrhythmias, particularly ventricular tachycardia, which may be evident on continuous ECG monitoring (McKenna et al. 1980, 1981)
3. Adverse haemodynamic features with a high left ventricular end-diastolic pressure and cardiac enlargement
4. Severe electrocardiographic or echocardiographic changes
5. Rapid symptom progression

Prospective studies suggest that ventricular tachycardia occurs in most subjects who succumb to sudden death. Its occurrence may be predicted in patients with:

1. Syncope
2. Left ventricular end-diastolic pressure of 20 mm or more
3. Left ventricular hypertrophy on the electrocardiogram
4. Septal thickness of 20 mm or more and systolic anterior motion on echocardiogram (McKenna et al. 1981)

Treatment

Treatment is generally used for symptomatic relief. Unfortunately there is little present evidence that there is an improvement in prognosis, although it may be improved to some extent by surgery. There is some evidence to suggest that β-adrenoceptor blocking compounds may slow the progression of the disease.

Medical Measures

GENERAL SYMPTOMS AND ARRHYTHMIAS

β-*Blocking Compounds.*   Angina, dyspnoea and palpitation are improved in some 70% of patients by β-adrenoceptor blocking compounds. The most widely used has been propranolol, a non-selective β-blocker with no intrinsic sympathomimetic activity. There may be less effect on diastolic function with selective β-blockers. The addition of β-adrenoceptor blocking compounds slows the isovolumic relaxation time and reduces the outflow systolic gradient both at rest and, more particularly, on exercise. The left ventricular end-diastolic volume is usually increased, with a resulting reduction in left ventricular end-diastolic pressure. The initial dose is usually low (40 mg b.i.d.) so that hypotension and bradycardia may be avoided. The dose is increased to maximum tolerated doses in incremental steps. Unfortunately although these compounds reduce symptoms, the incidence of arrhythmias is unaffected (McKenna et al. 1980).

Calcium Channel Blocking Compounds.   Verapamil has been shown to improve symptoms and to increase exercise tolerance, with a possible reduction in myocardial hypertrophy (Rosing et al. 1979; Kaltenbach et al. 1979). Unfortunately the incidence of cardiac arrhythmias is unaffected.

Disopyramide.   This may induce a similar haemodynamic improvement. The mechanism of these changes is thought to be secondary to a negative inotropic effect. Disopyramide may also be effective in reducing ventricular arrhythmias. Its effect on prognosis remains unknown (Polliok 1982).

Amiodarone.   This is effective in suppressing ventricular arrhythmias in patients with hypertrophic obstructive cardiomyopathy (McKenna et al. 1981). This compound may also be of use in cardioverting patients who have established atrial fibrillation.
   The onset of atrial fibrillation in patients with obstructive cardiomyopathy often requires emergency treatment. Early anticoagulation is recommended to avoid systemic emboli. Electrical cardioversion with anticoagulant cover may restore atrial activity, although the arrhythmia may continue to be troublesome. Digoxin may be used to slow the ventricular rate and can be administered in combination with β-adrenoceptor blockade.

CARDIAC FAILURE

Congestive cardiac failure may occur in the late phase, particularly in those cases with widespread ventricular involvement. There is usually no systolic gradient at this stage in the disease process. Digoxin and diuretic therapy should be used in the usual way.

Surgical Management

Surgical resection of the hypertrophied septum may be required to relieve symptoms which show no significant response to medication. This is indicated in patients who have a systolic gradient of more than 50 mmHg. In the presence of gross papillary muscle hypertrophy, mitral valve replacement may be required. The effect of surgical treatment on the long-term prognosis remains unclear (Morrow et al. 1975).

Congestive Cardiomyopathy

Congestive cardiomyopathy is a form of heart muscle disease in which there is impaired pump activity with dilatation of the ventricles and reduced systolic function (Goodwin 1979). Descriptive terms have been applied to this condition, such as congestive heart failure of unknown cause (Goodwin et al. 1961), end dilated cardiomyopathy (Roberts and Ferrans 1978) and congestive dilated cardiomyopathy. These descriptive terms emphasise that this condition represents a non-specific syndrome rather than a precise disease entity. Patients present with ventricular dilatation and poor ejection leading to forward manifestations of cardiac failure and an increased filling pressure at rest or during exercise.

Pathophysiology

The left ventricle is dilated and there is only modest hypertrophy; the heart is flabby and dilated, with patchy fibrosis. There are no specific histological, enzymological or ultrastructural changes. Variation in the size of the muscle fibres is apparent and vacuolation is present (Davies et al. 1977). Peters et al. (1977) suggested that there was a reduced number of cardiac enzymes, including cytosol malate dehydrogenase, but with increased lactic dehydrogenase and myofibrillar calcium activated ATPase.

Clinical Presentation

Symptoms

Patients present with progressive cardiac failure, dyspnoea and fatigue. The manifestations of left ventricular failure usually precede right ventricular failure, and the presenting illness may be precipitated by respiratory infection or a change of cardiac rhythm from sinus to atrial fibrillation.

Signs

Peripheral cyanosis and a low volume arterial pulse suggest a low cardiac output. Atrial fibrillation is a common arrhythmia. An elevated JVP and hepatic enlargement may accompany associated right heart failure. The cardiac apex is displaced and there may be evidence of right ventricular hypertrophy. Additional third or fourth heart sounds may be present, and mitral or tricuspid regurgitation may occur secondary to ventricular regurgitation.

Diagnosis

The diagnosis is made by exclusion of other specific causes of cardiac failure. Evidence of valvular heart disease, congenital heart disease, hypertensive heart disease, constrictive pericarditis, cor pulmonale and coronary heart disease should be sought. The rare secondary specific heart muscle diseases should be excluded.

In some situations it may be difficult to exclude an underlying primary cause. Hypertensive heart disease may be difficult to diagnose when left ventricular failure has supervened and blood pressure becomes normal. A previous history of hypertension should be excluded and target organ involvement sought. When the cardiac output is reduced, valvular disease may be obscured and it may be difficult to decide whether mitral and tricuspid regurgitation is due to primary valvular disease or to ventricular dilatation. Coronary heart disease usually presents with recurrent episodes of myocardial infarction or alternatively with a long history of angina pectoris, although the presentation may occasionally be silent.

Associations

1. *Alcohol.* Although there is evidence that acute alcoholic intoxication may cause cardiac arrhythmias and reduce the ventricular contractile performance (Regan et al. 1969) there is no specific proof that chronic alcohol ingestion leads to dilated cardiomyopathy in the absence of additional nutritional problems. There is enough of an association, however, to suggest that alcohol be totally withdrawn.

2. *Pregnancy and puerperium.* Although the cause of cardiomyopathy in pregnancy is unknown, it is suggested that further pregnancy be avoided.

3. *Myocarditis.* Viral myocarditis may lead to chronic left ventricular dysfunction with cardiac failure and an end-result indistinguishable from dilated cardiomyopathy. These changes may be the consequence of an autoimmune reaction on the part of the myocardium previously injured by a toxin or infective agent. Nutritional factors may also be important (Eckstein et al. 1982).

Complications

Complications include mural thrombi with resulting systemic or pulmonary embolism, particularly if there is atrial fibrillation. Recurrent pulmonary embolism may result when venous thrombosis is present. This may lead to right heart failure or to non-specific symptoms of fever, dizziness or transient hypotension. The typical clinical and radiological signs of pulmonary infarction may occur.

Investigations

1. *Electrocardiography.* Low voltage QRS complexes with occasional Q waves may be seen, together with non-specific T wave flattening and ST depression. Intraventricular conduction defects (bundle branch block) occur in some 10% of cases (Gau et al. 1972).

2. *Chest X-ray* frequently reveals generalised cardiac enlargement with all the chambers involved. There is pulmonary congestion with upper lobe blood diversion.

3. *Echocardiography* shows increased systolic and diastolic dimensions of the left ventricle, and a reduced ejection fraction. The mitral valve is displaced towards the posterior left ventricular wall.

4. *Cardiac catheterisation.* Left ventricular angiography confirms the presence of an increased left ventricular end-diastolic volume and a reduced ejection fraction. The coronary arteries are often dilated. Pressure studies confirm the presence of an elevated left ventricular end-diastolic pressure and pulmonary hypertension. Valvular gradients are absent.

5. *Transvenous endomyocardial biopsy* may be helpful in the diagnosis of specific causes of dilated cardiomyopathy (Nippoldt et al. 1982). Biopsy may also be used in patients with neoplasm to guide adriamycin therapy (Caves et al. 1973). At present endomyocardial biopsy is regarded as a research investigation rather than a routine clinical tool in the diagnosis of dilated cardiomyopathy.

Treatment

Specific causes of myocardial disease should be excluded by careful clinical examination, laboratory investigations and biopsy findings where appropriate. Where no other specific measures can be offered, the standard therapy for the treatment of congestive cardiac failure should be introduced:

1. *Restriction of physical activity:* Abstinence from alcohol and improvement in overall nutritional status should be achieved.

2. *Diuretic therapy:* The selection is made depending on the degree of cardiac failure. Most patients will require a loop diuretic. Long-term usage may

lead to over-diuresis with resulting metabolic alkalosis and raised blood urea and creatinine. Routine measurement of the serum electrolytes and assessment of the patient's sense of well-being are required. In refractory failure, combination therapy with an aldosterone antagonist such as spironolactone should be continued, and combinations of loop diuretic and thiazide may also be required.

3. *Digoxin therapy* is especially useful in the presence of atrial fibrillation. Considerable controversy remains concerning its use in cardiomyopathy in the presence of sinus rhythm.

4. *Vasodilators* should be introduced according to the haemodynamic findings; whether a venous, mixed or arteriolar dilator is used depends on the haemodynamic subset of the patient.

5. *Anticoagulant therapy* should be considered in all patients with cardiomyopathy in view of the high incidence of recurrent pulmonary or systemic emboli. Indications are significant cardiomegaly and a low cardiac output.

6. *Anti-arrhythmics*:   In patients with congestive cardiomyopathy, a high incidence of ventricular extrasystoles and ventricular tachycardia have been noted. The choice of anti-arrhythmic therapy is influenced by the negative intropic properties of most of the established agents. There is increasing evidence that amiodarone may offer an appropriate anti-arrhythmic spectrum for use in those patients with cardiomyopathy and may lead to an improvement in symptoms and long-term prognosis. The use of β-adrenoceptor blocking compounds has been suggested. This therapy remains controversial as the original observations have not been confirmed; it cannot be recommended as routine practice at the present time (Swedberg et al. 1980).

Prognosis

Once cardiac failure develops, most patients die within 1–5 years. The individual prognosis remains variable (Fuster et al. 1981).

Restrictive Cardiomyopathy

Pathophysiology

Restrictive cardiomyopathy is an uncommon condition in western countries. The commonest cause is amyloid disease; however, it may also be secondary to myocardial fibrosis, hypertrophy or infiltrative disease and is associated with haemochromatosis, glycogen deposition, endomyocardial fibrosis, fibroelastosis, eosinophilia, neoplastic infiltration and myocardial fibrosis which may be of unknown cause. Contractile function is relatively unimpaired and ventricular systolic emptying is good. Ventricular filling, however, is markedly impaired due to reduced compliance (excessive rigidity) during diastole (Chew et al. 1975).

Clinical Presentation

The findings are similar to those associated with chronic constrictive pericarditis. Differentiation between these two conditions is important as surgical treatment may reverse the haemodynamic problem in constrictive pericarditis, whereas treatment is disappointing in restrictive cardiomyopathy.

Symptoms

Patients present with weakness, tiredness and dyspnoea due to an inability to increase their cardiac output on exercise. Chest pain is usually not a problem except where amyloid involvement of the coronary arteries is present.

Signs

In severe disease, marked right heart failure and its sequelae develop. Clinical findings may include raised jugular venous pressure, additional heart sounds and systolic murmurs of functional valvular regurgitation.

Investigations

The echocardiogram usually confirms thickening of the left ventricular wall, with an increased left ventricular muscle mass.

Haemodynamics

The atrial pressure tracings show a prominent 'y' descent followed by a rapid rise in plateau phase, and the 'a' wave is also prominent. A rapid 'x' descent also occurs. The left ventricular end-diastolic pressure is usually greater than the right and this difference is accentuated on exercise. The pulmonary artery pressure is usually more than 50 mmHg (Tyberg et al. 1981).

Management

The treatment of restrictive cardiomyopathy is supportive, with specific measures being directed towards any underlying systemic disease. Standard cardiac failure measures should be introduced, although the results of treatment tend to be disappointing since the prognosis is uniformly poor.

References

Braunwald E, Ebert PA (1962) Haemodynamic alterations in idiopathic hypertrophic subaortic stenosis induced by sympathomimetic drugs. Am J Cardiol 10: 389–395

Caves PK, Stinson EB, Billingham M, Shumway N (1973) Percutaneous transvenous endomyocardial biopsy in human heart recipients. Ann Thorac Surg 16: 325–336

Chew CC, Ziady GM, Raphael MJ, Oakley CM (1975) The functional defect in amyloid heart disease. The stiff heart syndrome. Am J Cardiol 36: 438–442

Davies MJ, Brooksby IAB, Jenkins BS, Cankovic-Darracott S, Swanton RH, Coltart DJ, Webb-Peploe MM (1977) Left ventricular endomyocardial biopsy. II. The value of light microscopy. Cathet Cardiovasc Diagn 3: 123–130

Doi YL, McKenna WJ, Gehrke J, Oakley CM, Goodwin JF (1980) M-mode echocardiography in hypertrophic cardiomyopathy: diagnostic criteria and prediction of obstruction. Am J Cardiol 45: 6–14

Eckstein RE, Mempel W, Bolte HD (1982) Reduced suppressor cell activity in congestive cardiomyopathy and in myocarditis. Circulation 65: 1224–1229

Fuster V, Gersh BJ, Giuliani ER et al. (1981) The natural history of idiopathic dilated cardiomyopathy. Am J Cardiol 47: 525–531

Gau GT, Goodwin JF, Oakley CM, Olsen EGJ, Rahmjoola SH, Raphael MJ, Steiner RE (1972) Q waves and coronary arteriography in cardiomyopathy. Br Heart J 34: 1034–1041

Goodwin JF (1979) Cardiomyopathy: an interface between fundamental and clinical cardiology. Proceedings of the VIII World Congress of Cardiology. Excerpta Medica, Amsterdam, pp 103–116

Goodwin JF (1980) An appreciation of hypertrophic cardiomyopathy. Am J Med 68: 797–800

Goodwin JF (1982) The frontiers of cardiomyopathy. Br Heart J 48: 1–18

Goodwin JF, Krikler DM (1976) Arrhythmias as a cause of sudden death in hypertrophic cardiomyopathy. Lancet II: 937–940

Goodwin JF, Hollman GH, Gordon H, Bishop A (1961) Clinical aspects of cardiomyopathy. Br Med J I: 69–79

Henry WL, Clark CE, Glancy DL, Epstein SE (1973) Echocardiographic measurement of the left ventricular outflow gradient in idiopathic hypertophic subaortic stenosis. N Engl J Med 288: 989–993

Kaltenbach M, Hopf R, Kober G, Bussmann WD, Keller M, Petersen Y (1979) Treatment of hypertrophic obstructive cardiomyopathy with verapamil. Br Heart J 42: 35–42

Lorell B, Paulus WJ, Grossman W et al. (1982) Modification of abnormal left ventricular diastolic properties in patients by nifedipine with hypertrophic cardiomyopathy. Circulation 65: 499–507

Maron BJ, Lipson LC, Roberts WC, Savage DD, Epstein SE (1978) "Malignant" hypertrophic cardiomyopathy: identification of a subgroup of families with unusually frequent premature death. Am J Cardiol 41: 1133–1140

McKenna WJ, Chetty S, Oakley CM, Goodwin JF (1980) Arrhythmia in hypertrophic cardiomyopathy: exercise and 48 hour ambulatory electrocardiographic assessment with and without beta-adrenergic blocking therapy. Am J Cardiol 45: 1–5

McKenna WJ, England D, Doi YL, Deanfield JE, Oakley C, Goodwin JF (1981) Arrhythmia in hypertophic cardiomyopathy. 1. Influence on prognosis. Br Heart J 46: 168–172

Morrow AG, Reitz BA, Epstein SE et al. (1975) Operative treatment in hypertrophic subaortic stenosis. Techniques and the results of pre- and post-operative assessments in 83 patients. Circulation 52: 88–102

Murgo JP, Alter BR, Dorethy JF, Altobelli SA (1980) Dynamics of left ventricular ejection in obstructive and non-obstructive hypertrophic cardiomyopathy. J Clin Invest 66: 1369–1382

Nippoldt TB, Edwards WD, Holmes DR et al. (1982) Right ventricular endomyocardial biopsy: clinicopathologic correlates in 100 consecutive patients. Mayo Clin Proc 57: 607–618

Peters TJ, Wells G, Oakley CM, Brooksby IAB, Jenkins BS, Webb-Peploe MM, Coltart DJ (1977) Enzymic analysis of endomyocardial biopsy specimens from patients with cardiomyopathies. Br Heart J 39: 1333–1339

Polliok C (1982) Haemodynamic and clinical improvement after disopyramide. N Engl J Med 307: 997–999

Regan TJ, Levinson GE, Oldewurtal HA, et al. (1969) Ventricular function in noncardiacs with alcoholic fatty liver. Role of ethanol in the production of cardiomyopathy. J Clin Invest 48: 397–400

Roberts WC, Ferrans VJ (1978) Pathology of myocardial diseases. In: Hurst JW, Logue RB, Schiant RC, Wenger NK (eds) The heart, arteries and veins, 4th edn. McGraw-Hill, New York, pp 1516–1521

Rosing DR, Kent KM, Maron BJ, Epstein SE (1979) Verapamil therapy: a new approach to the pharmacologic treatment of hypertrophic cardiomyopathy. II. Effects on exercise capacity and symptomatic status. Circulation 60: 1208–1213

Savage DD, Seides SF, Maron BJ, Myers DJ, Epstein SE (1979) Prevalence of arrhythmias during 24-hour electrocardiographic monitoring and exercise testing in patients with obstructive and nonobstructive hypertophic cardiomyopathy. Circulation 59: 866–875

Shabetai R (1983) Cardiomyopathy: How far have we come in 25 years? How far yet to go? J Am Coll Cardiol 1: 252–263

Simon AL, Ross J Jr, Gault JH (1967) Angiographic anatomy of the left ventricle and mitral valve in idiopathic hypertophic subaortic stenosis. Circulation 36: 852–867

Swedberg K, Hjalmerson A, Waagstein F, Wallentin I (1980) Beneficial effects of longterm betablockade in congestive cardiomyopathy. Br Heart J 44: 117–133

Tyberg TI, Goodyer AVN, Hurst JW et al. (1981) Left ventricular filling in differentiating restrictive amyloid cardiomyopathy and constrictive pericarditis. Am J Cardiol 47: 791–796

15 Cor Pulmonale

Definition

Cor pulmonale or pulmonary heart disease can be defined as "hypertrophy of the right ventricle from diseases affecting the function and/or structure of the lungs except when those pulmonary changes result from disease primarily affecting the left side of the heart." (WHO 1963)

Aetiology

There are many possible causes of cor pulmonale (Table 15.1). The vast majority of patients have bronchitis and emphysema, with lung changes which result in a reduction in arterial oxygen tension (PaO_2) and an increase in arterial carbon dioxide ($PaCO_2$).

Table 15.1. Causes of cor pulmonale

1. Disorders of gas exchange
   a) Diseases of the air passages and alveoli: Chronic bronchitis, asthma, emphysema
      Pulmonary fibrosis
      Pulmonary infiltration, granuloma
      Cystic disease
   b) Disorders of the thoracic cage: Kyphoscoliosis
      Thoracoplasty
      Neuromuscular disease
   c) Disorders of the respiratory control mechanisms: Obesity
      Idiopathic hypoventilation
      Cerebrovascular disease
2. Mechanical disturbance of pulmonary circulation
   a) Pulmonary microembolism
   b) Primary pulmonary hypertension

Symptoms and Signs

Most patients present with symptoms of lethargy, chronic dyspnoea and wheeze, all of which may be severe during an acute exacerbation. The signs are similar to those of right heart failure from other causes (see Chap. 9), though respiratory wheeze is more marked and peripheral oedema may be gross. The presence of oedema is generally a poor prognostic sign (Burrows and Earle 1969; Mitchell et al. 1964). Its accumulation reflects sodium and water retention precipitated by renal anoxia and hyperaldosteronism. In addition, redistribution of water from the intracellular to the extracellular compartment may occur. Such a situation is suggested when oedema appears with little increase in body weight, and its reduction with therapy may correspondingly be achieved without significant weight loss. This redistribution may be initiated by extracellular acidosis secondary to increasing hypercapnia, loss of central respiratory drive and a decline in PaO_2 with right ventricular decompensation.

Treatment

The treatment of cor pulmonale is directed towards the reversal of the acute exacerbation and the management of the long-term problem.

Acute Exacerbation

1. Appropriate antibiotics are given for respiratory tract infection.

2. Bronchodilators such as salbutamol and theophylline or ipratropium should be given when wheeze is present. The vasodilating and inotropic properties of the β_2-agonist salbutamol and the phosphodiesterase inhibitor theophylline may be of value.

3. Corticosteroid therapy may be indicated for relief of bronchospasm.

4. Expectorants, mucolytics or cough suppressants may be required in individual cases, and respiratory physiotherapy may also be of value.

5. Digoxin should be used in the presence of atrial fibrillation, but may not have major effects if sinus rhythm is present (Green and Smith 1977).

6. Modest doses of loop diuretics should be given with potassium supplements. Spironolactone should be introduced when oedema is evident.

7. Respiratory stimulants are indicated if drowsiness supervenes following the introduction of oxygen therapy.

8. If secondary polycythaemia is marked (haematocrit greater than 65%) then venesection may be occasionally undertaken (Dayton et al. 1975).

9. *Oxygen Therapy.* This is the mainstay of management and is given by

nasal catheters with careful monitoring of the blood gases. In those patients with chronic carbon dioxide retention, the use of a high concentration of oxygen may be associated with respiratory arrest when the anoxic drive is reduced. Low concentration oxygen should be used in the initial stages in all patients who have carbon dioxide retention. Oxygen therapy should be commenced at 1.5 litres; if this is tolerated it can then be increased to 2 litres/minute. Oxygen therapy should be continuous whenever possible. If it fails to raise the PaO_2 above 50 mmHg in the presence of an excessive rise in $PaCO_2$, intermittent positive pressure ventilation may be required. Patients should be selected who have been previously stable and have some degree of recoverable function. It is often difficult to wean patients with severe bronchitis and emphysema from the ventilator, and this results in major long-term management problems.

Long-Term Management

Long-term management requires the maintenance of diuretic and bronchodilator therapy. Following stabilisation of the acute illness, long-term oxygen therapy including domicillary oxygen can be considered, since it has been suggested in several studies that this may improve prognosis (Nocturnal Oxygen Therapy Trial Group 1980; Medical Research Council Working Party 1981). Oxygen therapy appears to arrest the pathophysiological changes, with maintenance of blood oxygen levels and reduction in raised pulmonary arterial pressures. The use of compounds with vasodilating properties is currently being investigated as an alternative method of reducing pulmonary vascular resistance and right ventricular hypertrophy. The role of these agents in long-term management remains unclear.

Pulmonary Thromboembolism

Pulmonary thromboembolism is a common condition, being found in 10%–64% of routine autopsies. Many incidents are of no clinical significance and are not accompanied by recognisable clinical events. The incidence of major pulmonary thromboembolism remains unknown. It is, however, recognised as the commonest cause of in-hospital death in postsurgical patients.

Pathophysiology

Acute pulmonary thromboembolism leads to the rapid development of cor pulmonale following obstruction of the pulmonary circulation by thrombi embolised from distal sites, most commonly the legs or pelvic veins. Major predisposing factors are:

1. Recent surgery or trauma
2. Prolonged bed rest
3. Malignancy
4. Paralysis
5. Congestive cardiac failure
6. Acute myocardial infarction
7. A history of previous venous thrombosis or pulmonary emboli

Rare causes of acute cor pulmonale include:

1. Amniotic fluid embolus after Caesarean section
2. Bone marrow or fat embolism after trauma
3. Air embolism

   The pulmonary vascular bed must be obstructed to some 80% of its cross-sectional area to increase pulmonary artery pressure and to precipitate cor pulmonale (Fishman 1980). As well as because of mechanical obstruction by embolic material, the pulmonary artery pressure rises as a result of release of vasoactive substances, particularly histamine, serotonin and prostaglandins. These compounds lead to vascular contraction and also bronchial smooth muscle constriction. The haemodynamic consequences parallel the degree of pulmonary arterial obstruction and arterial hypoxia. Pulmonary hypertension may occur, but in the acute episode the pulmonary artery pressure is seldom above 40 mmHg systolic. The other right-sided intracardiac pressures are also elevated.

Clinical Presentation

There is no single combination of symptoms which is specifically diagnostic of pulmonary embolism (McIntyre et al. 1972). Central chest pain (88%), dyspnoea (84%), pleuritic chest pain (74%) and cough (53%) are frequent. Syncope and sudden profuse sweating may accompany massive embolism; however, the classical triad of pleuritic pain, dyspnoea and haemoptysis occurs in only some 25% (Fishman 1980). Tachypnoea is the most common sign and is associated with cyanosis, tachycardia and fever. Third or fourth heart sounds and a loud pulmonary second sound are present when the embolism leads to significant haemodynamic upset. Atypical presentations are common and may include the sudden development of expiratory wheeze.

   The investigations employed in acute pulmonary embolism, and the typical findings, are shown in Table 15.2.

Table 15.2. Investigations in acute pulmonary embolism

Electrocardiography	This is highly variable. Non-specific findings are frequent, e.g. conduction defects. The S1, Q3 and T3 may indicate cor pulmonale. P pulmonale (P wave height > 2.5 mm) is common. Right axis deviation uncommon.
Blood gas estimation	Arterial oxygenation (PaO_2) usually < 90 mm. This is a sensitive but non-specific finding.
Biochemistry	CPK and LDH may be raised. Fibrin and fibrinogen degradation products are increased; this is again sensitive but not specific. Fibrinopeptide A and fibrinolytic fibrin fragment E are increased but this is non-specific.
Chest X-ray	Usually abnormal; often non-specific changes with pleural effusion. Oligaemic areas and change in vessel size may be evident, with loss of lung volume. Occasionally there is an increase in pulmonary artery size.
Radionuclides	Most widely used and most accurate non-invasive test. *Perfusion scintigraphy* is sensitive, normal perfusion excluding pulmonary thromboembolic disease. However, it is non-specific and requires exclusion of: a) extraluminal compression b) bronchopulmonary anastomoses c) regional hypoxia. *Ventilation scans.* These complement the perfusion scan and show normal ventilation in areas with inadequate perfusion. These perfusion defects may be single or multiple.
Pulmonary angiography	This shows good sensitivity, reproducibility and specificity. Its use is, however, limited, as it is an invasive test and requires good facilities and experienced investigators.

Management

Prophylaxis

Those patients at high risk for development of deep venous thrombosis and pulmonary thromboembolic disease should be managed by early and vigorous mobilisation. Prophylactic anticoagulant therapy is administered as low-dose subcutaneous heparin, giving 5000 units of high potency heparin 12 hourly. This has significantly reduced the incidence of venous thrombosis in patients having abdominal or gynaecological operations but has been less successful in patients undergoing hip or prostatic surgery (Kakkar et al. 1975).

Acute Pulmonary Thromboembolic Disease

In general terms the management depends on the degree of circulatory compromise.

ANTICOAGULANT THERAPY

Early introduction of anticoagulant therapy is indicated unless there is some specific contra-indication, such as a bleeding tendency. Full heparinisation is required, 5–10 000 units being given in an intravenous bolus dose followed by 1–2000 units hourly by constant infusion. Heparin therapy is continued until the cardiopulmonary status is stabilised. This will usually require at least 7 days of therapy. Oral anticoagulant therapy is then introduced and continued for at least 6 weeks. Therapy, however, may be indicated for 3–6 months (Kernahan and Todd 1966).

Heparin. Heparin is one of a heterogeneous group of mucopolysaccharides or glycosaminoglycans which have a strongly acidic charge. Its anticoagulant action is immediate and is mediated indirectly by means of the plasma co-factor antithrombin III, an α_2-globulin and a protease inhibitor which neutralises several of the activated clotting factors. It forms an irreversible complex with thrombin, and it is this action which underlies the use of full anticoagulation with heparin following the onset of thrombosis or embolism.

When given in low concentration, heparin increases the anti-thrombin III activity, particularly against factor XA and thrombin. The stimulation of this activity is the rationale behind the use of low-dose heparin given subcutaneously in the prophylaxis of deep venous thrombosis in high-risk patients.

Heparin is not absorbed by the gastrointestinal tract and is given parenterally, either subcutaneously for low-dose therapy or by intravenous bolus or constant infusion. Following its administration it apparently follows first order kinetics, its half-life being dependent on dose. It is metabolised by a heparinase to inactive metabolic products. The half-life is prolonged in patients with renal failure or hepatic disease.

Heparin is usually given by continuous infusion following a loading dose of 5–10 000 units. The infusion rate is 1000 units/h, with the rate being determined from the measurement of the activated partial thromboplastin time, which should be prolonged twofold from the control or pre-treatment level. If constant infusion pumps are not available, then intermittent intravenous therapy may be given; after a loading dose of 10 000 units, 5–10 000 units are given 4–6 hourly, with haematological screening being performed 1 h before each dose. For low dose prophylaxis prior to surgery, 5000 units subcutaneously should be given 2 h before the operation, with further dosing every 4–12 h after it. A similar regime may be employed in non-surgical patients who are at high risk for the development of deep venous thrombosis.

Heparin may have various side-effects:

1. *Haemorrhage.* This may be best avoided by careful control using the partial thromboplastin time. It is contra-indicated when there is a history of any active bleeding, haemophilia, the presence of purpura, existing thrombocytopenia and suspicion of intracranial haemorrhage. Caution must be exercised when there is severe hypertension or any evidence of occult neoplasm.

2. Occasional *sensitivity reactions* may occur if there is a history of allergy; in such patients heparin should be used cautiously.

3. *Thrombocytopenia* may rarely complicate continued therapy.

If subcutaneous injections are continued for prophylactic use, deep subcutaneous sites should be used, which slows absorption to prolong activity. Small bore needles should be used to reduce the risk of haemorrhage. The injectate volume should be small at varying sites, and pressure should be applied after administration.

If heparin activity requires reversal, protamine sulphate should be given. This is a low molecular weight protein which has a strongly basic charge and a high arginine content. One milligram of protamine should be given for every 100 units remaining — injection being given slowly as it may be associated with dyspnoea, flushing, bradycardia and hypotension.

Oral Anticoagulants. Warfarin is the most widely used oral anticoagulant. It is a 4-hydroxy coumarin derivative. Its pharmacological activity is the result of inhibition of blood clotting by interference with hepatic synthesis of vitamin K-dependent clotting factors. Its onset of action is influenced by the half-lives of the clotting factors in the circulation, and therefore therapeutic effects are delayed for at least 8–12 h after oral administration. The drug is usually given by a loading dose over a 72-h period followed by a maintenance dose which is determined on the basis of the value of the one-stage pro-thrombin acitivity. The administration of the loading dose prolongs the time that the concentration of drug in plasma remains above that which suppresses the synthesis of the clotting factors.

The activity of warfarin may be influenced by both physiological and pharmacological factors, including vitamin K deficiency, hepatic disease, congestive cardiac failure, a prior history of alcoholism and hypermetabolic states.

Following absorption, warfarin is almost totally bound (99%) to plasma albumin and has a half-life of some 35 h. The volume of distribution is 11%–12% of body weight. The contra-indications to its use are similar to those for heparin.

Warfarin is available as 2 mg, 5 mg and 10 mg tablets for standard use. A loading dose may be 10 mg, 10 mg and 5 mg over a 3-day period.

Toxic effects are mainly related to the development of haemorrhage; this can arise at any site, with ecchymoses or haematoma formation and gastrointestinal, uterine or urinary tract bleeding. These problems are obviously increased if there is lack of close long-term supervision.

Long-term management demands good supervision at an anticoagulant clinic which has adjacent laboratory facilities to allow rapid haematological screening and thus make possible appropriate dose adjustments. Patients should be given detailed instructions, both oral and written, concerning their drug regime and the importance of compliance. The possibility of drug interaction should be explained, placing particular emphasis on commonly prescribed drugs with high protein-binding properties.

Severe *complications* may occur, with major bleeding intra-abdominally or intracranially. In the presence of any significant haemorrhage, warfarin should be discontinued and vitamin K administered. In the presence of severe bleeding, 50 mg vitamin K_1 may be given by the intravenous route. Fresh whole blood or frozen plasma may be required, or alternatively the administration of the vitamin-K dependent clotting factors.

Prior to *elective surgery*, warfarin should be discontinued for at least 2 days and serial thrombotests performed. Where prophylactic anticoagulant cover is required, e.g. for prosthetic valves, subcutaneous heparin may be substituted and continued for 5–7 days post-surgery, at which time warfarin can be re-introduced.

OXYGEN THERAPY

High flow oxygen should be introduced by a close-fitting mask or nasal prongs, with frequent analysis of blood gases.

THROMBOLYTIC THERAPY

In patients with a major haemodynamic upset, thrombolytic therapy with streptokinase or urokinase should be considered. Serial haemodynamic and angiographic studies have suggested an earlier reduction in pulmonary artery pressure, with more rapid clearance of filling defects and an improved symptomatic response. Thrombolytic therapy should be followed by controlled heparin and warfarin therapy (National Cooperative Study 1973). The thrombolytic drugs which are in most common use are streptokinase and urokinase, although newer agents with more specific actions and possibly less systemic effects are being produced.

Streptokinase. This drug stimulates the conversion of endogenous plasminogen to plasmin, a proteolytic enzyme which hydrolyses fibrin. It is prepared from group C β-haemolytic streptococci and interacts with the pro-activator of plasminogen, which catalyses the conversion of plasminogen to plasmin. Fibrin in haemostatic plugs is lysed. The use of streptokinase may be complicated by allergic reactions and anaphylactoid response. Antistreptococcal antibodies cross-react and reduce the activity which prolongs the thrombin time.

Streptokinase is administered intravenously using a loading dose of 250 000 units which neutralises any antibodies from previous streptococcal infections. The pretreatment thrombin time and prothrombin time are measured. If heparin has been given previously, the thrombin time should be twice normal before the commencement of therapy. The loading dose is covered with the administration of hydrocortisone 100 mg and an antihistamine may also be given. Following the loading dose, the therapy is continued at a rate of 100 000 units hourly and therapy is continued for 24–72 h. The treatment is adjusted to the thrombin time within the range of twice to five times normal. It is continued for 24 h in the management of pulmonary embolism and for 72 h if associated deep venous thrombosis is present. Short time, high concentration infusion regimes have been recommended in the treatment of myocardial infarction.

Following the administration of streptokinase, the serum plasminogen and fibrinogen will be reduced and there will be an increase in fibrin degradation products. Heparin can be introduced when the thrombin time is less than twice normal and warfarin can be introduced in conventional fashion.

Urokinase. This is a proteolytic enzyme originally isolated from urine but now obtained from human renal cell cultures. Urokinase activates plasminogen, with a resulting action on plasmin. Urokinase is given in a dosage of 4400 IU/kg over 10 min and 4400 IU/kg/h over 12 h. Heparin can thereafter be introduced, along with oral anticoagulation.

The use of thrombolytic therapy is contra-indicated in those conditions which preclude the use of anticoagulants. In addition, therapy should be withheld in the presence of healing wounds, recent trauma, malignancy, pregnancy and cerebrovascular disease.

If bleeding complications accompany the use of streptokinase or urokinase, aminocaproic acid is used to reverse the increased fibrinolysis. The recommended standard dose is 6 g 4–6 times daily. Although it can be given intravenously in a dose of 1.25 g/h, the dosage should not exceed 30 g/24 h. The dose should be reduced if renal function is impaired, and rapid intravenous injection should be avoided as dizziness, nausea and diarrhoea are occasional unwanted effects.

Surgical Management

Pulmonary Embolectomy. This procedure may be required in selected patients with major coronary artery obstruction. Cardiopulmonary bypass is necessary, and the operative mortality is high. Surgery should probably only be considered in those patients with massive embolisation and whose haemodynamic status remains compromised despite maximum medical therapy (Alpert et al. 1975).

Prophylactic Surgery. Surgery may also be of value to reduce the recurrence of embolism in patients with confirmed deep venous thrombosis. The inferior vena cava may be clipped or tied, or an "umbrella" to filter out emboli may be inserted below the level of the renal veins, though this intervention is rarely required.

Long-Term Prognosis

Less than 10% of patients with even massive embolism die in the acute phase. However, a significant mortality occurs within some 60 min of onset of symptoms. Twenty-five per cent of deaths occur during the following 48 h. Defects demonstrated on lung scan and serial pulmonary angiograms may last for many weeks or months.

References

Alpert JS, Smith RE, Ockene IS, Askenazi J, Dexter L, Dalen JE (1975) Treatment of massive pulmonary embolism: The role of pulmonary embolectomy. Am Heart J 89: 413–418

Burrows B (1974) Arterial oxygenation and pulmonary haemodynamics in patients with chronic airways obstruction. (Proceedings of Conference on the Scientific Basis of Respiratory Therapy) Am Rev Resp Dis 110: 64–70

Burrows B, Earle RH (1969) Course and prognosis of chronic obstructive lung disease. A prospective study of 200 patients. N Engl J Med 280: 397–404

Dayton LM, McCullough RE, Scheinhorn DJ, Weil JV (1975) Symptomatic and pulmonary response to acute phlebotomy in secondary polycythemia. Chest 68: 785–790

Fishman AP (1980) Pulmonary thromboembolism. Pathophysiology and clinical features. In: Fishman AP (ed) Pulmonary diseases and disorders. McGraw-Hill, New York, p 809

Green LA, Smith TW (1977) The use of digitalis in patients with pulmonary disease. Ann Intern Med 87: 459–465

Kakkar UV, Corrigan TP, Fossard DP (1975) Prevention of fatal postoperative embolism by low dose heparin: An international multicenter trial. Lancet II: 45–51

Kernahan RJ, Todd C (1966) Heparin therapy in thromboembolic disease. Lancet I: 621–623

McIntyre KM, Sasahara AA, Sharma GV (1972) Pulmonary thromboembolism: Current concepts. Adv Intern Med 18: 199–218

Medical Research Council Working Party (1981) Long-term domicillary oxygen therapy in chronic hypoxic cor pulmonale complicating chronic bronchitis and emphysema. Lancet I: 681–686

Mitchell RS, Webb NC, Filley GF (1964) Chronic obstructive lung disease. III. Factors influencing prognosis. Am Rev Resp Dis 89: 878–896

National Co-operative Study (1973) The urokinase-pulmonary embolism trial. Circulation 47 (Suppl 11): 1–101

Nocturnal Oxygen Therapy Trial Group (1980) Continuous or nocturnal oxygen therapy in hypoxemic chronic obstructive lung disease: a clinical trial. Ann Intern Med 93: 391–398

World Health Organization (1963) Chronic cor pulmonale. A report of the expert committee. Circulation 27: 594–615

Subject Index